AF813930

Dynamics of Linseed and its Valorization

Rajni Chopra • Anupama Singh
Harinder Singh Oberoi
Editors

Dynamics of Linseed and its Valorization

Springer

Editors
Rajni Chopra
Department of Food Science
and Technology
National Institute of Food Technology
Entrepreneurship and Management
Kundli, Haryana, India

Anupama Singh
Department of Food Engineering
National Institute of Food Technology
Entrepreneurship and Management
Kundli, Haryana, India

Harinder Singh Oberoi
National Institute of Food Technology
Entrepreneurship and Management
Kundli, Haryana, India

ISBN 978-981-96-8926-2 ISBN 978-981-96-8927-9 (eBook)
https://doi.org/10.1007/978-981-96-8927-9

© The Editor(s) (if applicable) and The Author(s), under exclusive license to Springer Nature Singapore Pte Ltd. 2025

This work is subject to copyright. All rights are solely and exclusively licensed by the Publisher, whether the whole or part of the material is concerned, specifically the rights of translation, reprinting, reuse of illustrations, recitation, broadcasting, reproduction on microfilms or in any other physical way, and transmission or information storage and retrieval, electronic adaptation, computer software, or by similar or dissimilar methodology now known or hereafter developed.
The use of general descriptive names, registered names, trademarks, service marks, etc. in this publication does not imply, even in the absence of a specific statement, that such names are exempt from the relevant protective laws and regulations and therefore free for general use.
The publisher, the authors and the editors are safe to assume that the advice and information in this book are believed to be true and accurate at the date of publication. Neither the publisher nor the authors or the editors give a warranty, expressed or implied, with respect to the material contained herein or for any errors or omissions that may have been made. The publisher remains neutral with regard to jurisdictional claims in published maps and institutional affiliations.

This Springer imprint is published by the registered company Springer Nature Singapore Pte Ltd.
The registered company address is: 152 Beach Road, #21-01/04 Gateway East, Singapore 189721, Singapore

If disposing of this product, please recycle the paper.

Preface

The idea for this edited volume, *Dynamics of Linseed and Its Valorization*, emerged from a profound need to explore the dynamics of linseed, an important oilseed crop. Linseed has gained significant attention recently due to its exceptional nutritional profile and its health benefits. However, despite its growing popularity and demand in the food industry, there is a lack of comprehensive literature that consolidates all the relevant information in one place. This book aims to fill that gap by combining various insights and expertise from leading scholars and academicians.

This book is organized into four sections, each focusing on a different aspect of linseed. The first section addresses linseed/flaxseed cultivation, characteristics, and challenges in oil extraction, providing a foundation for understanding linseed cultivation practices and its oil's characteristics. The subsequent sections delve into the nutritional attributes of linseed oil, its stability, by-product utilization, and application in the food industry. Each chapter builds on the previous one to create a cohesive and comprehensive exploration of the subject. Our contributors from various disciplines and backgrounds offer unique perspectives, enriching the book's narrative.

The journey of compiling and editing this book has been both challenging and rewarding. From the initial idea when Prof. Rajni Chopra one of the editors whose interests in linseed was sparked while studying Food and Nutrition during master's and started working on linseed oil. Coming from a farming family, she had even cultivated the crop herself, which further deepened her connection towards this nutritionally important oilseed crop. That was when she realized the nutritional importance and challenges in using it as an edible oil. The whole process, from the ideation of writing the edited book to the final manuscript, involved meticulous planning, extensive research, and close collaboration with the contributors. One of the significant challenges we faced was overlapping content received from the authors, but through persistent effort and teamwork, we overcame it and brought this project to final shape.

We would also like to acknowledge the support of NIFTEM-Kundli, whose resources and encouragement were crucial throughout this project.

Finally, we extend our heartfelt thanks to our families and friends for their unwavering support and understanding while bringing this book to life. Their encouragement and patience were vital to the successful completion of this project.

We hope this book will be a valuable reference resource for researchers, students, and working professionals in the food processing industry. The diverse perspectives and comprehensive coverage of linseed processing and its nutritional benefits will contribute significantly to ongoing discussions and future research.

Kundli, Haryana, India

Rajni Chopra
Anupama Singh
Harinder Singh Oberoi

Acknowledgments

Completing this edited volume would not have been possible without the support and contributions of all the authors who contributed immensely to giving shape to this book.

First and foremost, I would like to express my deepest gratitude to my co-editors, Dr. Harinder S Oberoi and Dr. Anupama Singh, for their motivation throughout the process. Their tireless efforts and unwavering commitment ensured that the highest standards were maintained in every chapter of this book.

I am also deeply grateful to all the contributing authors, especially my Scholars, Aishwarya Dhiman, Himanshi Madan, Snigdha Homroy, Sayani Mavai, Monika Chand, Binanshu Talwar, Abdul Wahid P, Priyanka Kumari Singh and Aniket Kamboj for their dedicated efforts in the subject matter, which added significant value to the overall discourse. This book would not have come to fruition without their selfless efforts and willingness to share their knowledge and research.

I extend my special thanks to the Department of Science and Technology (DST) for funding a significant research project on the linseed crop and its use in value-added food products, which inspired me to fulfill my dream of writing a book covering all aspects of linseed crop.

Additionally, I am thankful to the editorial and production team at Springer Nature, particularly Dr. Swayi and Dr Nandini Viswanathan, whose professionalism and attention to detail have greatly enhanced the quality of this book. Their patience and support throughout the publication process have been greatly appreciated.

On a personal note, I extend my heartfelt thanks to my family and friends. Their continuous encouragement and understanding, especially during this project's more demanding periods, gave me the strength to persevere. I am particularly grateful for their unwavering support from my husband Mr Amit Kumar and my son Arnav Kumar, for their constant support and motivation throughout journey.

Finally, I thank all the readers and scholars who engage with this work. Your interest and feedback are what truly give this book its purpose.

To all who have contributed in various ways to the completion of this edited book, I offer my sincerest thanks.

Contents

Editors and Contributors

About the Editors

Rajni Chopra is currently working as Professor in the Department of Food Science and Technology, National Institute of Food Technology Entrepreneurship and Management (NIFTEM) Kundli. She holds a PhD in Biochemistry from the Central Food Technological Research Institute (CFTRI), Mysore. Her research interests are value addition to underutilized oil seed crops, designer lipids, oil-based nutraceuticals, oil meal/cake-based proteins and encapsulated oil powder. She has more than 25 years of teaching and research experience; is also associated with several professional societies; has published numerous research papers, review papers, and patents; and has received fellowships and awards, including the Dr. S. Husain Zaheer Memorial Award for excellence in research contribution by Oil Technologists Association of India. She is a reviewer for various reputed journals.

Anupama Singh is the Dean Faculty Affair, Professor, and Head of the department of Food Engineering, at the National Institute of Food Technology Entrepreneurship and Management (NIFTEM) Kundli, India. Her areas of research interest are biowaste utilization, sustainable food processing novel technologies (post-harvest), product development, and value addition. She has been nominated for prestigious international scholarships and invited to be visiting faculty at an international university, providing her extensive international exposure. She has presented her research at national and international conferences, published in peer-reviewed journals, and delivered numerous lectures at various conferences. She is a reviewer for various journals/book proposals and a recipient of several prestigious awards including the Nutritional Leadership Excellence Award in March 2022.

Harinder Singh Oberoi, Director, NIFTEM-Kundli, is actively shaping the future of Food Technology in India. His unwavering commitment is to democratize access to Food Technology innovations and bring them within reach of the common man. He was earlier working as an Advisor to FSSAI, where he had initiated several impactful activities like 40 state-of-the-art microbiology laboratories in 26 States/Union Territories across India. He played a crucial role in implementing the national initiative on rice fortification and restructured the Scientific Panels at FSSAI to enhance stakeholder involvement and foster collaboration between the scientific community and the food industry, and contributed significantly to the development of the Indian Food-o-copeia. He is renowned for his dynamic leadership and tireless efforts in advancing food safety and technology in India. Under his leadership, NIFTEM-Kundli is at the forefront of revolutionizing the food technology landscape in India, with a vision to make advancements in this field accessible and beneficial to all.

Contributors

Aditika Agarwal Department of Foods and Nutrition, Faculty of Family & Community Sciences, The Maharaja Sayajirao University of Baroda, Baroda, India

Reena Malongil Bapputty Department of Pediatrics, Case Western Reserve University, Cleveland, OH, USA

Monika Chand Department of Food Science and Technology, National Institute of Food Technology and Entrepreneurship and Management, Kundli, Haryana, India

Komal Chauhan Department of Foods and Nutrition, Faculty of Family & Community Sciences, The Maharaja Sayajirao University of Baroda, Baroda, India

Rajni Chopra Department of Food Science and Technology, National Institute of Food Technology Entrepreneurship and Management, Kundli, Haryana, India

Aishwarya Dhiman Department of Food Science and Technology, National Institute of Food Technology and Entrepreneurship and Management, Kundli, Haryana, India

Meenakshi Garg Department of Food Technology, Bhaskaracharya College of Applied Sciences, University of Delhi, New Delhi, India

Lalit Goswami Department of Civil Engineering, College of Engineering, Kyung Hee University, Yongin, Republic of Korea

Prabodh Halde Head Global Regulatory, Marico Ltd., Mumbai, India

Snigdha Homroy Department of Food Science and Technology, National Institute of Food Technology Entrepreneurship and Management, Kundli, Haryana, India

Shweta Jaiswal Department of Food Science and Technology, National Institute of Food Technology and Entrepreneurship and Management, Kundli, India

Shumaila Jan Department of Food Science and Technology, National Institute of Food Technology and Entrepreneurship and Management, Kundli, India

Deepak Joshi Department of Food Science and Technology, National Institute of Food Technology Entrepreneurship and Management, Kundli, Haryana, India

Anju Kapoor Chaudhary Sarwan Kumar Himachal Pradesh Krishi Vishvavidyalaya, Palampur, Himachal Pradesh, India

Rashim Kumari Department of Agriculture, Guru Nanak Dev University, Amritsar, Punjab, India

Priyanka Kumari Singh Department of Food and Nutrition and Food Technology, Institute of Home Economics, University of Delhi, New Delhi, India

Neelam Lohiya Global Active Clay LLP, Ahmedabad, Gujarat, India

Himanshi Madan Department of Food Science and Technology, National Institute of Food Technology and Entrepreneurship and Management, Kundli, Haryana, India

Sheetal Mane Department of Food Engineering, National Institute of Food Technology Entrepreneurship and Management, Kundli, Haryana, India

Sayani Mavai Department of Food Science and Technology, National Institute of Food Technology Entrepreneurship and Management, Kundli, Haryana, India

Seungdae Oh Department of Civil Engineering, College of Engineering, Kyung Hee University, Yongin, Republic of Korea

Ankur Ojha Department of Food Science and Technology, National Institute of Food Technology and Entrepreneurship and Management, Kundli, India

Abdul Wahid P Department of Food Science and Technology, National Institute of Food Technology Entrepreneurship and Management, Kundli, Haryana, India

Arshia Prashar Chaudhary Sarwan Kumar Himachal Pradesh Krishi Vishvavidyalaya, Palampur, Himachal Pradesh, India

Deepa Sanglekar Department of Life Science and Food Science and Nutrition, University School of Science, Gujarat University, Ahmedabad, Gujarat, India

Shreya Saran Department of Food Science and Technology, National Institute of Food Technology and Entrepreneurship and Management, Kundli, India

Vidhi Shah Department of Life Science and Food Science and Nutrition, University School of Science, Gujarat University, Ahmedabad, Gujarat, India

Anupama Singh Department of Food Engineering, National Institute of Food Technology Entrepreneurship and Management, Kundli, Haryana, India

Gaurav Singh Department of Oil Technology, Harcourt Butler Technical University, Kanpur, Uttar Pradesh, India

Kinjulck Singh Agriculture College Campus, Padra Rewa, India

Sakshi Singh Department of Food Technology, Jamia Hamdard, New Delhi, India

Richa Soni Department of Life Science and Food Science and Nutrition, University School of Science, Gujarat University, Ahmedabad, Gujarat, India

Binanshu Talwar Department of Food Science and Technology, National Institute of Food Technology and Entrepreneurship and Management, Kundli, Haryana, India

Neetu Kumra Taneja Department of Interdisciplinary Science, National Institute of Food Technology Entrepreneurship and Management, Kundli, Haryana, India

Yachana Department of Food Science and Technology, National Institute of Food Technology Entrepreneurship and Management, Kundli, Haryana, India

Heena Yadav Department of Food Science and Technology, National Institute of Food Technology and Entrepreneurship and Management, Kundli, Haryana, India

Praveen Kumar Singh Yadav Department of Oil Technology, Harcourt Butler Technical University, Kanpur, Uttar Pradesh, India

Agricultural Practices in Linseed Cultivation (National and International)

Aishwarya Dhiman, Priyanka Kumari Singh,
Snigdha Homroy, Monika Chand, Binanshu Talwar,
Himanshi Madan, and Kinjulck Singh

Abstract

Linseed is an essential crop of great importance in the nutritional and industrial sector. It is an annual herbaceous winter crop, requiring cold and temperate conditions for optimal growth. The cultivation and yield of linseed are primarily dependent on selection of varieties, sowing period, environmental conditions, and management practices. A well-drained, fertile, medium to heavy soil, such as silty clay, clay loam, and silty loam soils are suitable along with a rain-fed area. The crop management practices vary with the selected linseed variety and geographical area. The genetic makeup of linseed has a significant effect on its degree of resistance to environmental stresses and nutritional profile, especially the omega-3 content, which is beneficial for human health. Low temperature during winters promotes the production of higher proportions of omega-3 fatty acids. Linseed cultivation also has positive effects on soil health. The residues fortify the soil with organic matter, thus, promoting the microbial activity and soil fertility. Additionally, it also aids in controlling soil erosion and restoring the soil nutrient balance. The harvesting practice for linseed largely depends on its sowing time and winter spread. Rising consumer demands can be addressed by application of diverse fertilizers and their combinations according to recommendations of soil health cards, adoption of organic and green manuring practices,

A. Dhiman · S. Homroy · M. Chand · B. Talwar · H. Madan
Department of Food Science and Technology, National Institute of Food Technology and Entrepreneurship and Management, Kundli, Haryana, India

P. Kumari Singh
Department of Food and Nutrition and Food Technology, Institute of Home Economics, University of Delhi, New Delhi, India

K. Singh (✉)
Agriculture College Campus, Padra Rewa, India

© The Author(s), under exclusive license to Springer Nature Singapore Pte Ltd. 2025
R. Chopra et al. (eds.), *Dynamics of Linseed and its Valorization*,
https://doi.org/10.1007/978-981-96-8927-9_1

incorporating leguminous crops in cropping systems and implementation of integrated nutrient management strategies. The chapter comprehensively focuses on the agricultural practices of linseed production at the global and national level (India).

Keywords
Linseed cultivation · Agricultural practices · Omega-3 fatty acids · Integrated nutrient management

1 Introduction

Linseed, a traditional oilseed, is rising in prominence owing to its edible and functional oil and high-quality fiber used in the textile industry. It serves as a valuable alternative for cropping systems owing to its adaptability to poor soil conditions and water scarcity. The high economic value of linseed is attributed to its beneficial seed oil quality, which is highly appreciated by consumers, the food industry, and the cosmetics and eco-materials sectors (Zanetti et al., 2013). Linseed is an annual, herbaceous winter crop with a short, slender taproot that grows vertically downward and branches out laterally. The depth of the root system is dependent on the plant type, climate, and soil factors. This crop has two distinct morphological types: the seed type and the flax type. The linseed varieties cultivated in India are primarily utilized for oil extraction purposes (Singh, 2016).

The Asian region, which accounts for a mere 0.19% of the global linseed area (2.27 million hectares), contributes 34.29% to the world's linseed production. However, the productivity in this region is only 85% of the global average yield of 986 kg/ha. The primary reason for the lower productivity in the Asian region is India's significantly low yield (Singh, 2016). India plays a crucial role in the global oilseed landscape, accounting for 19% of the total oilseed acreage and 9% of production. According to data from 2022, India ranks sixth in global linseed production—behind Kazakhstan, Canada, Russia, China, and the USA—but holds the fifth position in linseed acreage (Shakya et al., 2023a). The crop is cultivated across an area of 342,000 hectares in India, producing 153,700 tonnes. However, the average yield of 449 kg/ha remains considerably lower than the global average productivity of 1006 kg/ha. Madhya Pradesh leads for linseed cultivation, followed by Uttar Pradesh, Chhattisgarh, Bihar, Rajasthan, Odisha, Karnataka, and West Bengal. These states have substantial linseed acreage and yields, occupying prominent positions in both area and production. Madhya Pradesh and Uttar Pradesh together contribute approximately 70% of India's national linseed production. Many of the popular cultivars have also been developed in these regions. The demand for edible oils in India stands at 18.94 million tonnes, with a supply of only 10.08 million tonnes, leading to the need for edible oil imports to bridge the gap. To address this yield disparity, various agronomic practices have been implemented (Shakya et al., 2023; Singh, 2016).

The nutritional quality of linseed primarily depends on its oil content and fatty acid composition. Additionally, linseed seeds are a rich source of high-quality protein and soluble fiber, with significant potential as a source of phenolic compounds. The linseed variety influences the quality of the seeds, and respective varieties must be chosen to improve the linseed product quality. Assessment of linseed varieties in different environmental conditions becomes essential before planning an appropriate cultivation strategy (Bernacchia et al., 2014). Linseed seeds thrive optimally in temperate regions with moderate temperatures, high humidity, and well-drained, medium-to-heavy soils. Moreover, continental temperate climates tend to result in linseed crops with higher contents of polyunsaturated fatty acids and lower levels of oleic acid compared to crops grown in the Mediterranean and subtropical regions. Linseed also exhibits increased total oil content when cultivated in cooler temperature environments. Furthermore, linseed has a relatively high water requirement, needing 400 to 450 mm of water during its 140 days growth period. Increasing the plant-available soil moisture from 40% to 80% can nearly double the seed yield per plant while also improving the oil content marginally (Čeh et al., 2020). Seed quality and quantity are known to be influenced by genotypic characteristics, growing season conditions, geographic location, and agronomic management practices. Environmental factors that influence crop growth and development are crucial determinants of crop productivity. To address market demands, various techniques are employed to enhance linseed productivity. These include the use of diverse fertilizer types and combinations, optimization of fertilizer application methods, prevention of runoff and nutrient losses, utilization of nitrification inhibitors, adoption of organic and green manuring practices, incorporation of leguminous crops in cropping systems, addressing imbalanced nutrient use, and implementation of integrated nutrient management strategies (Bernacchia et al., 2014; Čeh et al., 2020). Soil Health Card-based crop-specific recommendations also aid to nutrient management.

This chapter elucidates the multifaceted agricultural practices of linseed crops on both the global and Indian level. It discusses the production scenarios, varied cultivation practices, examines factors affecting cultivation and yield, linseed varieties, and cropping cycles. Furthermore, it highlights the effective crop management and disease control strategies, their impact on soil health, and best practices for harvesting. This chapter shall provide a solid foundation for understanding and improving linseed cultivation.

2 Production Scenario Global/National

Linseed is one of the most versatile and useful crops that have been grown for thousands of years. It is cultivated as a commercial or subsistence crop across more than 30 countries. The global production landscape of linseed is predominantly controlled by a few key players, namely, Russia, Kazakhstan, and Canada (Biradar et al., 2016).

According to the FAO statistics from 2013, the global area harvested for linseed was 2,252,104 hectares. Canada maintained a significant cultivation area of 412,000 hectares, traditionally leading in linseed production, followed closely by the Russian Federation with 410,000 hectares and Kazakhstan with 384,300 hectares (Zuk et al.,

2015). Both Russia and Kazakhstan have exponential growth in production over the years. India, with 338,000 hectares, and China, with 312,890 hectares, also demonstrated substantial growth. Conversely, the USA exhibits much smaller cultivation area of 56,960 hectares and countries like Ukraine (55,000 hectares), Argentina (14,600 hectares), and Egypt (5000 hectares) show even lesser production. Among the European Union countries, the United Kingdom had the largest area of linseed cultivation, covering 34,000 hectares, followed by France with 8510 hectares and Belgium with 7900 hectares. Other countries such as Sweden, Germany, Romania, Italy, the Netherlands, the Czech Republic, and Poland primarily cultivated linseed for local niche markets and experimental purposes rather than for the global industry (FAO, 2013).

Over the decade, the evolving landscape of linseed production have shown significant changes, transitioning from the 2013 to recent years, 2022, reflecting both challenges and growth in different regions. Russia stands out as the top producer, contributing a significant 47% to the world's linseed production, with an enormous yield of 1,766,559 tonnes, followed by Kazakhstan with 845,642.2 tonnes, accounting for 22% of global production, while Canada ranks third, producing 473,175 tonnes, representing 13% of global share of linseed production. Other notable contributors include China, India, and the USA, with production of about 290,000 tonnes (8%), 126,420 tonnes (3%), and 109,330 tonnes (3%), respectively. Ethiopia, France, and the United Kingdom also make significant contributions, albeit on a smaller scale, highlighting the geographic diversity in linseed production from Europe and North America to Asia and Africa (FAO, 2022).

The graph illustrates the global area harvested for linseed cultivation from 2012 to 2022 (Fig. 1). A general upward trend is observed, with a notable increase from approximately 2.4 million hectares in 2012 to over 4.5 million hectares in 2022. This upward trend indicates a growing recognition of linseed's value, driven by its multifaceted applications in the food, health, and industrial sectors.

The pie chart presents the top ten leading producers of linseed in world, showcasing their respective production volumes and percentage contributions to global production (in tonnes) (Fig. 2). Rise of shift toward plant based-dietary pattern, increase demand of herbal nutraceuticals and functional foods, advances in

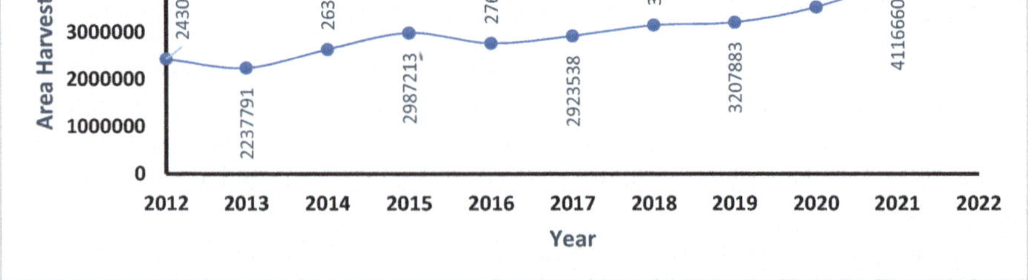

Fig. 1 Global linseed cultivation—area harvested (2012–2022)

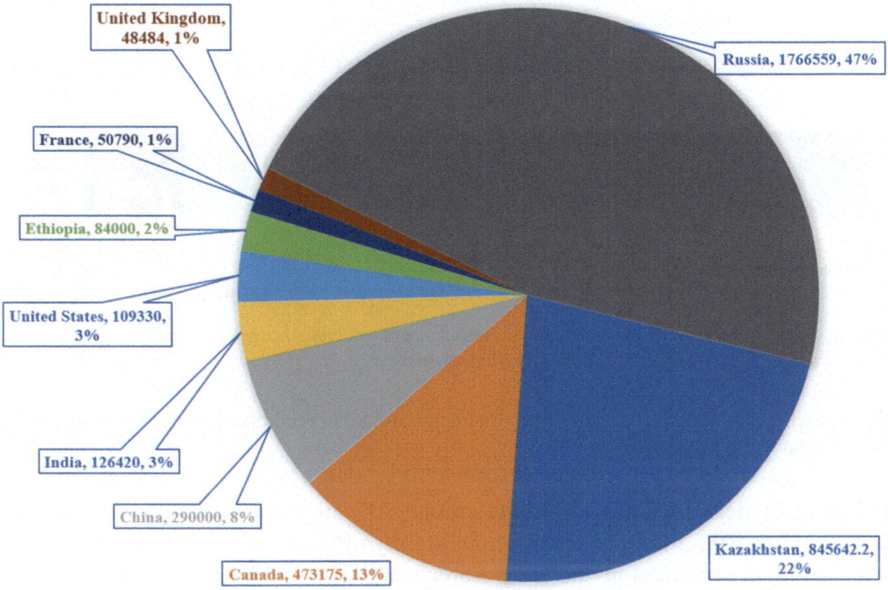

Fig. 2 Global linseed production: Top ten leading producers and their contribution (tonnes, %)

agricultural practices, improved seed varieties, and heightened demand for linseed oil and fiber are some of the factors contributing to this growth in production of linseed worldwide (Dixit et al., 2012).

2.1 Linseed Production in India

Linseed *(Linum usitatissimum),* a crucial rabi oilseed crop, holds significant economic and agricultural importance in India, it stands as the second most cultivated oilseed after rapeseed mustard, showcasing its pivotal role in the agricultural landscape (Saleem et al., 2020). In India, linseed is cultivated across an area of 3.420 lakh hectares, resulting in a production of 1.537 lakh tonnes. However, the average yield is 449 kg/ha, which is considerably lower than the global average productivity of 1006 kg/ha (Čeh et al., 2020). Due to its ability to grow in varied rainfed conditions, it occupies a greater importance among rabi oilseeds where it is grown mainly for seed used for extracting oil. De-oiled Linseed cake is a very good manure and animal feed. Linseed is also used in making paper and plastics. That is why it is also known as plastic crop.

The State-wise contribution to linseed production in India has been illustrated in Fig. 3. Madhya Pradesh is the leading state for linseed cultivation in India, followed by Jharkhand, Uttar Pradesh, Bihar, Rajasthan, Odisha, Nagaland, Chhattisgarh, Assam, and West Bengal. These states not only have significant acreage and yield but also hold prominent positions in terms of area and production. Madhya Pradesh

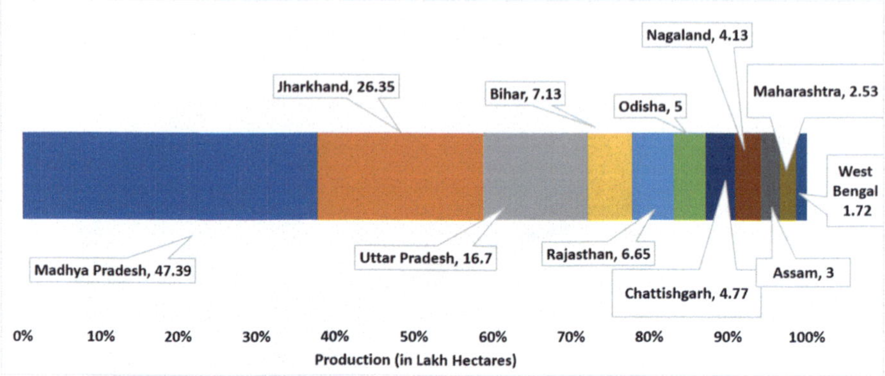

Fig. 3 State-wise contribution to linseed production in India (Seed division, GOI website (seednet.gov.in) & ICAR institutes)

and Uttar Pradesh together contribute around 70% of the national linseed production (DAC & FW, 2018). States such as Madhya Pradesh and Uttar Pradesh have achieved higher production due to favorable conditions and improved farming practices. In contrast, other regions show lower production due to lower yields caused by poor soil health (Shakya et al., 2023). Numerous varieties of linseed are cultivated in different regions suiting the climate, pluviometry and sunshine, hours of the region. The seed varieties cultivated in different regions of India with potential yield is tabulated in Table 1.

3 Cultivation Practices

3.1 Factors Affecting Cultivation Practices and Yield

Linseed (*Linumusitatissimum* L.) cultivation and yield are influenced by multiple factors, including genotype selection, environmental conditions, and management practices.

- *Genotype Selection:* The genus Linum has 20 species spread in warm temperate Europe and Asia and 50 species spread in America. The oil varieties that are relatively short branched usually bear large seeds and they are grown for high yield of linseed whereas the fiber varieties are taller, sparsely branched and usually bear small seeds. The transitional form is cultivated for both oil and fiber. To maximize yield, genotype selection is essential. The varieties vary in how they react to weather factors like temperature and precipitation. Oil content, composition, and linseed yield are also greatly influenced by environmental factors, including soil type, temperature and availability of water, and location. Studies have indicated that the use of cultivars such as Comtess and Altess can result in increased yields in areas with higher levels of precipitation and mid-heavy soils.

Table 1 Seed variety and yield cultivated in different regions of India

S. No	Seed variety	Yield potential (kg/ha)	States/regions
1.	LC-2063	41.00	Irrigated area of Punjab state
2.	Ruchi (LCK-5021)	39.84	UP (Except BKD), Bihar, WB JKD, Assam, and NEH region
3.	Himani (KL-214)	36.40	HP, J&K, Haryana, and Punjab
4.	Bhagsu (KL-215)	36.38	Himachal Pradesh, J&K, Uttaranchal, Punjab, Haryana
5.	SLS-73 (JLS-73)	38.82	BKD area of UP, MP, and Rajasthan
6.	JLS 67 Shival (Shival)	40.16	Bundelkhand of UP, MP, and Rajasthan
7.	Jawahar Linseed-41 (PKDL-41)	40.00	Area of MP state with limited irrigated facility
8.	PKV-NL-260 (NL-260)	37.67	Maharashtra
9.	MAU Azad Alsi-2	40.17	Chhattisgarh, Maharashtra, KNK, Odisha
10.	NDL 2004–05	42.00	UP
11.	NDL-2002	43.00	UP
12.	Arpita	35.67	Odisha
13.	Pratap Alsi-2	41.81	Rajasthan
14.	JLS-79	36.85	Madhya Pradesh
15.	Indu (LCK-1108)	39.0	Uttar Pradesh
16.	Divya (BAU-06-03)	39.81	Punjab, Haryana, HP, and Uttarakhand
17.	Him Palam Alsi-2(KL-263)	35.27	HP, Haryana, and J&K
18.	JLS-95	38.38	Bundelkhand part of Uttar Pradesh, Rajasthan, Madhya Pradesh, and Central Peninsular India (Zone-III)
19.	Sabour Tisi-1. (BAUP-101)	33.24	Uttar Pradesh excluding Bundelkhand, Bihar, Jharkhand, West Bengal, and Assam
20.	HIM PALAM ALSI-1 (KL-241		Himachal Pradesh
21.	JLS-66 (SLS 66)	42.85	Madhya Pradesh
22.	UteraAlsi (RLC-143)	34.01	Chhattisgarh, Odisha, Madhya Pradesh, Bihar, Jharkhand, and Assam
23.	NDL 2004–05	42.00	UP
24.	VarshaAlsi (RLC-148)	36.4	Rajasthan, Madhya Pradesh, Bundelkhand region of Uttar Pradesh, Odisha, Maharashtra, Chhattisgarh, and Karnataka
25.	Jawahar Linseed-66, (SLS-66)	42.80	Rainfed areas of MP

(continued)

Table 1 (continued)

S. No	Seed variety	Yield potential (kg/ha)	States/regions
26.	Surya (LCK-1404)	35.49	Jammu and Kashmir, Himachal Pradesh, Punjab, and Haryana
27.	TL-99		UP, Bihar, Jharkhand, WB, Assam, and Nagaland
28.	LSL-93	37.95	Maharashtra
29.	Azad Alsi-1 (LMS 9-2 K)	39.92	Bundelkhand of UP, MP, and Rajasthan
30.	Jawahar Linseed-66, (SLS-66)	42.80	Rainfed areas of MP

Source Economics, Statistics & Evaluation Division, Ministry of Agriculture & Farmers Welfare, (GOI, 2023)

The cultivation techniques and yield of linseed are significantly influenced by the variety, timing of sowing, and cultivation location. For example, in warmer Mediterranean climates, autumn sowing yields higher seed and oil yields than spring sowing (Čeh et al., 2020). In India, the linseed varieties are of two types: peninsular types, which have deep root system and alluvial types, which are shallow rooted and are characterized by profuse tillering. There are number of varieties available for cultivation in different cropping systems, situations, and for varied agro-climatic conditions in linseed. A considerable number of double purpose varieties have been developed, which have good seed and fiber yielding potentials. Varieties differ in maturity, growth habit, and seed size and color.

- *Environmental Conditions:* The yield and oil content of linseed are greatly influenced by temperature and the availability of water. While chilly and wet circumstances in the spring can prevent plant emergence, water scarcity and high temperature in the summer can have a detrimental impact on harvests (Čeh et al., 2020; Koubaa-Ghorbel et al., 2020). Research shows that colder temperatures increase the amount of omega-3 fatty acids in linseed, especially α-linolenic acid. Although it does well with irrigation, linseed is normally produced in rainfed environments. Studies show that even little watering during crucial phases greatly boosts productivity. For instance, compared to single irrigation regimes or no irrigation at all, two irrigations at 35 and 70 days after sowing (DAS) have demonstrated noticeably greater seed yields. This improved yield can be attributed to better plant stand, increased plant height, more branches per plant, and higher straw yield due to improved nutrient utilization facilitated by water (Koubaa-Ghorbel et al., 2020). The environmental factors most likely to affect yields were high temperature, due to its effect on development rate, and the consequent shortening of the growing cycle and perhaps water shortage. The foliage duration was more important than the maximum leaf area index.

- *Weed Management:* Herbicide use and manual weeding are two important strategies for minimizing weed competition, which can otherwise result in large production losses. Studies emphasize the significance of integrated weed control plans suited to crop and environmental circumstances.
  A significant obstacle to growing linseed is weeds, especially when resources are scarce. Twenty-five to forty-five days after sowing is the important period for crop-weed competition and weed infestations can result in yield losses of up to 42–45%. Herbicide application and early weed eradication are essential components of effective weed management. It has been discovered that a number of herbicides, including pre- and postemergence products, are effective at controlling weeds. Pendimethalin and imazethapyr, for example, have proven to be a good combination for controlling troublesome weeds and boosting seed output. Even though it takes a lot of work, hand weeding is still a very successful technique, especially when done twice during the crucial period (Čeh et al., 2020). Hand weeding is quite popular in small farms like India otherwise chemical control is followed. Hand weeding also allows proper aeration for the growth of root zone. A wheel hoe is often used in weeding between the rows.
- *Farming Practices:* Farming practices in linseed play a crucial role in determining the quality, yield, and profitability of the crop. For instance, the method and timing of tillage affect soil structure and nutrient availability. Planting density and proper spacing ensures optimal light, water, and nutrient availability for each plant. Other practices including crop rotation and diversifying plant types can help maintain soil fertility and reduce pest and disease incidents. Bund cleaning is also being practiced for maintaining field sanitation, which helps in eradicating alternate perennial hosts of the crop pests.
- *Nutrient and Fertilizer Management:* Proper fertilizer management is crucial for linseed growth. Nitrogen, phosphorus, and potassium are the primary nutrients required, with specific recommendations varying based on soil fertility and environmental conditions. Organic amendments, such as compost and manure, can also enhance soil health and crop productivity. Nutrient availability, particularly phosphorus and sulfur, is vital for linseed growth and yield. Adequate fertilizer application strategies are necessary to meet the crop's nutritional requirements, thereby enhancing yield and oil content. Linseed cultivation often occurs in nutrient and moisture-deprived conditions, leading to lower productivity. Improved varieties respond well to fertilizers, particularly nitrogen, phosphorus (P), and potassium (K). Phosphorus enhances root development and helps in utilizing subsurface moisture, while potassium is crucial for the healthy development of the linseed plant, with deficiencies leading to shorter stems and fiber length (Tiwari et al., 2018). Sulfur application significantly boosts seed and oil yield, with studies showing increased yields with sulfur levels up to 60 kg/h. Fertilizers like gypsum have proven effective in improving nutrient uptake and yields. The combination of full NPK doses with organic amendments like FYM (farmyard manure) further enhances seed yields (Sangma, 2019). The applica-

tion of nitrogen equivalent to 60 kg/ha through vermicompost in linseed proved to be highly effective in enhancing the growth and yield of linseed, positively influencing various parameters, from plant height to test weight (Janghel et al., 2023). The response to applied biofertilizer was greater in the absence of chemical fertilizer and the response decreased with increase in chemical fertilizer level (Lawania et al., 2015).

3.2 Linseed Varieties

Linseed varieties exhibit different responses to environmental factors and management practices. Selecting the appropriate variety is essential for maximizing yield and oil quality. For instance, the Comtess variety has been identified as yielding the highest oil content among various tested genotypes. The genetic makeup of linseed varieties influences their resistance to environmental stresses and their nutritional profile, particularly the omega-3 to omega-6 fatty acid ratio, which is beneficial for human health (Heller et al., 2015).

3.3 Cropping Cycle

The cropping cycle for linseed involves several critical stages, from seedbed preparation to sowing, growth, and harvesting. Proper timing and management of these stages are crucial for achieving optimal yields. Linseed can be grown in rotation with other crops to enhance soil fertility and reduce pest and disease incidence. The choice of preceding and succeeding crops in the rotation cycle can significantly influence linseed productivity (Singh et al., 2022). Intercropping of chickpea with linseed in 4:2 and 5:1 row arrangement was equally productive as sole chickpea and 50% economy in fertilizer dose to linseed can be achieved under intercropping system, thus providing an opportunity for diversification and achieving stability under rainfed situations. Intercropping systems were found more advantageous than sole cropping under reduced fertilizer application.

- *Seedbed Preparation:* A well-prepared seedbed ensures good seed-to-soil contact, which is essential for uniform germination and growth. Soil should be tilled to a fine texture to facilitate root development and nutrient uptake.
- *Sowing:* Sowing time and seed rate are critical factors. Early sowing in regions with a longer growing season can result in better establishment and higher yields. The recommended seed rate varies based on soil fertility and environmental conditions but generally ranges between 25 kg/ha and 40 kg/ha.
- *Growth Stages:* Linseed growth stages include germination, seedling, vegetative growth, flowering, and seed maturation. Each stage requires specific management practices to ensure healthy crop development. Adequate irrigation, pest, and disease control during these stages are vital for achieving high yields (Kumar et al., 2019).

3.4 Crop Management

Effective crop management practices, including pest and disease control, are essential for maintaining linseed health and productivity. Implementing agro-ecological approaches that focus on promoting soil health, diversifying vegetation, and creating landscape heterogeneity is recommended. Specific practices such as breeding for genetic resistance and applying seed treatments can also be beneficial (Vega et al., 2023). Additionally, managing plant diseases involves avoidance strategies like crop rotation and phytosanitary measures, alongside control methods such as developing resistant cultivars and increasing diversity in cropping systems.

- *Pest and Disease Control:* Linseed is susceptible to various pests and diseases, including aphids, cutworms, and fungal infections like powdery mildew and rust. Integrated pest management (IPM) strategies, combining chemical and biological controls, are effective in minimizing pest and disease impact (Čeh et al., 2020).
- *Integrated Disease Management (IDM):* The important diseases damaging linseed crop in India are mainly fungal, causing crop losses up to 80–100 percent under epidemic condition. Rust (*Melampsora lini* Erenb), wilt [*Fusarium oxysporum* f.sp. lini (Bolley) Snyder & Hansen], Alternaria blight (Alternaria lini Dey, Alternaria linicola Groves and Skolko), powdery mildew [*Oidium lini* Skoric, *Leveillula taurica* (Lev.) Arnaud] are the major ones. The minor diseases are *Macrophomina/Rhizoctonia* wilt/collar rot, *Sclerotium stem* rot, *Pythium* damping-off, *Botrytis* rot, anthracnose and *Dreschlera* blight. Strategies like regular scouting, accurate disease identification, and chemical control, are crucial for mitigating yield loss in linseed and other crops, emphasizing the need for proactive disease management practices.
- *Irrigation:* Irrigation management is critical, especially in regions with irregular rainfall. Overhead and drip irrigation systems can be used to ensure consistent water supply during critical growth stages, such as flowering and seed filling (Estela et al., 2007).

3.5 Effect on Soil Health

Soil health is a fundamental component of sustainable agriculture, with significant implications for agricultural productivity, ecosystem vitality, and food security. Linseed cultivation can have positive effects on soil health, particularly when integrated into crop rotation systems (Makkar et al., 2019). Linseed's deep root system helps improve soil structure and enhances nutrient cycling. Additionally, linseed residues contribute organic matter to the soil, promoting microbial activity and soil fertility.

- *Soil Erosion Control:* The extensive root network of linseed plants helps in soil stabilization, reducing the risk of erosion. This is particularly beneficial in regions prone to heavy rainfall and wind erosion.

- *Soil Nutrient Balance:* Linseed can enhance soil nutrient balance by fixing nitrogen and improving phosphorus availability through its root exudates. Crop rotation involving linseed and legumes can further boost soil nitrogen levels, benefiting subsequent crops (Klein et al., 2017).

Understanding and optimizing the factors affecting linseed cultivation practices and yield, selecting appropriate varieties, managing cropping cycles, and implementing effective crop management strategies are essential for maximizing linseed productivity. These practices also contribute to soil health and sustainability, making linseed a valuable crop in diverse agricultural systems.

4 Harvesting Practices

Harvesting procedures for flax are tailored to the type and intended application. When flax is grown for fiber, the stalks are plucked up by the roots before the seeds ripened and dried upright to separate the fibers from the stem. Harvesting of linseed crop at optimum stage is important. It is observed that when plant is harvested before the optimum harvesting time the yield is low. Despite having low strength, the former fiber is finely textured and soft. The optimum time to harvest linseed crop is at the yellow ripened stage of stem when the lowest two-thirds of the stem are defoliated (capsule maturity stage) to preserve fiber and seed quality (Husain et al., 2009). The linseed crop is harvested in 130–150 days. The linseed crop is harvested when the leaves are dried and the capsules turn brown. Along with this when the seeds become shiny the crop is harvested using a sickle. The crop is then beaten with sticks or tramped by the use of bullocks, this technique is known as threshing (Ahlawat, 2008). The harvest time is important for the dual-purpose production of flaxseed. This balance helps to avoid excess lignification, which helps to obtain a high seed yield (Rossini & Casa, 2003). After harvesting the crop, it should be allowed to dry in the field. Harvesting is then followed by winnowing, which is a process done to remove the straw from the seed with the help of a winnower or natural wind (Singh, 2016). The linseed crop harvesting is done at red ripe stage for grain as well as fiber purposes. After threshing, the moisture content of the crop should lie between 10% and 12% before storage. The maturation of linseed crop initiates in February. The harvesting also depends upon sowing time and winter spread. The harvesting is done at capsule maturity when fiber is required along with the seed (Maurya, 2020).

The harvest index is an agricultural concept, which measures the efficiency of conversion of total biomass turned into harvestable yield. The harvest index can be calculated by the ratio of economic yield to total biological yield. Apart from this, apparent harvest index can be calculated by the ratio of seed weight and mature plant weight times 100 (Tavarini et al., 2019). Linseed crop is harvested in the rabi season, starting in somewhere in the month of February and ending in the month of April in different states of India. Table 2 shows the harvesting calendar of linseed crop.

Table 2 Harvesting calendar of linseed crop (Singh, 2016)

Starting month	Week	State
February	1st	Karnataka
	4th	Andhra Pradesh
March	1st	Assma, Bihar, Madhya Pradesh, Chhattisgarh, Maharashtra, Uttar Pradesh, Orrisa, Jharkhand, West Bengal, Rajasthan, and Nagaland
	4th	Punjab
April	4th	Himachal Pradesh and J&K
Ending month		
March	2nd and 3rd	Karnataka
	4th	Rajasthan, Andhra Pradesh, Bihar, Maharashtra, Chhattisgarh, Madhya Pradesh, Orrisa
April	2nd and 3rd	West Bengal
	4th	Assam, Bihar, Uttar Pradesh, Jharkhand, Punjab
May	2nd and 3rd	Himachal Pradesh and J&K

5 Conclusion

Linseed is one of the oldest as well as most useful and versatile crop. It is cultivated in more than 30 countries worldwide and has an important contribution in agricultural productivity and economic stability. It has an array of applications in the food, feed, and industrial sector. The chapter had discussed the multifaceted aspects of its production, harvest, and varieties from a historical as well as geographical context in detail. The global and national production scenarios highlight the significance of this versatile crop with its widespread application in various industries. Obtaining the potential yield is still a challenge to many developing countries whereas climatic change is becoming an urgent issue to be addressed. The factors that influence cultivation practices and yield, such as genotypic characteristics, environmental conditions, and geographical morphology, are crucial for optimizing its production. The crop management and disease control strategies play a vital role in maintaining the quality and quantity of the crop. The integrated pest management approach, involving the use of biological, cultural, and chemical method has been observed to be most effective for preserving the quality of linseed. Additionally, methods such as regular monitoring, and use of resistant varieties, also form a crucial part of the crop management system. The application of such systems can ensure a better productivity and health of crop, while mitigating any economic loses. Furthermore, it is a valuable alternative for cropping systems owing to its adaptability to poor soil conditions. Effective harvesting practices are essential for ensuring the quality and economic value of the linseed crop. Proper timing, techniques, and postharvest handling are critical for preserving seed quality and minimizing losses. Advances in agriculture and storage technology can further improve the efficacy of linseed production.

References

Ahlawat, I. P. S. (2008). Linseed.'Agronomy—Rabi Crops' Production.

All India Normal Estimation of Area, Production and yield of linseed (Average 2017–18 to 2021–22) source economics, statistics & evaluation division, ministry of agriculture & farmers welfare, GOI, 2023.

Bernacchia, R., Preti, R., & Vinci, G. (2014). Chemical composition and health benefits of flaxseed. *Austin Journal of Nutrition and Food Sciences, 2*(8), 1045.

Biradar, S., Ajithkumar, K., Rajanna, B., Savitha, A., Shubha, G., Shankergoud, I., Chittapur, B., & Singh, P. (2016). Prospects and challenges in linseed (Linumusitatissimum L.) production: A review. *Journal of Oilseeds Research, 33*(1), 1–13.

Casa, R., Russell, G., Lo Cascio, B., & Rossini, F. (1999). Environmental effects on linseed (Linum usitatissimum L.) yield and growth of flax at different stand densities. *European Journal of Agronomy, 11*(3), 267–278.

Čeh, B., Štraus, S., Hladnik, A., & Kušar, A. (2020). Impact of linseed variety, location and production year on seed yield. *Oil Content and Its Composition. Agronomy, 10*(11), 1770. https://doi.org/10.3390/agronomy10111770

Department of Agriculture, Cooperation and Farmers Welfare (DAC & FW). (2018). *Agricultural statistics at a glance 2019*. Available at www.agricoop.nic.in & http://eands.dacnet.nic.in

Dixit, S., Kanakraj, S., & Rehman, A. (2012). Linseed oil as a potential resource for bio-diesel: A review. *Renewable and Sustainable Energy Reviews, 16*(7), 4415–4421. https://doi.org/10.1016/j.rser.2012.04.042

Estela, G., Schalamuk, S.-V. S., & Sarandón, S. J. (2007). Effect of different sowing patterns of oil linseed (Linumusitatissimum L.) crop on Brassica sp. as a strategy for sustainable weed management. *Biological Agriculture & Horticulture, 25*(2), 123–131. https://doi.org/10.1080/01448765.2007.9755041

FAO. (2013). *Food and agriculture organization of united nations*. Available at, http://faostat3.fao.org/faostat-gateway

FAO. (2022). *Food and agriculture organization of united nations*. Available at, https://www.fao.org/markets-and-trade/commodities/oilcrops/en/

Heller, K., Sheng, Q. C., Guan, F., Alexopoulou, E., Hua, L. S., Wu, G. W., Jankauskienė, Z., & Fu, W. Y. (2015). A comparative study between Europe and China in crop management of two types of flax: linseed and fibre flax. *Industrial Crops and Products, 68*, 24–31. https://doi.org/10.1016/j.indcrop.2014.07.010, https://desagri.gov.in/document-report/4-1-17-state-wise-yield-of-linseed/, https://doi.org/10.56739/jor.v34i2.137694.

Husain, K., et al. (2009). Production technology and industrial uses of dual purpose linseed (Linumusitatissimum): An overview. *Indian Journal of Agronomy, 54*(4), 374–379.

Janghel, V., Kher, D., Ahirwal, A., Prakash, A., Azad, A. R., & Chourasiya, P. (2023). Response of liquid biofertilizers on yield and economics of linseed (Linum usitatissimum L.). *Pharma Innovations, 12*(10), 1856–1860.

Klein, J., Zikeli, S., Claupein, W., & Gruber, S. (2017). Linseed (Linumusitatissimum) as an oil crop in organic farming: abiotic impacts on seed ingredients and yield. *Organic Agriculture, 7*(1), 1–19. https://doi.org/10.1007/s13165-016-0146-6

Koubaa-Ghorbel, F., Chaâbane, M., Turki, M., Makni-Ayadi, F., & El Feki, A. (2020). The protective effects of Salvia officinalis essential oil compared to simvastatin against hyperlipidemia, liver, and kidney injuries in mice submitted to a high-fat diet. *Journal of Food Biochemistry, 44*(4), e13160. https://doi.org/10.1111/jfbc.13160

Kumar, A., Pramanick, B., Mahapatra, B. S., Singh, S. P., & Shukla, D. K. (2019). Growth, yield and quality improvement of flax (Linumusitattisimum L.) grown under tarai region of Uttarakhand, India through integrated nutrient management practices. *Industrial Crops and Products, 140*, 111710. https://doi.org/10.1016/j.indcrop.2019.111710

Lawania, T. K., Singh, B. P., Gupta, D. K. S., & Adityendera, K. (2015). Effect of biofertilizer, nitrogen and sulphur on growth and yield of linseed (Linum usitatissimum L.). *Annals of Agricultural Research, 36*(1), 77–81. file:///C:/Users/Compeq/Downloads/ojsadmin,+77-81.pdf.

Makkar, C., Singh, J., & Parkash, C. (2019). Modulatory role of vermicompost and vermiwash on growth, yield and nutritional profiling of Linumusitatissimum L. (Linseed): a field study. *Environmental Science and Pollution Research, 26*(3), 3006–3018. https://doi.org/10.1007/s11356-018-3845-6

Maurya, A. K. (2020). 'Advances in essential oils and natural products', Advances in Essential Oils and Natural Products [Preprint], (November). https://doi.org/10.22271/ed.book.985

Rossini, F., & Casa, R. (2003). Influence of sowing and harvest time on fibre flax (Linumusitatissimum L.) in the Mediterranean environment. *Journal of Agronomy and Crop Science, 189*(3), 191–196. https://doi.org/10.1046/j.1439-037X.2003.00034.x

Saleem, M. H., Ali, S., Hussain, S., Kamran, M., Chattha, M. S., Ahmad, S., Aqeel, M., Rizwan, M., Aljarba, N. H., Alkahtani, S., & Abdel-Daim, M. M. (2020). Flax (Linumusitatissimum L.): A potential candidate for phytoremediation? *Biological and Economical Points of View. Plants, 9*(4), 496. https://doi.org/10.3390/plants9040496

Sangma, E. (2019). Impact of irrigation and nutrient management on growth and yield of flaxseed (Linumusitatissimum L.). *Trends in Biosciences, 10*(March), 5624–5626.

Shakya, L., Singh, A., Agnihotri, A., Muyal, J. P., Umar, S., Barwa, S., & Dhiman, S. K. (2023). Various approaches used to increase the growth and yield of linseed linseed crop. *International Journal of Plant And Environment, 9*(04), 291–300.

Singh, P. K. (2016). Status paper on linseed/Flax agriculture. In M. V. Hegde, A. A. Zanwar, & S. P. Adekar (Eds.), *Omega-3 Fatty Acids* (pp. 21–44). Springer. https://doi.org/10.1007/978-3-319-40458-5_3, https://doi.org/10.56739/jor.v34i2.137694

Singh, A. B., Meena, B. P., Lakaria, B. L., Thakur, J. K., Ramesh, K., Rajput, P. S., & Patra, A. K. (2022). Production potential, soil health and economics of soybean (Glycine max)-linseed (Linumusitatissimum) cropping system under various nutrient-management protocols. *Indian Journal of Agronomy, 67*(3), 269–275. https://doi.org/10.59797/ija.v67i3.28

Tavarini, S., et al. (2019). Evaluation of chemical composition of two linseed varieties as sources of health-beneficial substances. *Molecules, 24*(20), 3729. https://doi.org/10.3390/molecules24203729

Tiwari, U. S., Dubey, S. D., Pandey, R. K., & Husain, K. (2018). Effect of integrated nutrient management on yield, nutrient uptake and quality of Linseed (Linum ustiatissimum L) in central plane zone of U.P. *Journal of Pharmacognosy and Phytochemistry, 7*(4), 643–645.

Vega, D., Ibarra, S., Varela Pardo, R. A., & Poggio, S. L. (2023). Agroecological management of crop diseases: A review. *Agroecology and Sustainable Food Systems, 47*(7), 919–949.

Zanetti, F., Monti, A., & Berti, M. T. (2013). Challenges and opportunities for new industrial oilseed crops in EU-27: A review. *Industrial Crops and Products, 50*, 580–595. https://doi.org/10.1016/j.indcrop.2013.08.030

Zuk, M., Richter, D., Matuła, J., & Szopa, J. (2015). Linseed, the multipurpose plant. *Industrial Crops and Products, 75*, 165–177. https://doi.org/10.1016/j.indcrop.2015.05.005

Physicochemical Characteristics, Handling, and Storage of Linseeds

Monika Chand, Rajni Chopra, Yachana, Deepak Joshi, Abdul Wahid P, and Himanshi Madan

Abstract

Linseed, or flaxseed, is an oilseed renowned for its rich nutritional profile and numerous health benefits. Originating from the Mediterranean and southwest Asia, linseed has been cultivated for millennia. It is a small shiny, oval oil seeds in appearance and varying in color from yellow to brown. The seed's physical characteristics, such as angle of repose, bulk density, and true density, play an important role in handling linseeds at a larger scale. Linseeds are rich in bioactive compounds including phenolics, lignans, secoisolariciresinol diglucoside, flavonoids, and carotenoids, which contribute to its significant antioxidant properties. The seed's comprehensive nutritional profile includes carbohydrates, fats, proteins, dietary fiber, and essential vitamins and minerals like vitamins E, K, and B complex, along with magnesium, calcium, and phosphorus. Effective handling and storage practices are crucial for maintaining its quality and minimizing postharvest losses. This involves cleaning and drying, which can be achieved through both traditional and advanced methods. Proper storage conditions are vital to prevent microbial contamination, lipid oxidation, and physicochemical changes. Factors such as moisture content, temperature, and packaging materials significantly impact the seeds' shelf life and quality. This chapter explores best practices for handling and storage, providing a detailed understanding of the physicochemical characteristics of linseed and its handling.

Keywords

Linseed storage · Physicochemical properties · Postharvest handling · Nutritional composition · Lipid oxidation prevention

M. Chand · R. Chopra (✉) · Yachana · D. Joshi · Abdul Wahid P · H. Madan
Department of Food Science and Technology, National Institute of Food Technology Entrepreneurship and Management, Kundli, Haryana, India
e-mail: rajni.chopra@niftem.ac.in

© The Author(s), under exclusive license to Springer Nature Singapore Pte Ltd. 2025

R. Chopra et al. (eds.), *Dynamics of Linseed and its Valorization*,
https://doi.org/10.1007/978-981-96-8927-9_2

1 Introduction

Linseed, due to its rich nutritional profile and versatile use, has been cultivated for thousands of years. The mediterranean and southwest Asia are considered the genesis regions of linseed (Millam et al., 2005). The morphological structure of linseed includes three layers: cotyledon, endosperm, and spermoderm (outermost to innermost). Linseeds have a glossy appearance and the color varies broadly from yellow to brown. The seed length, width, and thickness vary from 4.27 to 4.64 mm, 2.22 to 2.38 mm, and 0.85 to 0.88 mm respectively. Other engineering properties such as angle of repose, bulk density, true density all vary with respect to variety and moisture content.

Linseeds are a rich source of bioactive compounds including phenolics, lignans, secoisolariciresinol diglucoside, flavonoids, and carotenoids that enhance its antioxidant properties (Mueed et al., 2022). These compounds contribute to the seeds' health-promoting effects, making them a valuable addition to the human diet. Linseeds are considered as a multicomponent system due to their excellent nutritional profile. The carbohydrate content varies from 22% to 29%, fat (25% to 40%), protein (16% to 20%), and dietary fiber (25% to 29%) (Goyal et al., 2014) (Qui et al., 2020; Kauser et al., 2023). Linseeds constitute several minerals, water, and fat-soluble vitamins, specifically vitamins E and K (Katoch & Bhatia, 2021). While in water-soluble vitamins, it has a vitamin B complex. Additionally, it is a rich source of magnesium, calcium, and phosphorous. A total of 30 g of seed provides 7–30% of RDA for certain minerals (Singh et al., 2011).

It is equally important to understand the intrinsic properties of the seeds for appropriate handling and storage practices. These practices are essential for maintaining seed quality and minimizing postharvest losses. Cleaning and drying are important steps prior to application of seeds in the final products. Cleaning enhances its quality and utility by removing unwanted impurities from seeds. Drying can be done through conventional and nonconventional methods. Solar drying, air drying, and oven drying have been traditionally used for a long time to remove moisture from seeds. Advanced drying techniques including freeze drying, vacuum drying, microwave drying, and infra-red drying have a tendency to reduce the time and enhance yield as well as control the nutrient losses. Storage of seeds is crucial to slow down the microbial contamination, lipid oxidation, and physicochemical changes (Prescha et al., 2014; Douny et al., 2016; Szumała & Wysocka, 2018). Several other factors such as moisture content, temperature, environmental, and microbial conditions help in maintaining quality during storage (Kiaya, 2014). This chapter explores the best practices for handling and storage, aiming to mitigate degradation and preserve the functional and nutritional value of the seeds in detail. Understanding the physicochemical characteristics of linseeds is critical for optimizing their utilization across various sectors.

2 Physical Properties of Linseed

2.1 Morphology

Linseed has a variety of physical characteristics that enhance its adaptability to a wide range of uses. The seeds have a smooth, glossy surface and are small, oval-shaped, ranging from golden yellow to reddish-brown in color. Linseeds are usually 4–6 mm long and 2–3 mm wide (Slominski et al., 2007). There are three layers of seeds: cotyledon, endosperm, and spermoderm (outermost to innermost) (Fig. 1). The external hull or the mucous epidermis is where mucilage (water-soluble polysaccharides) is located, also known as testa. This layer is tough and has negligible amounts of protein and fat. The inner layer or tegmen of the hull is soft and has some amount of oil and protein. The epidermal cells consist of a varying number of layers of parenchyma cells, often ranging from one to five layers. The cells are called ring cells and may contain tannin and chlorophyll, which are responsible for the color of the seeds. The sclerenchyma, which is generally colorless, is a single layer of cells located directly below the ring cells. The subsequent two layers are formed of transversely oriented cells with uneven alignment. Another cellular layer present is the endosperm, which has a high concentration of oil and protein. The embryo is enclosed inside it and is characterized by being dicotyledonous. Typically, the cotyledons are mostly white or yellowish in color and also contain oil. The embryo is developed along an embryonic axis, and at each end, there is a proliferating point. The shoot system consists of the apical meristem located at the uppermost part of the plant, while the root system is produced by the basal meristem situated at the lowermost part of the plant. The seed is attached to the ovary wall by a stalk called the funiculus (Zuk et al., 2015).

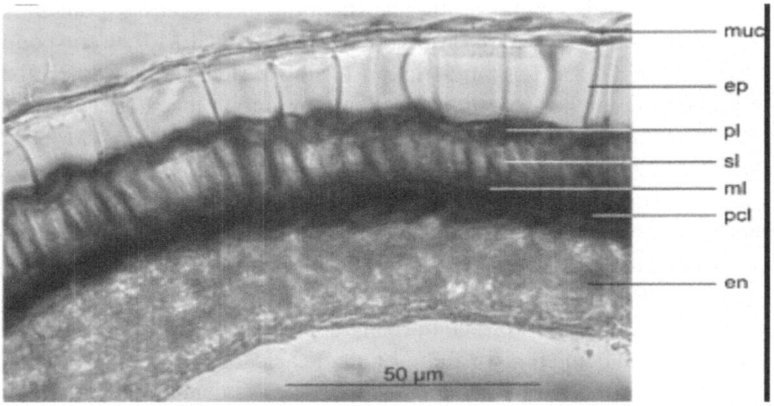

Fig. 1 Seed morphology of linseed adopted from Zuk et al. (2015) (*Linum usitatissimum* L.): embryo (em); seed coat (sc) also called the testa; cotyledons (seed leaves), (sl); endosperm (en); epicotyl (epc); hypocotyl (hy); radicle (ra); mucilage cell (muc); epidermis (ep); parenchymatous layer (pl); sclerite layer (sl); membraniform layer (ml); brown layer (bl); endosperm (en)

2.2 Engineering Properties

Linseeds encompass a diverse range of phytonutrients and essential fatty acids; this promising profile of linseeds makes it to count in superfoods. Knowledge of physical and mechanical properties of linseed aids in designing efficient harvesting, and processing equipment ensures quality control and fosters innovation in developing new food products. Linseed's nutritional value is significantly affected by numerous factors that include storage conditions and periods, process parameters, and environmental factors like moisture. Thus, studying the engineering properties of linseeds is important to preserves the rich nutritional and structural profile of the seed, such as size, mass, sphericity, surface area, bulk density, true density, porosity, angle of repose, and frictional properties. These properties are crucial for designing equipment for handling, processing, and storing (Selvi et al., 2006; Yalcin et al., 2010). Physicochemical properties of linseeds also get affected by environmental factors including the year of production, location, variety, seed maturity, cultivar modifications, and processing operations like fat extraction methods (Čeh et al., 2020; Piłat & Zadernowski, 2010). These factors not only affect the physical characteristics but also alter protein, oil, and ash contents, bioactive substances like tocopherols and sterols, as well as the fatty acid composition of linseeds, particularly affecting α-linolenic and oleic acids (Yalcin et al., 2010).

The seed length, width, thickness, arithmetic mean diameter (AM), and geometric mean (GM) diameter varied from 4.27 mm to 4.64 mm, 2.22 mm to 2.38 mm, 0.85 mm to 0.88 mm, 2.45 mm to 2.63 mm, and 2.00 mm to 2.12 mm, respectively (Coşkuner & Karababa, 2007). According to Pradhan et al. (2010), the AM and GM was found to be 2.67 and 2.21, respectively and angle of repose vary ranging from 21.57% to 33.38%. The density parameters including true density varies from 1000 kg/m^3 to 1111 kg/m^3, while bulk density varies from 726.6 kg/m^3 to 555.6 kg/m^3. Pradhan et al. (2010) reported bulk and true densities of 652.16 kg m^{-3} and 784 kg m^{-3}, respectively. In the current investigation, the synthesized binders exhibited densities of 37.5 kg m^{-3} for CEM I and 36 kg m^{-3} for CEM II, corresponding to a total porosity of 16.83 %. Static-friction testing further demonstrated that plywood presented the highest coefficient of friction among the substrates evaluated. The static coefficient of friction increased from 0.537 to 1.073, 0.515 to 0.933, 0.472 to 0.975, 0.499 to 0.877, 0.544 to 0.862, and 0.472 to 0. These were 824 for plywood, aluminum, stainless steel, galvanized iron, polypropylene knitted bag, and kraft paper surfaces, respectively. However, in another study the static coefficient of friction was found to be at least 0. 23 on the plastic sheet and maximum at 0.33 (Pradhan et al., 2010).

Notably, linseed is rich in oil, comprising about 30–45% of its weight, with the extracted linseed oil being high in alpha-linolenic acid, an omega-3 fatty acid (Daun et al., 2003). Its thermal properties include low thermal conductivity and a specific heat capacity of around 2.5 J/g·°C (Singh et al., 2011). Mechanically, linseed is relatively hard, withstanding milling and grinding processes, and exhibits moderate elasticity, making it suitable for use in composite materials and linoleum (Zuk et al., 2015). Additionally, linseed's hygroscopic nature allows it to absorb moisture from the air, affecting its storage stability, while its high fiber content enables it to form a mucilaginous gel when mixed with water (Oomah & Mazza, 1993). These properties make linseed valuable in food products, nutritional supplements, and industrial applications such as linseed oil for paints and varnishes, and the production of biodegradable plastics and composites. The physicochemical properties of linseeds are influenced by factors like variety. Varietal factors affecting linseed properties include plant height, seed weight, oil content (29.2–44.8%), protein content (19.80–21.72%), fatty acid composition, essential amino acids, and mineral composition (Narina et al., 2012).

2.3 Nutritional Composition

Linseed is well-known for its rich nutritive profile due to its high-quality carbohydrate, fat, protein, soluble dietary fibers, omega-3 polyunsaturated fatty acids (PUFA), lignans, vitamins, and minerals making it a multicomponent system (Goyal et al., 2014) (Fig. 2). Linseed's nutritional composition is affected by factors such as its environmental influences, particularly weather (temperature and rainfall regime), heredity, and seed preparation strategy (Kauser et al., 2023).

2.3.1 Carbohydrate

Linseeds are a rich source of nutrients, with carbohydrates constituting approximately 30% of their dry weight (Tarique et al., 2023). This percentage may vary, ranging around 22.6 grams per 100 grams of seeds. This variation can be attributed to several factors influencing the growth and processing of linseeds. Environmental conditions, such as temperature and rainfall patterns during cultivation, have been

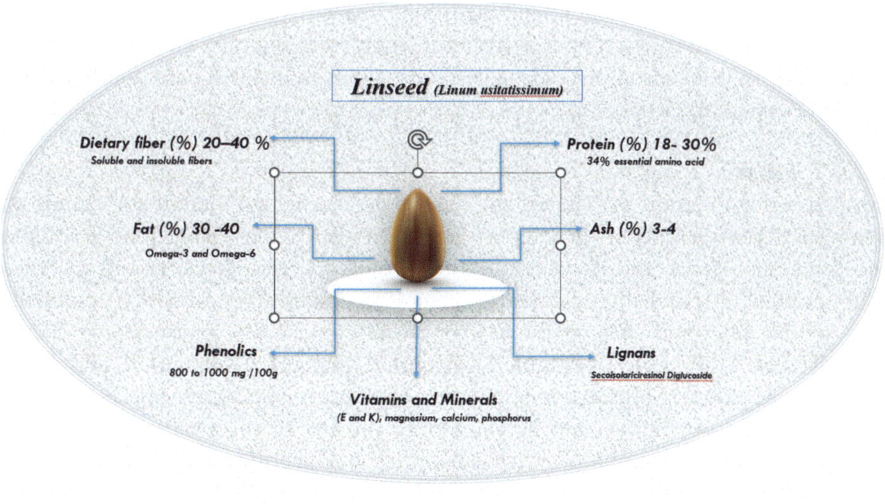

Fig. 2 Composition of linseed

shown to impact the final nutritional composition (Čeh et al., 2020). Additionally, the genetic makeup of the specific linseed variety can play a role in determining its inherent carbohydrate content (Kauser et al., 2023). Finally, the processing methods employed, such as grinding versus consuming whole seeds, can influence the accessibility and digestibility of the carbohydrate fraction.

2.3.2 Protein

Linseed is another proteinaceous crop in abundance, which is akin to soybean protein. It is however important to note that there is variability in the amount of protein in linseed with the amount ranging from 10% and 31% (Oomah & Mazza, 1993). Linseed has two major storage proteins, a predominant salt soluble protein with high molecular weight (11-12S; globulin; 18. 6% nitrogen) and a water-soluble basic protein with low molecular weight (1.6-2S; albumin; 17. 7% nitrogen) (Oomah et al., 2007). The amount of protein varies from genetic, environmental factors to the physical condition of the seeds. The crude protein level of dehulled and defatted linseed samples ranged significantly due to the growth of samples and processing techniques. Hull fraction has lower protein contents and that on dehulling, the protein content of linseed increases to 19. 2–21. 8% (Oomah & Mazza, 1993). Additionally, it has been noted that cool conditions often lead to seeds with high oil content and low protein content. The detailed amino acid profile is present in Table 2.

2.3.3 Fat

Linseed is an excellent source of healthy fat that exhibits various therapeutic properties (Kauser et al., 2023). The amount of fat varies from 25% to 45% of total seed weight as mentioned in Table 1. It is highly rich in unsaturated fat (87.8–89.8%) notably linolenic acid (C18:3). Linseed fat is one of the best plant sources of ω-3 fatty acid and ω-6 fatty acid (Goyal et al., 2014) (Qui et al., 2020; Kauser et al., 2023). However, the fat content and quality of linseed is affected by both environmental and hereditary factors. For instance, temperate regions with cool climates leads to higher concentrations of omega-3 fatty acids in linseed, particularly linolenic acid (Čeh et al., 2020).

2.3.4 Fiber

Linseed is rich in crude, acid detergent, neutral detergent, and total fibers (cellulose, lignin, and hemicellulose). It helps in forming bulk by increasing food's volume and, it retains water and prevents cardiovascular diseases, obesity, and diabetes (Rubilar et al., 2010). Linseed contains up to 40% dietary fiber, of which comprises 25% soluble fiber and 75% insoluble fiber (Kaur et al., 2018; Kauser et al., 2023). The variation in the ratio of soluble to insoluble fiber is between 20:80 and 40:60 (Goyal et al., 2014). Soluble fibers include gums, pectin, and β-glucan. For insoluble fiber, cellulose, lignin, and hemicellulose are the main constituents. Soluble fiber helps in decreasing blood sugar, absorbing triglycerides and cholesterol, and provides the gut's microorganisms with food (Kauser et al., 2023). This soluble part of the seed is responsible for 6% to 10.2% of mucilage content in linseed (Verma et al., 2014).

Table 1 Nutritional composition of linseed

S. no.	Moisture (%)	Ash (%)	CHO (%)	Protein (%)	Fat (%)	Crude fiber (%)	Dietary fiber (%)	References
1.	–	–	29	20	41	–	28	Kauser et al. (2023)
2.	5.98-6.22	3.21–3.60	–	16.02–18.50	33.25–38.38	23.3–26.80	–	Yaqoob et al. (2016)
3.	6.4	3.9	–	17.9	33.6	–	–	Bozan & Temelli (2008)
4.	6.71	3.21	25.12	20.21	36.55	7.05	–	Shaikh et al. (2020)
5.	6.5	2.41	26.1	19.67	36.7	5.49	–	Mancharkar et al. (2020)
6.	5.71	3.39	22.86	20.79	41.78	11.18	–	Sharma et al. (2020)
7.	6.96	3.72	28.88	18.29	42.16	–	27.3	Kaur (2023)
8.	5.42	3.67	–	17.33	36.76	10.77	25.8	Noreen et al. (2024)
9.	–	–	29	20	41	–	28	Goyal et al. (2014)
10.	6.5	–	28.9	20.3	37.1	4.8	27.5	Kajla et al. (2014)

Table 2 Amino acid profile of linseed (g/100 g)[a]

Amino acid	Bekhit et al., (2018)	Noreen et al., (2023)	Bernacchia et al. (2014)	Mueed et al. (2022)
ALA	5.4	6.49		4.59
ARG	11.8	13.92	9.2	10.63
ASP	–	6.51	9.3	–
ASN	12.5	–	–	9.76
CYS	3.8	0.11	1.1	3.80
GLU	26.3	8.45	19.6	26.92
GLY	7.0	2.11	5.8	6.14
HIS	2.9	6.90	2.2	2.45
ILE	5.2	6.28	4	5.21
LEU	6.8	4.86	5.8	6.82
LYS	4.1	2.78	4	4.18
MET	2.2	2.80	1.5	2.20
PHE	5.3	4.15	–	5.33
PRO	5.2	3.43	3.5	5.24
SER	5.8	6.70	4.5	5.88
THR	4.9	6.86	3.6	4.19
TRP	1.8	0.12	1.8	1.38
TYR	2.9	5.10	2.3	2.94
VAL	5.6	3.43	4.6	5.17

[a]*ALA* Alanine, *ARG* Arginine, *ASP* Aspartic acid, *ASN* Asparagine, *CYS* Cystine, *GLU* Glutamic acid, *GLY* Glycine, *HIS* Histidine, *ILE* Isoleucine, *LEU* Leucine, *LYS* Lysine, *MET* Methionine, *PHE* Phenylalanine, *PRO* Proline, *SER* Serine, *THR* Threonine, *TRP* Tryptophan, *TYR* Tyrosine, *VAL* Valine

Mucilage is a thick, gel-like substance mostly composed of complex polysaccharides such cellulose, pectins, arabinoxylans, and other polysaccharide variants. When this slimy material comes into touch with water, it becomes a viscous slime that forms a cover over the seeds (Chand et al., 2024). Linseed mucilage can bind 1600–3000 g of water per 100 g of solids. Polysaccharides in the seed coat of linseed are responsible for its high water-binding capacity (Katoch & Bhatia, 2021). Fifteen percent of the mucilage is in the shell or cover of the linseed (Kauser et al., 2023).

2.3.5 Vitamins and Minerals

Linseed contains several water and fat-soluble vitamins, specifically vitamin E, mainly in the form of γ-tocopherol: about 8.5–39.5 mg/100 g of seed (Katoch & Bhatia, 2021). Gamma-tocopherol is an antioxidant that protects cells from oxidation, controls sodium excretion urine, potentially lowering blood sodium levels, and lowers the risk of heart disease, some kinds of cancer, and Alzheimer's disease as well. The location, environment, variety, and extraction method affect the amount of tocopherol in linseed (Kauser et al., 2023). In fat soluble vitamins, linseed has vitamin E and vitamin K (Katoch & Bhatia, 2021), while in water soluble vitamins, it has vitamin B1 (0.23–0.53 mg/100 g), vitamin B2 (0.07–0.23 mg/100 g), vitamin

B3 (1.00–3.21 mg/100 g), vitamin B5 (0.57–0.6 mg/100 g), vitamin B6 (0.60–0.61 mg/100 g), vitamin B9 (112 mg/100 g), vitamin C (0.50 mg/100 g), and biotin (6.00 mg/100 g) (Bernacchia et al., 2014; Goyal et al., 2014; Kajla et al., 2014).

Linseeds are a good source of minerals like magnesium, calcium, and phosphorus. Given that 30 g of the seed provides 7–30% of the Recommended Dietary Allowances (RDAs) for certain minerals, it is crucial (Singh et al., 2011). Several bodily metabolic processes are aided by these minerals. The total amount of minerals in 100 g of linseed varies; zinc: 3.30–4.00 mg/100 g, manganese: 2.30–3.00 mg/100 g, copper: 1 mg/100 g, phosphorus: 581.46–622 mg/100 g, magnesium: 406.60–431 mg/100 g, iron: 5.00–5.13 mg/100 g, and sodium: 16.44–27 mg/100 g are all abundantly found in it (Goyal et al., 2014; Bernacchia et al., 2014; Noreen et al., 2024). Whereas, the potassium, calcium, phosphorus, and iron were found to be 170.0 mg, 750.0 mg, 370.0 mg, and 2.7 mg in 100 g of linseeds, respectively (Kajla et al., 2014).

2.4 Chemical Composition

There are various bioactive compounds that are responsible for therapeutics as well as functional property. Linseed has great antioxidant qualities that are evident as phenolic compounds, particularly in o-coumaric acid, ferulic acid, vanillic acid, lignans, and SDGs. Linseed contains a good amount of vitamin E, mostly in the form of gamma-tocopherol, which is about 8.5–39.5 mg/100 g of seed (Katoch & Bhatia, 2021). The tocopherol present has antioxidant effects that help protect linseeds from going rancid. To assist in stabilizing the radical created by auto-oxidation, tocopherol activity generates tocopherol dimmers and tocoquinone derivatives. The DPPH were found to be 3.25–8.40 μmol TE/g; FRAP, 32.22–61.65 μmol TE/g; and ORAC 38.43–88.16 μmol TE/g (Qiu et al., 2020). While, Noreen et al., (2024) reported DPPH, 35.68%–66.76% and FRAP, 608.9–5031 μM Fe^{2+}/g. Additionally, its phenolics, lignan, and SDG compound shield the body from generating free radicals, owing to their antioxidant property (Kauser et al., 2023).

2.4.1 Phenolic Compounds

Phenolic compounds have several health benefits including cardiovascular disease prevention, and anti-inflammatory. Phenolic compounds in linseed depend on genetic makeup, agronomic practices applied, and the prevailing climatic factors (Tavarini et al., 2019). Linseed is rich in phenolic acids; it contains 800–1000 mg of these compounds per 100 g of seed. Phenolic acids esterified can go up to 300–500 mg/100 g of seed (Shahidi & Naczk, 2003). The researches have indicated that the concentration of soluble and insoluble phenolic acids in linseed flour is 54% and 29%, respectively, of the total phenolic acids (Charlet et al., 2002). Qui et al. (2020) has reported total phenolic content as 235.15–389.65 mg GAE/100 g, while Bozan and Temelli (2008) reported it as 1670 mg GAE/100 g. The ferulic acid (14.96–46.98 μg/g) is the most common abundant phenolic acid, followed by caffeic acid (11.29–13.06 μg/g) and p-coumaric acid (7.66–10.59 μg/g) (Qui et al.,

2020). Whereas Mueed et al. (2022) has reported ferulic acid (161 mg/100 g), caffeic acid (4 mg/100 g), and p-coumaric acid (87 mg/100 g). Bernacchia et al. (2014) reported ferulic acid as 10.9 mg/g. Other phenolic compounds identified in linseed include: vanillic acid, hydroxycinnamic acid derivatives, p-coumarin-4-β-glucoside, ferulic acid-4-β-glucoside and the flavonoid, herbacetin diglucoside (Struijs et al., 2007) (Siger et al., 2008).

2.4.2 Lignan

Lignan's function as both estrogenic substances and hydroxyl radical sequestrators are responsible for their health advantages (Rubilar et al., 2010) (Durazzo et al., 2018). Linseeds can be regarded as one of the richest sources of lignan precursors in the diet. Lignan precursors, when consumed, are metabolized by bacteria that naturally inhabit the human gut into the enterolignans; enterodiol, and enterolactone. Two compounds of linseed lignan secoisolariciresinol (SECO) and its diglucoside (SDG) are said to have other health benefits that are said to be linked to their consumption and some of them include antioxidants (Adlercreutz, 2007). The quantity of lignans in linseed varies between 10–2600 mg (Goyal et al., 2014). Qui et al. (2020) reported total SDG as 61.98–144.66 μg/g and total SECO as 76.54–243.69 μg/g, while Mueed et al. (2022) reported total SDG as 1300 mg/100 g and total SECO as 156 mg/100 g.

2.4.3 Flavonoids

Flavonoids are the other bioactive compounds that contribute significantly to their antioxidant properties. Linseed has total flavonoid content of 37.9–64.0 (mg/100 g) (Oomah et al., 1995). Bernacchia et al. (2014) reported the total flavonoid content to be in the range of 35–70 (mg/100 g) and 35 to 71 mg/100 g (Johnsson et al., 2002). The total flavonoids contents may vary according to extraction methods and range from 1.5 mg/g to 5 mg/g (Hannah et al., 2017). The primary flavonoids present in linseeds include kaempferol (12–15 mg/100 g), quercetin (8–10 mg/100 g), and isorhamnetin (5–7 mg/100 g). Kaempferol concentrations differed markedly among linseed cultivars, spanning 2.79–28.51 mg 100 g^{-1}. The flavones apigenin and luteolin were present at 1–2 mg 100 g^{-1} and 0.5–1 mg 100 g^{-1}, respectively. Remarkably, yellow-seeded linseeds can accumulate luteolin at much higher levels, about 33.65 mg 100 g^{-1} - according to Özkaynak Kanmaz and Ova (2015). Flavanones like naringenin (3–4 mg/100 g) and eriodictyol (2–3 mg/100 g) contribute to the antioxidant capacity of linseeds. Isoflavones such as genistein (1–2 mg/100 g), daidzein (0.5–1 mg/100 g), and glycitein (0.2–0.5 mg/100 g) are present in smaller quantities but still contribute to the health-promoting effects of linseeds. Chalcones like isoliquiritigenin (0.1–0.3 mg/100 g) and flavan-3-ols such as epicatechin (2–3 mg/100 g) and catechin (1–2 mg/100 g) further add to the flavonoid profile of linseeds. Additionally, anthocyanidins like cyanidin (0.5–1 mg/100 g) and delphinidin (0.3–0.6 mg/100 g) are found in trace amounts (Gai et al., 2023). These compounds contribute to the anti-inflammatory, antioxidative, and potential anticancer properties of linseeds, making them a valuable addition to a healthy diet.

2.4.4 Carotenoids

Linseed is available in various colors due to its carotenoid content, which acts as a pigment giving the seeds their distinctive colors. These carotenoids, precursors of vitamin A, display a range of colors including red, orange, and yellow (Kauser et al., 2023). Carotenoids found in linseed include lutein (Lut.), beta-carotene (β-Car.), and zeaxanthin (Zea.). Linseed contains 0.7–3.1 mg/kg of carotenoids, whereas linseed oil contains 77 mg/kg of carotene (Farag et al., 2021; Mueed et al., 2022). Mohamed Ahmed et al. (2023) reported carotenoid content of 0.13–0.61 mg/g, and Fujisawa et al. (2008) reported 65.4–156.3 μg/g. The total carotenoid content ranges from 36.29 to 152.36 μg/100 g dry weight (DW), zeaxanthin ranges from 2.99 to 21.96 μg/100 g DW, and beta-carotene ranges from 5.92 to 52.03 μg/100 g DW (Fujisawa & Misawa, 2010). These antioxidants help protect unsaturated lipids in linseed from photooxidation (Mueed et al., 2020; Kauser et al., 2023). Among all carotenoids, beta-carotene exhibits the highest provitamin A activity (Kauser et al., 2023) and has been reported to have a content of 5.18 mg/100 g (Mueed et al., 2022).

2.5 Postharvest, Storage, and Packaging

Postharvest handling and storage is an important part in maintaining the quality and nutritional value of linseeds. Langyan (2023) emphasized the need for proper storage conditions to preserve the nutritional properties of linseeds including omega-3 fatty acids and bioactive compounds. Key factors influencing seed quality include storage, temperature, relative humidity, moisture content, germination, and fungal infection. Proper packaging and specific recommendations for safe storage are crucial for preventing seed deterioration (Mundhada (2022) Chauhan (2009)) (Fig. 3). All these studies collectively underscore the importance of proper postharvest handling and storage practices in preserving the quality and nutritional value of linseed.

2.5.1 Cleaning and Drying

The cleaning process is essential for improving the usability and quality of linseed during processing, typically involving four main stages. The initial stage focuses on removing large impurities such as husks, stones, and large debris, which can be done through hand-picking, sieving, or using screens. The secondary stage targets smaller impurities, including destoning, using mechanical equipment such as air aspirators, magnetic separators, and gravity separators. Air aspirators use airflow to remove physical impurities and deteriorated seeds, magnetic separators eliminate metal contaminants, and gravity separators, based on density, effectively remove unwanted particles. Additionally, color sorting is performed to identify and remove rotten seeds, and fine sieves are used to eliminate any remaining small unwanted particles. The third phase involves dehulling, which employs various equipment utilizing impact, abrasion, and mechanical forces to remove the seed coat or hull. The fourth and final step involves using aspirators to remove even the tiniest particles, ensuring that the linseed is as pure and clean as possible before proceeding to the next processing stage. This comprehensive cleaning process ensures the linseed

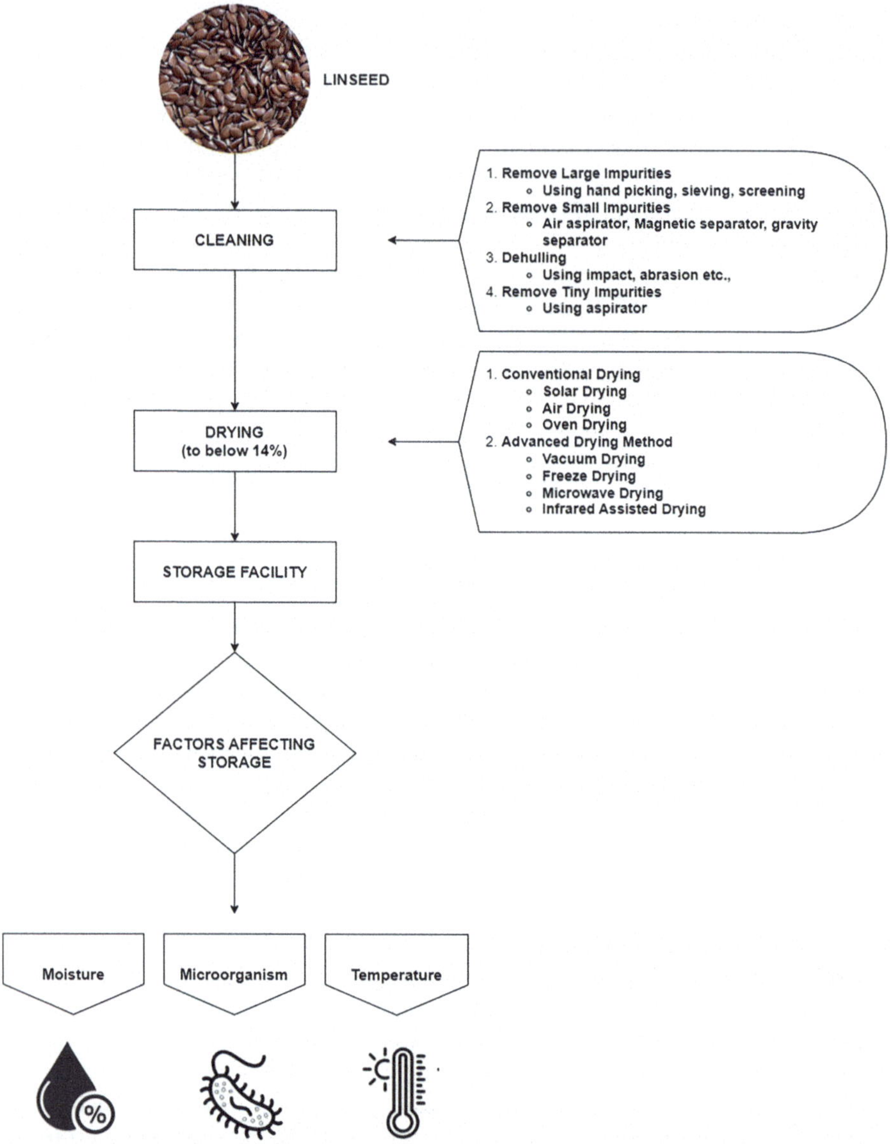

Fig. 3 Diagrammatic representation of postharvest and storage of linseed

is free from impurities, thus enhancing its quality and making it suitable for various applications.

The drying process plays a crucial role in ensuring better efficiency and quality of the husking process and the shelf life stability of linseeds. Drying reduces the moisture content to a level below 14%, which extends the shelf life and prevents infestation. Proper drying of flaxseeds contributes to achieving an effective husking process and guarantees the quality of the husking method and equipment. Efficient separation technologies are employed after drying to separate flax seed husks and kernels, underscoring the importance of the drying step. Seed drying methods using direct or indirect heat reduce moisture content; however, excessive drying at high temperature can cause deteriorative effect on the seeds. It is widely acknowledged that drying before processing enhances the quality and quantity of oil obtained (McDowell et al., 2017). The regulated drying process can damage the cellular structure and expand the microchannels of matrix substances, facilitating the release of bioactive compounds and enhancing oil content. Thus, integrating efficient cleaning and drying processes ensures that linseed is thoroughly prepared for further processing, maximizing its quality and suitability for various applications.

2.5.2 Conventional Drying Methods

Conventional drying methods are techniques that have been around for centuries to remove moisture from substances. These methods rely on natural elements like sunlight and air circulation or use simple tools to achieve drying. Solar drying is a common drying technique followed since ages where linseeds are spread out in the sun to dry. This method is environmentally friendly and cost-effective, utilizing solar energy to dry the seeds naturally. Traditionally, the oil from linseed is majorly used in the production of linoleum, varnishes, and paints due to its properties of drying and hardening after exposure to air and sunlight (Coşkuner & Karababa, 2007). Air drying: Air-drying is a method where linseeds are placed in a food dehydrator, which circulates warm air to dry the seeds efficiently. This method is convenient and ensures consistent drying but is slow as compared to other drying methods. The temperature of the air could be set at a particular temperature (Nair et al., 2012). Oven drying: Oven drying is another method where linseeds are placed in an oven at a low temperature to remove moisture. This method is quicker than air-drying and ensures uniform drying of the seeds. The oven is heated at 150 °C causing more protein denaturation and increasing amounts of the volatiles, such as alkanes, pyrazines, and aldehydes. The release of oil from oven drying is less compared to other drying methods (Zhang et al., 2018).

2.5.3 Advanced Drying Methods

Advanced drying methods are a step up from conventional techniques, offering faster drying times, more precise control, and often better quality preservation of the dried material. These methods utilize various technologies to remove moisture efficiently. Vacuum drying led to a reduction in the extraction yield of oil in comparison to the native extraction method. The decrease in the yield can be attributed to the loss of oil due to the evaporation of moisture under vacuum conditions Zhang et al. (2018). However, the extraction rate of the vacuum-dried sample (0.053 l/h) is lower compared to the extraction rate of the native sample (0.084 l/h).

Freeze drying is a method that involves freezing the linseeds and then gradually reducing the surrounding pressure to allow the frozen water in the seeds to sublimate. This process results in dried linseeds with minimal damage to their nutritional content. The study revealed that freeze drying and microwave drying techniques exhibited superior extraction rates and yields of oil (46.36% and 46.16%, respectively) when compared to native linseed (33.90%) Zhang et al. (2018). Freeze drying yielded a higher percentage (46.2%) compared to the oven drying method (40.95%) (Zhang et al., 2018).

Microwave drying is a quick method where linseeds are placed in a microwave and dried using microwave radiation. This method is fast but requires careful monitoring to prevent overheating and ensure uniform drying. Microwave drying methods generally lead to high extraction and enhance increase in oil yield up to 46% (Zhang et al., 2018). During the microwave drying, protein reductions of 39%, 58%, and 63% were observed for power densities of 0.3, 0.6, and 1 W/g, respectively (Bouamrane et al., 2023). High amounts of denatured proteins were observed when microwave drying was done at 150 °C. In the case of microwave heating at 860 W, the amount and type of volatiles including alkanes, pyrazines, and aldehydes were significantly enhanced, and the microwave heating was observed to be more effective in terms of low heating power and short heating time (Hou et al., 2021).

Infrared-Assisted Spouted Bed Drying: Infrared (IR)-assisted spouted bed drying (SBD) is considered as a viable substitute for conventional hot air-drying methods when dealing with heat-sensitive components. The study conducted by Dehghan-Mabshadi et al. (2019) aimed to examine the impact of infrared-assisted steam distillation (IR-SBD) and the use of ultrasound-assisted extraction (UAE), solvent extraction (SE), and cold press (CP) on linseed oil quality. The fatty acids composition, acid values, drying rate, and oil peroxide value were evaluated by performing IR-assisted SBD and SBD at air temperatures of 40, 60, and 80 °C. It was discovered that the rate of drying increased with an increase in the air temperature in the presence of infrared radiation. The peroxide values (PVs) of SBD samples exhibited lower levels compared to those of IR-SBD samples at identical temperatures.

2.6 Factors Affecting Seed Storage Stability

The primary aim of storing seed is to slow down or stop the deterioration of seeds, which may be caused by climate and microbial activity, hence securing their nutritive value. The primary issue that affects the quality of oilseeds during storage is lipid oxidation, which results in an undesirable flavor and odor known as oxidative rancidity. In linseed, cyclolinopeptides, lignans, and tocopherols prevent this oxidation naturally that act as an antioxidant. Brühl et al. (2022) reported degradation of these cyclolinopeptides as well as tocopherols to their oxidized forms. When exposed to light, the intermediate product, methionine oxidizes to methionine sulfoxide and further to methionine sulfone when stored at a temperature of 60 °C for 25 days, with 12 h of light followed by 12 h of darkness. The nature of these by-products is toxic, and as a result, they have the potential to cause a wide variety of disorders that are harmful to human life (Frankel, 2014). At higher temperatures, the kinetics of oxidation change because the intermediate hydroperoxides decompose faster than compared to the lower temperatures. Darkness has been observed to slow the rate of oxidation of fatty acids in linseed, but no oxidation product was isolated. Linseed is very useful for health purposes as it contains large quantities of linolenic acid (omega 3) and another essential acid. Nevertheless, this unsaturated polyunsaturated fatty acid (PUFA) is sensitive to heat, light, and air. Thus, the storage period of linseed oil significantly reduces (Table 1) (Choo, Birch, & Dufour 2007a). Several studies (Prescha et al., 2014; Douny et al., 2016; Szumała & Wysocka, 2018) have examined the oxidation of linseed oil by assessing multiple markers of shelf life, including conjugated diene levels, free fatty acids, and peroxide value.

These indicators are used to analyze the oxidation of linseed lipids. Stored cereal or oilseeds' quality is directly influenced by exposure to oxygen, temperature, duration of storage period, moisture content, humidity level, and presence of light (Table 1). These factors not only facilitate the infestation by insects, pests, and the growth of microbes but also lead to chemical degradation, which results in a significant loss (Kiaya, 2014). Modifying these factors can help slow down the degradation process and maintain the stored seed's quality for a long time. The amount of moisture that is contained inside the seed is the most important component that determines how seeds or grains are stored. White et al. (1999) conducted a study and found that seeds with a moisture content of 9.5% developed mold after being stored for 6 months. Moisture content typically falls within the range of 35–45% at the point of physiological maturity. Nevertheless, in order to store the seeds for an extended period, the moisture content must fall within the range of 5–15%. A reduction of 1% in moisture content leads to a twofold increase in the shelf life of stored seeds. Higher moisture content leads to an elevation in the level of free fatty acids, resulting in a decline in the overall quality.

2.6.1 Moisture

The seeds of linseed exhibit an inverse logarithmic correlation between their lifespan and moisture content. White et al. (1999) found that the composition of linseed oil remained relatively stable during a 6-month storage period. There was just one alteration that was determined to be statistically significant, and that was an increase in the amount of palmitic acid. The palmitic acid content of Linola TM 947 went from 6.6% to 7.0%, while the palmitic acid content of Mc Gregor climbed from 5.9% to 6.1%. Both increases occurred in the same period. Despite this, they chose not to reveal the fundamental root of the problem. Linseed should be stored in dry circumstances with a moisture level of no more than 10% because the viscid component (mucilage) that is found on the outside of linseed becomes very sticky when it is exposed to moisture (Dexter et al., 2011). It is possible for linseed to become badly compacted and unfit for sale if it is kept in an environment that is wet or if it is exposed to snow or rain. Various techniques for drying seeds, including mechanical drying, continuous flow dryers, solar drying, radial drying bins, and tray drying, are used to effectively reduce the amount of moisture present in the seeds. The seeds, however, are susceptible to damage if they are subjected to excessive drying at high temperatures. This is an essential point to keep in mind (Yousaf et al., 2016).

2.6.2 Temperature

Elevated temperatures accelerate the respiration rate of stored seeds and exacerbate infestations by insect pests, hence further compromising the seed quality. The shelf life of most foods decreases by 50% for every 10 °C increase in temperature. An increase in temperature coupled with a simultaneous decrease to 5 °C results in a twofold increase in the longevity of the seed. This occurrence takes place within the temperature range of +273.15–323.15 K or within the range of 0–50 °C (Yousaf et al., 2016). In their 1974 study, El-Gharbawi et al. proved that there are 13–37% increments in TBA value, 2–2. 1–26. 7 and 1. 20–3. 65, respectively, after 14 weeks at a temperature of 28 °C. Moreover, these values also rose even higher to 73, 53. 4, and 5. 21 respectively, after 14 weeks at a 58 °C. However, the period of storage as well as the temperature did not significantly affect the iodine value. Tautorus and McCurdy (1990) discovered that linseed oil stored at 55 °C had a greater amount of oxidation products compared to the oil stored at 28 °C. However, the concentration of conjugated dienes was significantly greater in chemically randomized oils, excluding linseed oil. Nevertheless, there were no notable disparities in lipid oxidation at a temperature of 55 °C when comparing it to soyabean oil and canola oil. Consequently, the most effective method to prolong the lifespan of the stored seed is to decrease the temperature of the storage area. For the storage of linseed, it is recommended to maintain a temperature below 25 °C and a relative humidity below 15%. To extend the freshness of ground linseeds, it is recommended to refrigerate them and store them in containers that are airtight (Bernacchia et al., 2014). Malcolmson et al. (2000) conducted an investigation to determine the shelf life of milled linseed oil by measuring variables such as free fatty acids and peroxide. It was found that when milled linseed oil was kept at a temperature of 23 ± 2 °C, the oil remained stable for a period of 128 days. Furthermore, no noticeable disparity was seen in the sensory attributes of the freshly generated or preserved linseed samples. This may be explained by the presence of abundant antioxidative chemicals in linseeds, which effectively eliminate peroxyl radicals and inhibit lipid peroxidation (Kraushofer & Sontag, 2002).

2.6.3 Environmental Impacts

The weather conditions, particularly the amount of temperature and rainfall, not only affect the amount of oil produced but also have influence on the composition of fatty acids. Čeh et al. (2020) showed that the α-linolenic acid content in the Recital variety decreased from 53% to 47.4% over 2 consecutive years. This indicates that environmental factors play a significant role in determining the fatty acid profile. Although the aforementioned factors may result in losses, linseed seeds can remain viable for several months or even years if stored correctly. The chart issued by the Canadian Grain Commission serves as a guide for determining the precautions required to store linseed safely. . If the linseeds are kept inside the no spoiling zone, they may be securely stored for a period of 5 months. If the seed falls in an area prone to deterioration, it must be cooled and dried until it reaches a region where rotting does not occur. For long-term storage, it is recommended to preserve linseed with a moisture level not exceeding 8.5%. If the seed lot to be stored has poor physical quality due to chaffing and damaged seeds, it may be important to keep the moisture level below 8.5% for extended storage.

2.6.4 Microorganisms

Effective seed storage, whether on a large or small scale, necessitates safeguarding against physical elements such as rainfall, moisture, and temperature, as well as biotic factors including insects, pests, rodents, birds, and microorganisms. Dubey et al. (1985) carried out a study to assess the impact of six frequently isolated storage fungi. Among these, it was found that four fungi species, *Aspergillus repens, Aspergillus flavus, Alternaria alternata,* and *Torula allii* significantly affected the oil content of the seeds. This impact varied with a decrease of 5–71%. Also, these fungal species enhanced value by raising the saponification number and the free fatty acids content. Further, the percentage of iodine value was decreased by three fungi species *A. flavus, A. alternate* and *T. allii* whereas it was increased by two fungi species *Cladosporium herbarum* and *Fusarium culmorum.* There are other techniques of seed and grain preservation that can be adopted instead of chemical preservation including controlled chilling, aeration, and atmospheric storage among others. The methods of capturing insect pests and applying technologies for the detection and assessment of the level of infestation in bulk storage have been elaborated. The use of insect traps may be part of the management plan where they are needed. The use of physical control methods can be expensive and, in some cases, may not be effective in eliminating all the pests. The integration of at least one physical method in addition to chemical methods at low dosages is sometimes a viable and efficient way of treatment.

2.6.5 Storage Conditions

There could be multiple levels of storage: bagged, bulk, farm-level, outdoor, and hermetic (airtight) storage, which is specifically for linseeds. Hermetic storage is a long-standing method for storing items where the levels of oxygen decrease and the levels of carbon dioxide increase, which helps to control insect populations and prevent the growth of mold. This is achieved through the respiration of organisms in the stored seeds (Ellis & Hong, 2007). The storage method ensures complete elimination of any residual contaminants, but it requires the use of fumigation methods or meticulous regulation of air conditions to get optimal results. Linseeds may be kept in bags or bulk in silos. The bags are organized in pyramidal configurations or housed in warehouses, some of which are chilled. It is necessary to safeguard the surfaces where these bags are kept by using tar, concrete, or plastic in order to avoid termite infestations. Storage facilities must be supplied with a drainage ditch to effectively control the flow of rainfall. Using tarpaulins to cover the storage pyramids is essential to avoid the accumulation of precipitation on the bags. Silos are often used for the purpose of maintaining reserves for security. A silo is built on a circular shaped concrete platform, with walls made of galvanized screening and interior walls covered with a thick layer of plastic film. The silo is covered with galvanized metal sheets to protect the seeds from being preyed upon by rats. The linseeds housed in these silos must be dried thoroughly due to the near airtight nature of these structures. The storage capabilities of these silos vary from 0.5 to million metric tonnes (Omobowale et al., 2015).

2.7 Packaging

Packaging plays an important role in preserving the nutritional and qualitative properties of formulated products, particularly those rich in functional substances such as linseed (*Linum usitatissimum* L.). Effective postharvest practices are crucial to maintaining the integrity of these properties. The choice of packaging materials is essential as they can affect the porosity of the packaging, which in turn influences the storage conditions and quality of the linseed. Linseed can be stored in various types of packaging such as polyethylene-coated paper packaging and polypropylene plastic packaging. These packages are commonly used for storing agricultural and food products (Bechline et al., 2019). Polyethylene-coated paper packaging demonstrated superior lipid preservation for brown linseed, and it maintained color parameters comparable to the control, indicating that the grains were not altered by ozone exposure. Thus, polyethylene-coated paper packaging enhanced the preservation of color parameters and lipids. Bechline et al. (2019) evaluated the effects of different packaging types and ozonation on the quality of brown and golden linseed grains and oil over a 90-day storage period. Another study found that ozonation and packaging types did not affect the moisture content of the grains or the peroxide index of linseed oil. However, golden linseed exhibited a rise in free fatty acids and higher fungi count than brown linseed, suggesting greater contamination. Storage conditions and optimal packaging material together play an important role in preserving quality of linseeds (Duan et al., 2024).

3 Conclusion

The physicochemical properties of linseed reveal linseed as a nutritionally rich multicomponent system, which contributes to its therapeutic benefits. Along with its superior protein quality, omega three rich fat, and soluble and insoluble dietary fiber, it has various bioactive compounds that provide its antioxidant properties. These compounds including phenolics, flavonoids, lignans, and SDGs give linseed its unique oxidative properties and help in reducing oxidative stress. Linseed has been used since ages for its oil and other products. Handling and processing methods such as proper cleaning, drying, storage, and packaging help preserve essential nutrients like omega-3 fatty acids, phenolic compounds, and lignans for a longer time. By implementing these practices, the quality, safety, and health benefits of linseed can be preserved, ensuring it remains a valuable nutritional resource. Understanding these physical and engineering properties of linseeds helps to handle the linseeds at larger scale and increase productivity and efficiency in industrial scale.

References

Abdul-Hamid, A., & Luan, Y. S. (2000). Functional properties of dietary fibre prepared from defatted rice bran. *Journal of the Science of Food and Agriculture, 80*(6), 711–717. https://doi.org/10.1002/(SICI)1097-0010(20000501)80:63.0.CO;2-Z

Bekhit, A. E.-D., Shavandi, A., Jodjaja, T., Birch, J., Teh, S., Mohamed Ahmed, I. A., Al-Juhaimi, F. Y., Saeedi, P., & Bekhit, A. A. (2018). Flaxseed: Composition, detoxification, utilization, and opportunities. *Biocatalysis and Agricultural Biotechnology, 13*, 129–152. https://doi.org/10.1016/j.bcab.2017.11.017

Bechlin, T. R., Granella, S. J., Christ, D., Coelho, S. R. M., & Viecelli, C. A. (2019). Evaluation of grain and oil quality of packaged and ozonized linseed. *Journal of Stored Products Research, 83*, 311–316. https://doi.org/10.1016/j.jspr.2019.07.014

Bernacchia, R., Preti, R., & Vinci, G. (2014). Chemical composition and health benefits of linseed. *Austin Journal of Nutrition and Food Sciences, 2*(8), 1045.

Bouamrane, O. L., Mekhaneg, B., Panigrahi, S. S., Hemis, M., & Singh, C. B. (2023). Fluidization-bed drying and microwave radiation effects on drying rate, fatty acid, protein, and germination of linseed. *Journal of Food Process Engineering, 47*(1), e14524. https://doi.org/10.1111/jfpe.14524

Brenes, M., Garcia, A., Dobarganes, M. C., Velasco, J., & Romero, C. (2002). Influence of thermal treatments simulating cooking processes on the polyphenol content of virgin olive oil. *Journal of Agriculture and Food Chemistry, 50*, 5962–5967.

Brestenský, M., Nitrayová, S., & Patras, P. (2023). The effects of heat treatment on the quality of fat in linseeds and chia seeds. *Czech Journal of Food Sciences, 41*(1), 21–28.

Brühl, L., Bonte, A., N'Diaye, K., & Matthäus, B. (2022). Oxidation of cyclo-lino peptides in linseed oils during storage. *European Journal of Lipid Science and Technology, 124*(12), 2200137. https://doi.org/10.1002/ejlt.202200137

Bozan, B., & Temelli, F. (2008). Chemical composition and oxidative stability of flax, safflower and poppy seed and seed oils. *Bioresource Technology, 99*(14), 6354–6359. https://doi.org/10.1016/j.biortech.2007.12.009

Coşkuner, Y. & Karababa, E. (2007) Physical Properties of Coriander Seeds (Coriandrum sativum L.). *Journal of Food Engineering, 80*, 408–416. https://doi.org/10.1016/j.jfoodeng.2006.02.042

Carrasco-Pancorbo, A., Neususs, C., Pelzing, M., Segura-Carretero, A., & Fernandez Guitierrez, A. (2007). CE- and HPLC–TOF-MS for the characterization of phenolic compounds in olive oil. *Electrophoresis, 29*, 806–821.

Čeh, B., Štraus, S., Hladnik, A., & Kušar, A. (2020). Impact of linseed variety, location and production year on seed yield, oil content and its composition. *Agronomy, 10*(11), 1770. https://doi.org/10.3390/agronomy10111770

Daun, J. K., & DeClercq, D. R. (1994). Sixty years of Canadian linseed quality surveys at the grain research laboratory. In *55th proceedings of Lin Institute of United States*, 192–200.

Daun, J. K., Barthet, V. J., Chornick, T. L., & Duguid, S. (2003). Structure, composition, and variety development of linseed.

Dehghan-Manshadi, A., Peighambardoust, S. H., Azadmard-Damirchi, S., & Niakousari, M. (2019). Effect of infrared-assisted spouted bed drying of linseed on the quality characteristics of its oil extracted by different methods. *Journal of the Science of Food and Agriculture., 100*(1), 74. https://doi.org/10.1002/jsfa.9995

Dexter, J. E., Jhala, A. J., Yang, R.-C., Hills, M. J., Weselake, R. J., & Hall, L. M. (2011). Harvest loss and seed bank longevity of lin (Linum usitatissimum) implications for seed-mediated gene flow. *Weed Science, 59*(1), 61–67. https://doi.org/10.1614/WS-D-10-00047.1

Douny, C., Razanakolona, R., Ribonnet, L., Milet, J., Baeten, V., Rogez, H., Scippo, M. L., & Larondelle, Y. (2016). Linseed oil presents different patterns of oxidation in real-time and accelerated aging assays. *Food Chemistry, 208*, 111–115. https://doi.org/10.1016/j.foodchem.2016.04.010

Drouillard, J.S., Farran, T. B., Blasi, D. A., LaBrune, H. J., Montgomery, S. P., Sindt, J. J., & Higgens, J. J. (2000, March). Modulation of Immune Response in Feeder Cattle with Linseed. In *Proceedings of the 58th Lin Institute*, (pp. 53–62).

Duan, Y., Xie, X., Kang, D., Li, Q., Gao, Y., Zhang, S., & Yu, X. (2024). Effect of storage conditions and packaging on the quality of linseed in Chinese dried noodles during long-term storage. *International Journal of Food Science and Technology., 59*(5), 3074–3086.

Dubey, G. L., Vayas, K. M., & Dubey, O. (1985). Physico-chemical properties of linseed oil as affected by various seed-borne fungi. *Journal of Phytopathology, 113*(1), 66–70. https://doi.org/10.1111/j.1439-0434.1985.tb00827.x

El-Gharbawi, M. I., Fahmay, A., & Abd-Allah, M. A. (1974). Comparative study on stability of linseed oil and oils extracted from wild weed seed growing with lin. *Annals of Agricultural Science, 190*, 57–67.

Ellis, R. H., & Hong, T. D. (2007). Quantitative response of the longevity of seed of twelve crops to temperature and moisture in hermetic storage. *Seed Science and Technology, 35*(2), 432–444. https://doi.org/10.15258/sst.2007.35.2.18

Epaminondas, P. S., Araújo, K. L. G. V., Nascimento, J. A., Silva, M. C. D., Rosenhaim, R., Soledade, L. E. B., Queiroz, N., Souza, A. L., Santos, I. M. G., & Souza, A. G. (2011a). Influence of toasting and the seed variety on the physico-chemical and thermo-oxidative characteristics of the linseed oil. *Journal of Thermal Analysis and Calorimetry, 106*, 545.

Epaminondas, P. S., Araújo, K. L. G. V., Nascimento, J. A., Silva, M. C. D., Rosenhaim, R., Soledade, L. E. B., et al. (2011b). Influence of toasting and the seed variety on the physico-chemical and thermo-oxidative characteristics of the linseed oil. *Journal of Thermal Analysis and Calorimetry, 106*(2), 545–550.

Frankel, E. N. (2014). *Lipid oxidation*. Woodhead Publishing.

Ganorkar P. M., & Jain, R. K. (2014). Effect of linseed incorporation on physical, sensorial, textural and chemical attributes of cooki.

Gerstenmeyer, E., Reimer, S., Berghofer, E., Schwartz, H., & Sontag, G. (2013). Effect of thermal heating on some lignans in lin seeds, sesame seeds and rye. *Food Chemistry, 138*(2–3), 1847–1855.

Gruia, A., Raba, D. N., Dumbrava, D., Moldovan, C., Bordean, D., & Mateescu, C. (2012). Fatty acids composition and oil characteristics of linseed (Linum Usitatissimum L.) from Romania. *Journal of Agroalimentary Processes and Technologies, 18*(2), 136–140.

Goyal, A., Sharma, V., Upadhyay, N., Gill, S., & Sihag, M. (2014). Flax and flaxseed oil: an ancient medicine & modern functional food. *Journal of Food Science and Technology, 51*(9), 1633–1653. https://doi.org/10.1007/s13197-013-1247-9

Hanaa, M. H., Ismail, H. A., Mahmoud, M. E., & Ibrahim, H. M. (2017). Antioxidant activity and phytochemical analysis of linseeds (Linum usitatisimum L.). *Minia Journal of Agricultural Research and Development, 37*(1), 129–140.

Imran, M., Anjum, F. M., Ahmad, N., Khan, M. K., Mushtaq, Z., Nadeem, M., & Hussain, S. (2015). Impact of extrusion processing conditions on lipid peroxidation and storage stability of full-fat linseed meal. *Lipids in Health and Disease, 14*(1), 92. https://doi.org/10.1186/s12944-015-0076-4

Imran, M., Nadeem, M., Manzoor, M. F., Javed, A., Ali, Z., Akhtar, M. N., Ali, M., & Hussain, Y. (2016). Fatty acids characterization, oxidative perspectives and consumer acceptability of oil extracted from pre-treated chia (Salvia hispanica L.) seeds. *Lipids in Health and Disease, 1*, 162.

Katoch, M., & Bhatia, N. S. (2021). Linseed and its basic composition. *International Journal of Advances in Agricultural Science and Technology, 8*(6), 10–26. https://doi.org/10.47856/ijaast.2021.v08i6.002

Kaur, S. (2023). Linseed: An emerging functional food. *The Pharma Innovation Journal, 12*(6), 3025–3035.

Kasote, D. M., Badhe, Y. S., & Hegde, M. V. (2013). Effect of mechanical press oil extraction processing on quality of linseed oil. *Industrial Crops and Products, 42*, 10–13. https://doi.org/10.1016/j.indcrop.2012.05.015

Kauser, S., Hussain, A., Ashraf, S., Fatima, G., Ambreen, Javaria, S., ... Korma, S. A. (2023). Flaxseed (Linum usitatissimum); phytochemistry, pharmacological characteristics and functional food applications. *Food Chemistry Advances, 4*, 100573. https://doi.org/10.1016/j.focha.2023.100573

Kajla, P., Sharma, A., & Sood, D. R. (2014). Flaxseed—a potential functional food source. *Journal of Food Science and Technology, 52*(4), 1857–1871. https://doi.org/10.1007/s13197-014-1293-y

Kiarie, E., Nyachoti, C. M., Slominski, B. A., Blank, G. Growth performance, gastrointestinal microbial activity, and nutrient digestibility in early-weaned pigs fed diets containing flaxseed and carbohydrase enzyme1,2. *J Anim Sci.* 2007 Nov 1;85(11):2982–93.

Kiaya, V. (2014). *Post-harvest losses and strategies to reduce them.* ACF International. https://www.actioncontrelafaim.org/wp-content/uploads/2018/01/technical_paper_phl__.pdf

Kraushofer, T., & Sontag, G. (2002). Determination of some phenolic compounds in lin seed and nettle roots by HPLC with coulometric electrode array detection. *European Food Research and Technology, 215*(6), 529–533. https://doi.org/10.1007/s00217-002-0606-y

Kumar, M., Bangar, S. P., & Panesar, P. S. (Eds.). (2024). *Oilseed meal as a sustainable contributor to plant-based protein: Paving the way towards circular economy and nutritional security.* Springer Nature.

Malcolmson, L. J., Przybylski, R., & Daun, J. K. (2000). Storage stability of milled linseed. *Journal of the American Oil Chemists' Society, 77*(3), 235–238. https://doi.org/10.1007/s11746-000-0038-0

Mancharkar, H. A., Ghatge, P. U., & Sawate, A. R. (2020). Studies on Physico-chemical and mineral evaluation of linseed. *The Pharma Innovation Journal, 9*(3), 476–478.

McDowell, D., Elliott, C. T., & Koidis, A. (2017). Pre-processing effects on cold pressed rapeseed oil quality indicators and phenolic compounds. *European Journal of Lipid Science and Technology, 119*(9), 1600357.

Millam, S., Obert, B. & Pret'ová, A. (2005). Plant cell and biotechnology studies in Linum usitatissimum – a review. Plant Cell Tiss Organ Cult 82, 93–10. https://doi.org/10.1007/s11240-004-6961-6

Moknatjou, R., Hajimahmoodi, M., Toliyat, T., Moghaddam, G., Sadeghpour, O., Monsef-Esfahani, H., & Shams-Ardekani, M. R. (2015). Effect of roasting on fatty acid profile of brown and yellow varieties of linseed (Linum usitatissimum L.). *Tropical Journal of Pharmaceutical Research, 14*, 117–123.

Moussa, E., Shereen, A., Manal, A., Mehanni, A., & Rasha, A. (2014). Nutritional value and fatty acid composition of household cooking on fish fatty acids profile using atherogenicity and thrombogenicity indices. *Journal of Food Chemistry and Nutrition, 2*, 27–41.

Mridula, D., Barnwal, P., & Singh, K. K. (2015). Screw pressing performance of whole and dehulled linseed and some physico-chemical characteristics of linseed oil. *Journal of Food Science and Technology, 52*, 1498–1506.

Mueed, A., Shibli, S., Korma, S. A., Madjirebaye, P., Esatbeyoglu, T., & Deng, Z. (2022). Linseed bioactive compounds: Chemical composition, functional properties, food applications and health benefits-related gut microbes. *Foods, 11*(20), 3307. https://doi.org/10.3390/foods11203307

Nykter, M., Kymäläinen, H. R., Gates, F., & Sjöberg, A. M. (2006). Quality characteristics of edible linseed oil. *Agricultural and Food Science, 15*, 402–413.

Noreen, S., Tufail, T., Khalid, Z., Khan, A. U., & Pane, Y. S. (2024). Health benefit of flaxseed (Linum usitatissimum): A mini review. *Food Research, 8*(5), 107–116. https://doi.org/10.26656/fr.2017.8(5).310

Narina, S. S. S., Hamama, A. A., & Bhardwaj, H. L. (2012). Nutritional and mineral composition of flax sprouts. *Journal of Agricultural Science, 4*(11), 60–67. https://doi.org/10.5539/jas.v4n11p60

Noreen, S., Perveen, S., Shafiq, N., Aslam, S., Iqbal, H. M. N., Ashraf, S. S., & Bilal, M. (2023). Laccase-loaded functionalized graphene oxide assemblies with improved biocatalytic properties and decolorization performance. ScienceDirect. https://doi.org/10.1016/j.colsurfb.2023.113452

Oomah, B. D., Kenaschuk E. O., Cui W, Mazza G. Variation in the composition of water-soluble polysaccharides in flaxseed. *J Agric Food Chem.* 1995 Jun;43(6):1484–8.

Omobowale, M., Mijinyawa, Y., Armstrong, P., Igbeka, J., & Maghirang, E. (2015). Performance evaluation of termite-mound clay, concrete and steel silos for the storage of maize grains in the humid tropics. *Journal of Stored Products and Postharvest, 6*(7), 56–65. https://doi.org/10.5897/JSPPR2015.0187

Oomah, B. D., & Mazza, G. (1993). Flaxseed proteins—a review. *Food Chemistry, 48*(2), 109–114. https://doi.org/10.1016/0308-8146(93)90043-F

Oomah, B. D., Kristensen, M., Bach Knudsen, K. E., Tømmeraas, K., Draget, K. I., Henriksson, G., Ebringerová, A., & Astrup, A. (2007). Extracted linseed fibres affect weight development: A rat feeding trial. *Food Chemistry, 103*(4), 1171–1178. https://doi.org/10.1016/j.foodchem.2006.10.028

Physicochemical Characteristics of Linseed Oil and Flour March 2010 *Polish Journal of Natural Science 25*(1):106–113. https://doi.org/10.2478/v10020-010-0008-8 Beata PiłatBeata PiłatRyszard ZadernowskiRyszard Zadernowski

Pradhan, R. C., Meda, V., Rout, P. K., Naik, S., & Dalai, A. K. (2010). Supercritical CO2 extraction of fatty oil from flaxseed and comparison with screw press expression and solvent extraction processes. *Journal of Food Engineering, 98*(4), 393–397. https://doi.org/10.1016/j.jfoodeng.2009.11.021

Popa, V. M., Gruia, A., Raba, D. N., Dumbrava, D., Moldovan, C., Bordean, D., & Mateescu, C. (2012). Fatty acids composition and oil characteristics of linseed (Linum Usitatissimum L.) from Romania. *Journal of Agroalimentary Processes and Technologies, 18*(2), 136–140.

Prescha, A., Grajzer, M., Dedyk, M., & Grajeta, H. (2014). The antioxidant activity and oxidative stability of cold-pressed oils. *Journal of the American Oil Chemists' Society, 91*(8), 1291–1301. https://doi.org/10.1007/s11746-014-2479-1

Qu, Q., Yang, X., Fu, M., Chen, Q., Zhang, X., He, Z., & Qiao, X. (2016). Effects of three conventional drying methods on the lipid oxidation, fatty acids composition, and antioxidant activities of walnut (Juglans regia L.). *Drying Technology, 34*(7), 822–829. https://doi.org/10.1080/07373937.2015.1081931

Raghuwanshi, V. P., Agrawal, R. S., & Mane, K. A. (2019). Linseed as a functional food: A review. *Journal of Pharmacognosy and Phytochemistry, 8*(3), 352–354.

Schorno, A. L., Manthey, F. A., & Hall, C. A. (2010). Effect of particle size and sample size on lipid stability of milled linseed (Linum usitatissimum L.). *Journal of Food Processing and Preservation, 34*, 167–179.

Shaikh, R. P., Gadhe, K. S., & Syed, S. J. (2020). Studies on physico-chemical and functional properties of linseed flour. *Journal of Pharmacognosy and Phytochemistry, 9*(1), 2309–2312.

Sharma, H. P., Sharma, S., & Nema, P. (2020). Physico-chemical and functional properties of flour prepared from native and roasted whole linseeds. *Journal of Pharmacognosy and Phytochemistry, 9*(5), 1428–1433.

Selvi, K. Ç., Pınar, Y., & Yeşiloğlu, E. (2006). Some physical properties of linseed. *Biosystems Engineering, 95*(4), 607–612. https://doi.org/10.1016/j.biosystemseng.2006.08.008

Singh, K. K., Mridula, D., Rehal, J., & Barnwal, P. (2011). Linseed: A potential source of food, feed and fiber. *Critical Reviews in Food Science and Nutrition, 51*, 210–222.

Singh, K. K., Jhamb, S. A., & Kumar, R. (2012). Effect of pretreatments on performance of screw pressing for linseed. *Journal of Food Process Engineering, 35*(4), 543–556.

Singh, G. D., Singh, A., Abhineet, S. K., Singh, P. K., & Singh, H. (2018). Evaluation of physical characteristics of linseed varieties. *IJCS, 6*(5), 509–512.

Slominski, B. A., Davie, T., Rogiewicz, A., Jia, W., Nyachoti, C. M., Jones, O., ... & Dribnenki, P. (2007). Quality characteristics of newly developed flaxseed: Chemical evaluation. In JOURNAL OF DAIRY SCIENCE (Vol. 90, pp. 589-590).

Szumała, P., & Wysocka, I. (2018). Effect of gelation and storage conditions on the oxidative stability of microemulsion and nanoemulsion delivery systems. *European Journal of Pharmaceutical Sciences, 124*, 17–25. https://doi.org/10.1016/j.ejps.2018.08.021

Szydłowska-Czerniak, A., Tymczewska, A., Momot, M., & Włodarczyk, K. (2020). Optimization of the microwave treatment of linseed for cold-pressing linseed oil – Changes in its chemical and sensory qualities. *LWT, 126*, 109317. https://doi.org/10.1016/j.lwt.2020.109317

Tautorus, C. L., & Mccurdy, A. R. (1990). Effect of randomization onoxidative stability of vegetable oils at two different temperatures. *Journal of the American Oil Chemists' Society, 67*(8), 525–530. https://doi.org/10.1007/BF02540760

Thompson, L. U., & Cunnane, S. C. (2003). *Linseed in human nutrition* (No. Ed. 2, pp. vi+–458).

Tuncel, N. B., Uygur, A., & Karagül Yüceer, Y. (2017). The effects of infrared roasting on HCN content, chemical composition and storage stability of linseed and linseed oil. *Journal of the American Oil Chemists' Society, 94*(6), 877–884.

Verma, P., & Mishra, S. (2014). Linseed: Functional food components and therapeutic role. *Journal of Medical Science And clinical Research, 2*, 2274–2282.

Wang, X., Yang, B., Yang, G., & Zhou, S. (2023). Effects of heat treatment on key quality and nutritional components of linseed meal. *Journal of food science and Biotechnology, 42*(7), 95–103.

Wanyo, P., Meeso, N., Kaewseejan, N., & Siriamornpun, S. (2015). Effects of drying methods and enzyme aided on the fatty acid profiles and lipid oxidation of Rice by-products. *Drying Technology, 34*(8), 953–961. https://doi.org/10.1080/07373937.2015.1087407

Wei, C., Zhou, Q., Han, B., Chen, Z., & Liu, W. (2019). Changes occurring in the volatile constituents of linseed oils (FSOs) prepared with diverse roasting conditions. *European Journal of Lipid Science and Technology, 121*(1), 1800068.

White, N. D. G., Mills, J. T., Kenaschuk, E. O., Oomah, B. D., & Dribnenki, P. (1999). Quality changes occurring in stored Solin, high linolenic acid and standard linseed (Linum usitatissimum L.). *Canadian Journal of Plant Science, 79*, 35–42. https://doi.org/10.4141/P98-065

Wiesenborn, D., Kangas, N., Tostenson, K., Hall, C., & Chang, K. (2005). Sensory and oxidative quality of screw-pressed linseed oil. *Journal of the American Oil Chemists' Society, 82*, 887–892.

Yaqoob, N., Bhatti, I. A., Anwar, F., Mushtaq, M., & Artz, W. E. (2016). Variation in physico-chemical/analytical characteristics of oil among different linseed (Linum usittatissimum L.) cultivars. Italian. *Journal of Food Science, 28*(1), 83–89.

Yousaf, N., Saleh, A. R., & Aftab, A. (2016). Z Postharvesting techniques and maintenance of seed quality. In S. Araújo (Ed.), *New challenges in seed biology–Basic and translational research driving seed technology* (pp. 113–135). IntechOpen. https://doi.org/10.5772/64994

Yalcin, H., Ozturk, I., Tulukcu, E., & Sagdic, O. (2010). Influence of the harvesting year and fertilizer on the fatty acid composition and some physicochemical properties of linseed (Linum usitatissimum L.). *Journal für Verbraucherschutz und Lebensmittelsicherheit, 6*(2), 197–202. https://doi.org/10.1007/s00003-010-0631-x

Zhang, Z. S., Li, D., & Zhang, L. X. (2013). Effect of heating on the fatty acid composition and oxidation products of linseed oil. *Asian Journal of Chemistry, 25*, 10082–10086.

Zhang, Z., Liu, Y., & Che, L. (2018). Effects of different drying methods on the extraction rate and qualities of oils from demucilaged linseed. *Drying Technology, 36*(13), 1642–1652. https://doi.org/10.1080/07373937.2017.1421220

Zuk, M., Richter, D., Matuła, J., & Szopa, J. (2015). Linseed, the multipurpose plant. Industrial Crops and Products, 75(Part B), 165–177. https://doi.org/10.1016/j.indcrop.2015.05.005

Application of Linseed in Food and Its Health Benefits

Komal Chauhan, Richa Soni, Aditika Agarwal, Deepa Sanglekar, and Vidhi Shah

Abstract

Linseed is popular as a food product in two main forms: whole seeds or its extracted edible oil. Although not commonly used in home cooking, increased awareness of its nutritional benefits has led to growing linseed consumption to address lifestyle-related health issues. Linseed stands out for its high omega-3 fatty acids, particularly alpha-linolenic acid, which support heart health. It is also rich in dietary fiber, aiding digestion and lignans with antioxidant properties. Linseed provides complete protein and essential vitamins and minerals such as magnesium, phosphorus, and copper. Linseed can be incorporated into various foods, including ground seeds, oil, capsules, milk, and gum. The chapter explores numerous food applications of linseed, including baked goods, cereals, snacks, dairy alternatives, dressings, and functional foods. Including linseed in food products enhances nutritional value and aligns with developing health-promoting sustainable foods.

Keywords

Linseed · Linolenic acid · Lignans · Food application · Fiber · Seeds

K. Chauhan · A. Agarwal
Department of Foods and Nutrition, Faculty of Family & Community Sciences, The Maharaja Sayajirao University of Baroda, Baroda, India
e-mail: komal.chauhanfn@msubaroda.ac.in

R. Soni (✉) · D. Sanglekar · V. Shah
Department of Life Science Food Science and Nutrition, University School of Science, Gujarat University, Ahmedabad, India
e-mail: richasoni@gujaratuniversity.ac.in

© The Author(s), under exclusive license to Springer Nature Singapore Pte Ltd. 2025

R. Chopra et al. (eds.), *Dynamics of Linseed and its Valorization*,
https://doi.org/10.1007/978-981-96-8927-9_3

1 Introduction

Over the past two decades, the incidence of cardiovascular disease risks, cancer, and other noncommunicable diseases (NCDs) have been on a sharp rise (Kalra et al., 2023). Individuals now exhibit an increasingly premature comorbidity and casualty trend (1990 vs. 2020) (Bennett et al., 2020; Manderson & Jewett, 2023). The youth show greater susceptibility to lifestyle-associated disorders, and scientific reports have highlighted a rise in the global share of NCD risk (Wang et al., 2023). These critical developments, alongside scientific discourse on therapeutic nutrition, and the rise of high throughput omics technology, have catalyzed the characterization of many phytochemicals for their concealed health benefits. Scientific efforts have expanded from identifying their healing properties to commercializing many underutilized crops and food products.

Oilseeds have a strong foothold in our agrarian country. Linseed (*Linum usitatissimum*), also called "flaxseed" in common parlance, holds immense significance to humans and animals. This crop plant's metamorphosis, especially in India, is specifically remarkable. It was earlier grown in India as a fodder crop for animals, primarily so because of its rich fiber content. The plant-based diet advocated nowadays indispensably places the nuts and seeds at focus backed with growing evidence of health benefits, disease reduction, and unequivocal sustainability for our planetary system. With the rapid advancements in food and medicinal sciences, this seed is now publicized as a "super food." But now one cannot imagine the plethora of applications this tiny nutrient-packed functional food or super food possesses.

Although its health benefits have been documented in ancient doctrines such as the Ayurveda and the principles of traditional Chinese medicine, flaxseed has not been in staple consumption for most of human history (Goyal et al., 2014). However, due to the identification of its fatty acids, cyclopeptides, phytosterol components, and their medicinal properties, flaxseed oil is now being touted as an "underrated superfood" (Mishra & Poonia, 2021). Likewise, dietary supplements and cosmetic products now show a centered focus on incorporating flaxseed oil (Shahada et al., 2024) (Table 1).

Linseeds are also revered for their remarkable versatility in culinary applications. These tiny seeds are a powerhouse of nutrients, rich in alpha-linolenic acid (53.4 g alpha-linolenic acid (ALA)/100 g linseed oil), dietary fiber (18.5 g), and lignans, making them an excellent addition to the functional food sector (Vp et al., 2019). With a subtle, nutty flavor, flaxseeds enhance the taste and texture of various foods, from baked goods to smoothies. The integration of flaxseeds into everyday foods exemplifies the innovative strides taken toward nutritionally enriched diets and underscores their growing significance in the food industry. This chapter discusses the health implications and potential food applications of linseed. The chapter covers some of the popular ways in which linseed can be incorporated into food products for a balanced consumption of this "superfood."

Table 1 Dietary sources of EFAs

Plant sources of essential fatty acids (EFA)	ALA content (g)	LA content (mg)	EPA content (mg)	DHA content (mg)
Pumpkin seeds (1tbsp)	0.051	#	–	–
Walnuts (1tbsp)	1.076	4.471	–	–
Soyabean oil (1tbsp)	1.231	#	–	–
Walnut oil (1tbsp)	1.414	#	–	–
Flaxseeds (1tbsp)	2.350	#	–	–
Flaxseed oil (1tbsp)	7.249	#	–	–
Almonds (100 g)	0.03	13,183	–	–
Peanuts (100 g)	0.003	11,584	–	–
Spinach (100 g)	0.2	75.06	–	–
Spirulina seaweed (dried) (100 g)	0.8	#	–	–
Soyabean, dry (100 g)	1.6	9754	–	–
Wheat flour (100 g)	0.05	0.7	–	–
Oats, germ (100 g)	1.4	#	–	–
Rice, bran (100 g)	0.2	#	–	–
Chicken mushroom (100 g)	0.03	111	–	–
Animal sources of EFA (per 100 g)				
Milk, whole (Buffalo)	0.035	132	–	–
Milk, whole (cow)	0.021	106	–	–
Paneer	0.233	206	–	–
Egg, poultry (whole boiled)	0.029	1169		
Chicken, wing (skinless)	0.028	623	–	–
Pork, ham	0.163	1598	–	–
Salmon	–	119	406	1192
Sardine	–	42.33	297	317
Tuna	–	23.05	90.6	345
Silver carp	–	194	171	125
Pomfret, black	–	51.5	244	565

Adapted from (Gebauer et al., 2006; Whelan & Rust, 2006; Williams & Burdge, 2006) and Indian Food Composition Tables, 2017)

2 Nutritional Profile of Linseed and the Associated Health Benefits

Flaxseed supplementation offers multiple health benefits, including lipid-lowering effects, decreased gut transit time, enhanced satiety, and improved cholesterol excretion (Nestel et al., 1997). Flaxseed fibers are metabolized by gut microbiota into short-chain fatty acids (SCFAs), such as propionate, which reduce cholesterol synthesis. The microbiome also metabolizes plant lignans like secoisolariciresinol diglucoside (SDG) and cinnamic acid glucoside, forming bioactive compounds (Sirotkin, 2023; Xu et al., 2012). FLC aids glycemic control, while ALA in flaxseed modulates LCFA metabolism, potentially impacting T2D by affecting GLUT-4 receptors due to changes in cell membrane fluidity (Das, 2005), which relates to diabetes and CVD risk.

2.1 Omega-3 Fatty Acids

Linseed, rich in ALA, supports heart health and protects cardio-metabolic and brain functions (NIH, 2022; Nijssen et al., 2023; Ros & Hu, 2013). Although essential fatty acids (EFAs) like ALA are found in various sources, flaxseed remains one of the richest plant-based options, offering advantages over marine sources (Williams & Burdge, 2006). With the right formulations, ALA-rich linseed products can enhance EFA intake.

2.2 Protein

Linseed provides up to 23% protein content, including essential amino acids, making it a valuable source for protein supplementation (Kaushik et al., 2016). Rich in arginine, glycine, and leucine, linseed protein supports cardiovascular health (Zhubi-Bakija et al., 2021; Chiavaroli et al., 2018). ICMR-NIN suggests incorporating ω-3 PUFA-rich foods like linseed into diets to help prevent noncommunicable diseases (ICMR-NIN Expert Group Report, 2020). Linseed cyclopeptides, also known as linusorbs or LOs, are compounds that have anticarcinogenic, immunomodulatory, and anti-inflammatory effects. LOs 23 and 32, for example, induce apoptosis in cancer cells via extrinsic and intrinsic pathways and arrest the cell cycle at the G1-S phase (Okinyo-Owiti et al., 2015; Zou et al., 2018). Linusorbs specifically target abnormal cells, sparing healthy cells, which provides an advantage over conventional cancer treatments (Sung et al., 2020).

2.3 Polysaccharides and Dietary Fiber

Linseed is high in both soluble and insoluble fibers, promoting digestion and gut health. The flaxseed mucilage (FM) or gum (LM) in linseed has unique properties, enhancing viscosity and water-binding properties in various products. Dietary fibers account for 20% of flaxseed's kernel weight, offering prebiotic and antioxidant benefits (Ding et al., 2014). LM can serve as a hydrocolloid in foods, cosmetics, and pharmaceuticals due to its functional properties (Bekhit et al., 2018). Its fibers aid bowel movements and weight management, while lignan metabolites like SCFs help regulate lipid absorption, benefiting gut health (Akila et al., 2023; Lange et al., 2023).

2.4 Lignans

Flaxseed contains phytoestrogens with antioxidant properties, primarily SDG, enterolactone, and enterodiol. Gut bacteria metabolize SDG, yielding mammalian lignans absorbed into the bloodstream, where they may exhibit anticarcinogenic properties (Rowland et al., 2003; Yuan et al., 2008). SDG offers antioxidant, anti-inflammatory, and anticarcinogenic effects through multiple pathways, influencing estrogen receptor activity and inhibiting cancer cell growth (De Silva & Alcorn, 2019). Lignans may also restrict tumor vascularization and inhibit metastatic potential (Thomasset et al., 2007; Menendez et al., 2011).

2.5 Vitamins and Minerals

Linseed is rich in folic acid, biotin, and vitamins B_1, B_2, B_6, C, and E, with γ-tocopherol supporting antioxidant functions (Morris, 2007). It also contains minerals like potassium, magnesium, calcium, and iron, beneficial for cardiovascular health and reducing stroke risks (Carter, 1993; Noreen et al., 2023). High potassium levels, inversely associated with platelet aggregation, further enhance linseed's health benefits.

Linseed, or flaxseed, has been the focus of numerous studies due to its broad spectrum of health benefits. These studies reveal promising results in areas ranging from cardiovascular and digestive health to hormonal balance and blood sugar control, among others. Numerous studies link linseed's high ALA content to reduced cardio-metabolic risks. A randomized control trial (RCT) on 21 coronary artery disease (CAD) patients consuming 30 g of flaxseed daily for 12 weeks showed an improved flow-mediated dilation (FMD) and reduced levels of C-reactive protein (CRP), IL-6, and TNF-α, suggesting a positive impact on inflammatory markers (Khandouzi et al., 2018). Another study showed significant reductions in total cholesterol, triglycerides, and LDL in patients consuming 20 g roasted powdered flaxseed with B_{12} (Agarwal, 2018). Yari et al. (2020a) found that patients with nonalcoholic fatty liver disease who consumed 30 g flaxseed powder saw significant improvements in total cholesterol and triglycerides. Furthermore, Yari et al. (2020b) noted that flaxseed, especially when combined with hesperidin, significantly reduced blood pressure, triglycerides, and insulin resistance in metabolic syndrome patients. Linseed's fiber content also aids weight management. Kuang et al. (2023) found that individuals consuming defatted flaxseed flour had significant weight and BMI reductions, particularly among those with specific genetic variants related to satiety. Animal studies on high-fat diets supplemented with flaxseed polysaccharide (FP) demonstrated reduced body weight and abdominal fat, potentially linked to leptin modulation, satiety improvement, and adiponectin upregulation, suggesting an anti-obesity effect via gut–brain axis interactions (Luo et al., 2019). Linseed helps stabilize blood sugar, beneficial for diabetes management. Meta-analyses indicate significant improvements in HbA1c, fasting blood glucose, and other glycemic parameters in patients with Type 2 diabetes mellitus (Xi et al., 2023; Villarreal-Renteria et al., 2022; Mahdavi et al., 2021). In an RCT on prediabetics, groups consuming 20 g and 40 g flaxseed daily showed significant reductions in fasting glucose, systolic blood pressure, and HOMA-IR scores, supporting its role in blood sugar regulation (Javidi et al., 2016).

Linseed's fiber also supports digestion, as shown by studies on flaxseed polysaccharide (FSP) supplementation in high-fat diet-fed mice, which improved metabolic syndrome by enhancing beneficial gut bacteria such as *Akkermansia* and *Bifidobacterium* (Yang et al., 2020). Similarly, flaxseed dietary fibers have prebiotic effects, supporting gut health through fermentation into SCFs (Thumann et al., 2019; Waghmode et al., 2020). Livingston et al. (2023) found that flaxseed-fed mice displayed increased microbial diversity and reduced inflammation, with improvements likely linked to linseed's fiber, lignans, and other bioactives.

Linseed is rich in lignans, which have antioxidative and estrogenic effects. In an RCT involving 99 prediabetic individuals, daily intake of 20 g or 40 g flaxseed powder for 12 weeks led to reductions in fasting glucose and HOMA-IR, highlighting its positive effect on glucose control (Javidi et al., 2016). Another study on prostate cancer patients consuming 200 mg phytoestrogens (including flaxseed) noted a trend toward reduced estradiol levels in patients with specific ERβ genotypes, pointing to potential benefits in hormonal health (Ahlin et al., 2023).

2.6 Application of Flaxseeds in Food

Flaxseeds come in various forms, each offering distinct applications and health benefits. These include whole flaxseeds, flaxseed meal, flaxseed oil, capsules, flaxseed flour, lignans, sprouted flaxseeds, flaxseed milk, flaxseed gum, and flaxseed fiber. As a versatile dietary ingredient, flaxseed powder is widely used for its high fiber and protein content, making it ideal for items such as bread, cereal, and energy bars, and as a plant-based egg substitute in baking (Ndou et al., 2018).

Whole flaxseeds are often used in baking or as a topping for salads and yogurt; however, they must be chewed or ground to release their nutritional benefits, as their outer shell can hinder digestion (Tarpila et al., 2005). Ground flaxseed, or flaxseed meal, is easily absorbed and can be added to smoothies and baked goods, acting as a vegan-binding agent (Prasad, 2000a, b). Flaxseed oil, extracted through cold pressing, is rich in ALA, an omega-3 fatty acid, and should be used in cold dishes to retain its nutritional properties (Hall et al., 2006). For convenience, flaxseed oil is available in capsule form, providing an easy way to consume omega-3 s

(Demark-Wahnefried et al., 2001). Flaxseed flour, created by grinding flaxseeds into a fine powder, serves as a substitute in gluten-free and low-carb baking (Cunnane et al., 1993). Additionally, flaxseed gum acts as a thickening and emulsifying agent in the food industry, commonly found in products like sauces and ice creams (Cui & Mazza, 1996). Finally, flaxseed fiber, derived from the seed coat, supports digestion and is often included in fiber-enriched foods (Cunnane et al., 1993).

There are several straightforward ways to incorporate flaxseed into baked goods. One approach is to finely grind flaxseed and then blend it into the batter or dough (Ahmad et al., 2021). These methods can improve the nutritional profile and texture of baked goods. Another option is to substitute flaxseed oil for other oils or fats in the recipe, which can enhance both the flavor and nutritional content of the baked items. In vegan baking, flaxseed can also serve as a replacement for eggs. Ground flaxseed can be used in recipes instead of eggs because it forms a gel-like consistency when mixed with water (Bryant & DeClue, 2021). This approach can potentially reduce the fat and cholesterol content in baked goods while preserving a comparable texture and structure (Viana et al., 2023). Due to its numerous health benefits and versatility, flaxseed has gained popularity as an ingredient in the baking industry. Many baked goods, including bread, muffins, cookies, cakes, and more, can incorporate flaxseed (Cakmak et al., 2021; Kumari & Morya, 2021; Kumari & Khetarpaul, 2019; Nassef et al., 2023; Saka et al., 2022; Sunwar, 2022; Taglieri et al., 2020; Wirkijowska et al., 2020; Yawale et al., 2022).

Dairy products are usually considered the most basic food for all ages and are an indispensable part of the human diet showing a high consumption rate. The commonly consumed dairy products include milk, curd, ice cream, yogurt, butter, buttermilk, and kulfi (a frozen milk product originating from the Indian subcontinent (Givens, 2018). Dairy products are rich in protein and fat (around 70% being saturated) but poor in fibers. On the other hand, flaxseeds are an excellent source of PUFA, fibers, and lignans. Hence, flaxseed and its components are excellent ingredients for incorporation into dairy products for developing nutritious and healthier composites of dairy products (Mueed et al., 2022) (Table 2).

3 Case Studies of Linseed Application in Food Products

The current expansion of linseed-based foods is widely witnessed across countries owing to an array of associated health benefits. This functional food offers limitless possibilities for inclusion into the daily dietary routine for meeting ALA requirements. The nutritionally rich properties of linseed, specifically higher quantity of proteins, healthy fats, and lignans, have made it attain an unprecedented stance in

Table 2 Diverse application and health benefits of flaxseeds

Application	Flaxseed component/ product name	Effect/role	References
Nutritional enhancement	Omega-3 fatty acids	Cardiovascular health and reduces inflammation	Kailash Prasad (2009)
	Dietary fiber	Digestive health, help in weight management, and regulate blood sugar levels	Bloedon and Szapary (2004)
	Protein source	Plant-based diets and an alternative protein source in food products	Dev and Quensel (1988)
	Lignans	Cancer-preventive effects	Thompson et al. (2006)
Functional food ingredients	Bakery products	Boost nutritional content and improve texture	Rubilar et al. (2010)
	Cereals and granola	Increases the fiber and nutrient density into staple breakfast	Morris (2007)
Functional properties in food processing	Emulsification	Food formulations, improving texture and stability	Mazza and Biliaderis (1989)
	Hydration and binding	Enhance water retention and binding properties	Shearer and Davies (2005)
	Shelf-life extension	Reserving the freshness and extending the shelf life of food products	Herchi et al. (2014)
Dietary supplements	Flaxseed oil	Health benefits as it contains omega-3 fatty acids	Singh et al. (2011)
	Powdered flaxseed	Meal replacement products and providing a convenient way to increase nutrient intake	Schumann et al. (2000)
Health and wellness products	Functional foods	Specific health benefits, such as heart health, digestive health, and weight management	Kristensen et al. (2012)
	Medical nutrition	For patients requiring high fiber and omega-3 fatty acids in their diets	Pan et al. (2009)
Animal feed	Livestock and poultry	To enhance the nutritional quality of meat and eggs, particularly increasing omega-3 fatty acid content	Bedigian (2004)
Gluten-free products	Gluten-free baking	Providing structure and moisture to products	Ganorkar and Jain (2013)
	Binding agent	Replace eggs in gluten-free and vegan recipes, enhancing texture and cohesion	Alu'datt (2013)
Meat alternatives	Meat extenders	Enhance nutritional value	Fuentes-Zaragoza et al. (2010)

(continued)

Table 2 (continued)

Application	Flaxseed component/ product name	Effect/role	References
Dairy alternatives	Flaxseed milk	Suitable for those with lactose intolerance or following a vegan diet	Parikh et al. (2019)
	Yogurts and creams	Offering a nutrient boost and improved texture	Mousavi et al. (2019)
Fortified foods	Infant formulas	Provide essential fatty acids important for brain development	Craig and Mangels (2009)
	Elderly nutrition	Improving heart health and digestive function	Kajla et al. (2015)
Flavor and aroma enhancement	Spices and seasonings	Add a nutty flavor to dishes	Herchi et al. (2014)
	Beverage flavoring	Enhance the taste profile	da Silva et al. (2018)
Nutraceuticals and functional foods	Cholesterol-lowering product	Lower cholesterol levels, leveraging their soluble fiber content	Kris-Etherton et al. (2002)
	Blood sugar regulation	Managing blood sugar levels	Pan et al. (2009)
Baking and cooking ingredients	Flaxseed flour	Adding nutritional benefits and altering texture	Hussain et al. (2008)
	Oil substitutes	Providing a healthier fat alternative with added omega-3 benefits	Hall et al. (2006)
Edible oils and dressings	Salad dressings	Unique flavor profile	Morris (2007)
	Cooking oils	Low-heat recipes and as a finishing oil for its health benefits	Lemay et al. (2002)
Innovative applications	Edible films and coatings	Biodegradable edible films and coatings for food packaging	Liu et al. (2018)
	Bioactive components	Enhanced health benefit	Oomah et al. (1994)

the current times. Linseed for human consumption is in four forms, namely, oil, whole seeds, ground, and defatted oilseed meal (Parikh et al., 2018). On the commercial scale, linseed being functionally beneficial is made available globally, in packaged food items such as cereals, bread, biscuits, fortified bars, soups, snacks, etc. (Bekhit et al., 2018). Further insight on food applications of linseed has been provided in the Table 3.

Table 3 Food applications of linseed

Type of sector	Linseed form and usage	Supplementation dose	Resultant effect	Reference
Dairy products	Lignans (SDG) in milk, yogurt, cheese, and whey-based drinks	200 mg/200 mL for milk, 100 mg/2x 200 mL for yoghurt, 1 g/10 L for cheese, 10 mg/100 mL for whey drinks	↑ SDG stability on temperature pasteurization of milk whey, yoghurt, and ripened cheese, post 6 months ↓SDG (up to 25%) due to ↓pH of whey drinks, ↓SDG recovery (6%) in edam cheese due to lactic acid bacteria and enzymes	Hyvärinen et al. (2006)
	Linseed mucilage	0.2% using *Lactobacillus delbrueckii* subs. Bulgaris and probiotic *Lactiplantibacillus plantarum* AG9	↑Physicochemical properties (viscosity, syneresis, water-holding capacity and texture) and ↑ antioxidant properties	Sungatullina et al. (2024)
	Micro-encapsulated linseed oil powder in spray-dried almond milk	0, 2, or 4 g flaxseed oil/100 g	↓ Oxidation values in 2% LO, ↑ ω-3 fatty acid	Bueno et al. (2022)
	Linseed oil in ice cream	12%	Stabilized the air cells by oil flocculates and strengthened foam structure	Goh et al. (2006)
	Linseed additive in butter	0.8,1.2,1.6%	Microstructure suspension formation, ↑plasticity, ↑ structure recovering ability, ↓structure destruction	Ivanov et al. (2011)
Bakery items	Linseed flour in yeast bread and muffins	Bread with15, 25, and 30% substitutions of flaxseed flour for wheat flour and 33, 50, and 66% for muffins	↑ Tenderness, nutty flavor, crunchiness, and desirable whole grain appearance in 30% flaxseed bread and ↑foam stability, volume, and keeping quality in 50% flaxseed muffins	Lipilina and Ganji (2009)
	Linseed flour in cookies	Defatted linseed, sesame, chia, and poppy flours in 50 g wheat flour	↑ Crumbly tendency, ↑ positive sensory assessments in flax and sesame	Martínez et al. (2021)
	Milled linseed in bagels	Plain, sunflower sesame and cinnamon raisin bagels without linseed/ with 30 g milled flaxseed flavored per bagel	↑ Grain/flax aroma and plain flavored linseed and ↓ aroma and flavor, ↑ sweet aroma and taste having higher acceptance rate for cinnamon raisin than sunflower sesame and plain	Aliani et al. (2012)

	Linseed cake in sourdough bread	7.5% of flaxseed cake flour	Significant ↓ in ω-6:ω-3 ratio with ↑ of fortification level, ↑ acceptance	Sanmartin et al. (2020)
	Roasted linseed flour in biscuits	0, 10,25,40 g	Significant ↑ in fiber(6.7-fold higher than control) protein and mineral content, ↑ total phenolic content and radical scavenging activity, 25% was nutritionally, texturally, and sensorially most accepted	Man et al. (2021)
	Linseed flour and linseed cake in pasta	5%, 9%, 13%, 17%, 20%, and 23%	↑Protein, fat, and dietary fiber in pasta without affecting quality, ↓ cooking losses, 23% flour and 17% cake yielded good quality pasta	Zarzycki et al. (2020)
Miscellaneous foods	Linseed oil by-product (LOB) in low-fat salad dressing	0.5%, 1%, 1.5%	↑rheological, microstructural, and recoverable properties, no phase separation, maintain viscoelasticity	Tekin and Karasu (2020)
	Roasted ground linseed in globs	10–20 g/ glob	↑ Energy, protein, fat, ALA, crude fiber, calcium content, sensory attributes, good appeal, softness, chewiness, 20 g superiorly accepted on 9-point hedonic scale, up to 6 days room storage	Agarwal and Chauhan (2015)
	Linseed in energy bar	5–20%	↑ Protein, fat, iron, fiber, ω-3 content, good acceptability at 10% and 15%, cool storage up to 90 days	Mridula et al. (2011)

Interestingly, the sudden emergent drift for plant-derived proteins is noticed among consumers warding off from the animal proteins with an emergent demand for other arable crops such as the linseed to replace the planetary health diet recommendations toward requirement for nuts (Schön & Böhringer, 2023). Hence, there is a burgeoning need for linseed and its by-products because of their promising lipid composition, high protein, lignan, and balanced amino acid contents as an integral dietary component. Linseed ingredients are capable enough to intensify the functional characteristics of food products through emulsification, foaming, and viscosity. Moreover, they can be an egg substitute serving as bulk protein ingredient and as thickener for sauces and salad dressings providing an additional benefit of lignan and fiber components (Bekhit et al., 2018).

Addition of up to 10% flaxseed flour for bread making to wheat flour improved the dough's physical stability, increased water absorption, binding ability, fat, protein content, crumb softness, and decreased in carbohydrate contents (Codină et al., 2019; Koca & Anil, 2007). Nevertheless, in a study exceeding 30 g linseed supplementation level, adverse effects on the textural properties of wheat bread such as color and volume by interfering with gluten development were observed (Santiago et al., 2019).

Speaking of the sensory profile for consumer acceptance, linseed often nullifies the food flavors where incorporated. For example, development of rancid odors due to high oil content results in off taste. Therefore, determination of optimum level of linseed is of great concern to ward off any flavor concerns (Pohjanheimo et al., 2006). Overall acceptability scores of certain foods, such as bagels, muffins, and meat products are reduced on addition of weighty amounts of linseed, although possessing nutty mouth feel and aroma (Ramcharitar et al., 2005). For health reasons, flaxseed milk has been developed as an easy alternative to animal milk being advantageous in consumption and preservation owing to its high ALA content with negligible cholesterol and lactose (Parikh et al., 2019). Another remarkable trait of growth impediment of some food spoilage microorganisms sets linseed to a unique positioning (Xu et al. 2019).

Linseed has numerous reasons be it nutritionally complete or diverse food applications for enjoying a wider appeal among the consumers. However, the oxidative degeneration is a prime deterrent for a limiting usability. Antioxidant stability of linseed oil was significantly intensified through addition of lycopene, which prolonged the shelf life by 31% and stability kinetics during storage to 42% (Condori et al., 2020).

Usage of nano-emulsion or microencapsulated form of linseed serves to greatly enrich the bioavailability of ω-3 polyunsaturated fatty acids. Adoption of such technologies is common nowadays by the food and wellness industries to retain, increase solubility and bioavailability, of omega-3 from deterrent factors as heat, light, oxygen, water, and digestion procedures for assisting in efficient target–oriented deliveries (Almasi et al., 2021). Generally, prior to being encapsulated, spray- or freeze-drying of linseed constituents with complex aggregation or coacervation treatment at times aids their shelf life to be longer (Yang et al., 2021). Nano-emulsion technology was established to yield linseed oil with enduring stability, solubility, rheological and nontoxic properties to its components when opted for consideration over synthetic antioxidants (likely to be toxic for humans) against factors such as heat, oxidative deterioration, and nutritive losses (Sharma et al., 2019).

Numerous animals, poultry, and fish-based studies have confirmed the effect of linseed supplementation on the quality of the animal feed given, which qualitatively improved the animal products as milk, meat, and eggs eventually. The impact of linseed ALA was determined on 30 randomized Holstein cows. It was found that ALA from the ground flaxseed significantly (($p < 0.001$) enhanced the total ω-3 PUFA levels and the milk ALA/ALA intake ratio and thereby reduced the ratio of ω-6 PUFAs to ω-3 PUFAs in milk (Huang et al., 2022). Broiler chicken fed with flaxseed meal resulted in enriched ω-3 fatty acids quantity in poultry meat with improved atherogenic and thrombogenic health indices (Kumar et al., 2019). Seven percent flaxseed oil added in Tilapia fish was assessed for lipid composition in the fish meat. Results revealed enrichment in both nutritional as well as physiological quality of meat by favorably impacting the increment of ω-3 fatty acids and decrement of saturated and ω-6 fatty acids (Tonial et al., 2012). Various researches were undertaken with flaxseed to replace fat (Rangrej et al., 2015; Lim et al., 2010). Rheological characteristics of flaxseed oil were tested in muffins replacing fat/shortening at different levels (10%, 20%, 30%, and 40%). Increased flaxseed oil percentage brought down the saturated acid and *trans*-fat content and 20% flaxseed oil muffins scored superior in terms of the texture, color, mouth feel, and acceptability (Punia et al., 2020).

Linseed proteins (LP) were firstly isolated by Osborne in 1892. The two protein types called linins and colinins were first extracted and identified by Vassel and Nesbitt. They employed a multistep extraction method using different reagents, namely, petroleum ether, phosphate salt, glycol, sodium hydroxide, and finally acidified by HCl to the isoelectric point (pI), which was 4.75 pH (Vassel & Nesbitt, 1945). The positive or negative protein charges or repulsive forces in between determine the homogeneity of the linseed slurry and also uphold their solubility. But, as the pH of this matrix moves near pI, the net protein charge decreases, triggering them to combine and so are unable to maintain their solubility. This procedure of separation of LP from the main slurry is applied for countless usages. Another solubility affecting factor is heat. For example, it was noted that in oil extraction process their solubility reduced from 73.2 to 44.9%. Boiling too enhanced protein solubility owing to protein denaturation and leaching of non-protein-nitrogen fraction (Bekhit et al., 2018).

Certain distinctive functional properties are exhibited by LP. Primarily, among all is the robust emulsification capacity (EC), enabling formation of strong emulsions by surface coating the surrounding oil particles when used in several food processes. EC is greatly influenced by heat, pH, and extraction settings. Alkali-solubilized EC of LP scored superior in comparison to canola, gelatin, soy, or whey proteins and stood good in acidic and basic mediums. Hence, they can function as emulsification agent to produce bioactive compounds in nano-emulsions. LP in permutation with linseed mucilage had amplified emulsification properties, which may be reinforced through variations in LP confirmations (Ye et al., 2022).

Secondly, the LP holds a significant water and fat absorption capacity (AC). The AC can be defined as the amount of water or fat that can be held by protein present in a biological matrix without undergoing significant structural damage. This particular LP characteristic is formed by its polar amino acids, which are crucially responsible for huge retention of lipid content inside linseed kernel meanwhile sufficing for better mouth feel and good taste in terms of food outweighing soy protein and gelatin successfully. Simultaneously, this LP feature imparts its usage as a meat extender in cooking procedures for thwarting fat and weight loss of the food products (Ye et al., 2022).

Alternatively, LP has a noteworthy property of formation of stable foam or foaming capacity on being whipped or stirred at various pH and temperatures. Plant proteins better foam in the acidic mediums. At pH 2.0–6.0, the foam formation ability of LP was kept in a stable state. With a rise to pH 8, the foaming capacity increased although being unstable. But linseed is superiorly attributed to develop stable foams as compared to soy in all pH levels (Lan et al., 2020). Despite the well-documented health benefits of flaxseed, several strategic challenges limit its incorporation into human diets. First, the majority of flaxseed's observed health benefits have been reported in animal studies, with a limited number of clinical trials available to substantiate its therapeutic potential in humans. This shortage of clinical evidence makes it difficult to quantify flaxseed's efficacy across various health conditions.

Second, even in human cohorts with initially positive health outcomes—particularly in cardiovascular disease (CVD) studies—these benefits often diminish over time. In some long-term trials, there are no statistically significant differences between the experimental and placebo groups. Additionally, the precise mechanisms by which flaxseed exerts its effects remain unclear, and mixed results across studies have led to inconclusive findings on its overall benefits. These inconsistencies may stem from variations in control and experimental group characteristics, or from inadequate use of neutral placebos within trials (Kris-Etherton et al., 2003; Rodriguez-Leyva et al., 2010).

Lastly, the presence of anti-nutrients in flaxseed, such as cyanogenic glycosides and trypsin inhibitors, poses challenges for regular or high-volume consumption, especially when flaxseed is unprocessed or uncooked. Additionally, the nutritional variability across flaxseed cultivars, along with the inherent instability of flaxseed oil, may contribute to inconsistencies in health outcomes. Advances in processing technologies that reduce anti-nutrient content and stabilize flaxseed's nutritional components will be critical for overcoming these challenges (Cardoso Carraro et al., 2012; Nowak & Jeziorek, 2023). Nonetheless, an interesting number of studies have emerged regarding its therapeutic outcomes, which warrants further clinical trials with an enthusiastic approach. Based on prevailing evidence, following a healthy diet, supplemented with flaxseeds and regular physical activity, is presumed to be synergistically more effective in alleviating NCD risk.

4 Conclusion

Linseeds are a multi-nutritional crop, which is used as supplement of functional food due to the presence of bioactive and antioxidant-rich nutrients. The rich nutrient profile in terms of omega −3 fatty acids, proteins, polysaccharides, or dietary fiber, lignans, vitamins, and minerals has also been discussed at length with respect to their individual role in providing health benefits and efficacy in the disease management. The nutritional, medicinal, and therapeutic properties have made it a multi-fix for all health issues and it is no wonder why it has become so sought after by the food industry too. Their wide applicability has a found a way for numerous food products wherein linseed is a primary ingredient or even worthy of being a promising accessory generating an increased consumer demand and awareness. With this advanced technological development to tap its various forms, we are often faced with rancidity issues, which require immediate attention when used in oil or readily cooked forms, in turn making it an expensive exercise. Therefore, more scientific studies need to address these with natural antioxidants for longer storage of linseed or its by-products.

References

Agarwal, A. (2018). *Vitamin B12 and Omega-3 fatty acid interventions for cognition in elderly- A voice trial*. [Unpublished doctoral thesis]. The Maharaja Sayajirao University of Baroda.

Agarwal, A., & Chauhan, K. (2015). Formulation and organoleptic evaluation of flaxseed globs as a functional food. *Journal of Food Measurement and Characterization, 9*(3), 448–453. https://doi.org/10.1007/s11694-015-9252-5

Ahlin, R., Nørskov, N. P., Nybacka, S., Landberg, R., Skokic, V., Stranne, J., Josefsson, A., Steineck, G., & Hedelin, M. (2023). Effects on serum hormone concentrations after a dietary phytoestrogen intervention in patients with prostate cancer: A randomized controlled trial. *Nutrients, 15*(7), 1792. https://doi.org/10.3390/nu15071792

Ahmad, N., Nurul, A., Mohammad, Z., & Nurul Sham Izzuani, N. (2021). Effects of flaxseed (linum usitatissimum) as fat mimetics on physicochemical and sensory properties of muffin. *Journal of Academia, 9*(2), 183–191. https://ir.uitm.edu.my/id/eprint/53889

Akila, M., Sasikumar, S., Malgija, B., Rachael, M. S., & Freddy, A. J. (2023). In silico approach towards the anti-obesity effects of flaxseed components alpha Linolenic acid and Secoisolariciresinol Diglucoside by the inhibition of SOCS3–the inhibitor of leptin Signalling pathway.

Aliani, M., Ryland, D., & Pierce, G. N. (2012). Effect of flax addition on the flavor profile and acceptability of bagels. *Journal of Food Science, 77*, S62–S70. https://doi.org/10.1111/j.1750-3841.2011.02509.x

Almasi, K., Esnaashari, S. S., Khosravani, M., & Adabi, M. (2021). Yogurt fortified with omega-3 using nanoemulsion containing flaxseed oil: Investigation of physicochemical properties. *Food Science Nutrition, 9*, 6186–6193. https://doi.org/10.1002/fsn3.2571

Alu'datt, M. H., Rababah, T., Ereifej, K., & Alli, I. (2013). Distribution, antioxidant and characterisation of phenolic compounds in soybeans, flaxseed and olives. *Food Chemistry, 139*(1–4), 93–99.

Bedigian, D. (2004). Economic botany. *Flax: The genus Linum, 58*, 755–758.

Bekhit, A. E.-D. A., Shavandi, A., Jodjaja, T., Birch, J., Teh, S., Mohamed Ahmed, I. A., et al. (2018). Flaxseed: Composition, detoxification, utilization, and opportunities. *Biocatalysis and Agricultural Biotechnology, 13*, 129–152. https://doi.org/10.1016/j.bcab.2017.11.017

Bennett, J. E., Kontis, V., Mathers, C. D., Guillot, M., Rehm, J., Chalkidou, K., Kengne, A. P., Carrillo-Larco, R. M., Bawah, A. A., Dain, K., Varghese, C., Riley, L. M., Bonita, R., Kruk, M. E., Beaglehole, R., Ezzati, M., & Countdown, N. (2020). NCD Countdown 2030: Pathways to achieving sustainable development goal target 3.4. *The Lancet, 396*(10255), 918–934. https://doi.org/10.1016/S0140-6736(20)31761-X

Bloedon, L. A. T., & Szapary, P. O. (2004). Flaxseed and cardiovascular risk. *Nutrition Reviews, 62*(1), 18–27.

Bryant, H., & DeClue, B. (2021). *Egg replacements in Vegan Cookies*. https://griffinshare.fontbonne.edu/fcs-424-2021/3/.

Bueno, F., Chouljenko, A., Reyes, V., & Sathivel, S. (2022). Spray-dried almond milk powder containing microencapsulated flaxseed oil. *Drying Technology, 40*(16), 3496–3508. https://doi.org/10.1080/07373937.2022.2061507

Cakmak, H., Mama, M., & Yilmaz, S. M. (2021). Determination of the effects of flaxseed (Linum Usitatissimum L.) sprouts powder on the gluten-free cupcake quality. *Journal of Food Processing and Preservation, 45*(5).

Cardoso Carraro, J. C., Dantas, M. I. D. S., Espeschit, A. C. R., Martino, H. S. D., & Ribeiro, S. M. R. (2012). Flaxseed and human health: Reviewing benefits and adverse effects. *Food Reviews International, 28*(2), 203–230.

Carter, J. F. (1993). Potential of flaxseeds and flaxseed oil in baked goods and other products in human nutrition. *Cereal Foods World, 38*, 754–759.

Chiavaroli, L., Nishi, S. K., Khan, T. A., Braunstein, C. R., Glenn, A. J., Mejia, S. B., Rahelić, D., Kahleová, H., Salas-Salvadó, J., Jenkins, D. J. A., Kendall, C. W. C., & Sievenpiper, J. L. (2018). Portfolio dietary pattern and cardiovascular disease: A systematic review and meta-analysis of controlled trials. *Progress in Cardiovascular Diseases X, 61*(1), 43–53. https://doi.org/10.1016/j.pcad.2018.05.004

Codină, G. G., Istrate, A. M., Gontariu, I., & Mironeasa, S. (2019). Rheological Properties of Wheat–Flaxseed Composite Flours Assessed by Mixolab and Their Relation to Quality Features. *Food, 8*(8), 333. https://doi.org/10.3390/foods8080333

Condori, M. A. V., Chagman, G. J. P., Barriga-Sanchez, M., Vilchez, L. F. V., Ursetta, S., Pérez, A. G., & Hidalgo, A. (2020). Effect of tomato (*Solanum lycopersicum* L.) lycopene-rich extract on the kinetics of rancidity and shelf-life of linseed (*Linum usitatissimum* L.) oil. *Food Chemistry., 302*, 125327. https://doi.org/10.1016/j.foodchem.2019.125327

Craig, W. J., Mangels, A. R., & American Dietetic Association. (2009). Position of the American dietetic association: Vegetarian diets. *Journal of the American Dietetic Association, 109*(7), 1266–1282.

Cui, W., & Mazza, G. (1996). Physicochemical characteristics of flaxseed gum. *Food Research International, 29*(3–4), 397–402.

Cunnane, S. C., et al. (1993). High alpha-Linolenic acid flaxseed (Linum Usitatissimum): Some nutritional properties in humans. *British Journal of Nutrition, 69*(2), 443–453. http://ovidsp.ovid.com/ovidweb.cgi?T=JS&PAGE=reference&D=emed6&NEWS=N&AN=23105482

da Silva, T. L. T., et al. (2018). Sensory and technological evaluation of margarines with reduced saturated fatty acid contents using Oleogel technology. *JAOCS, Journal of the American Oil Chemists' Society, 95*(6), 673–685.

Das, U. N. (2005). A defect in the activity of Δ6 and Δ5 desaturases may be a factor predisposing to the development of insulin resistance syndrome. *Prostaglandins, Leukotrienes and Essential Fatty Acids, 72*(5), 343–350. https://doi.org/10.1016/J.PLEFA.2005.01.002

De Silva, S. F., & Alcorn, J. (2019). Flaxseed Lignans as important dietary polyphenols for cancer prevention and treatment: Chemistry, pharmacokinetics, and molecular targets. *Pharmaceuticals, 12*(2), 68.

Demark-Wahnefried, W., et al. (2001). Pilot study of dietary fat restriction and flaxseed supplementation in men with prostate cancer before surgery: Exploring the effects of hormonal levels, prostate-specific antigen, and histopathologic features. *Urology, 58*(1), 4752.

Dev, D. K., & Quensel, E. (1988). Preparation and functional properties of linseed protein products containing differing levels of mucilage. *Journal of Food Science, 53*(6), 1834–1837.

Ding, H. H., Cui, S. W., Goff, H. D., Wang, Q., Chen, J., & Han, N. F. (2014). Soluble polysaccharides from flaxseed kernel as a new source of dietary fibers: Extraction and physicochemical characterization. *Food Research International, 56*, 166–173. https://doi.org/10.1016/j.foodres.2013.12.005

Fuentes-Zaragoza, E., Riquelme-Navarrete, M. J., Sánchez-Zapata, E., & Pérez-Álvarez, J. A. (2010). Resistant starch as functional ingredient: A review. *Food Research International, 43*(4), 931–942.

Ganorkar, P. M., & Jain, R. K. (2013). Flaxseed – A nutritional punch. *International Food Research Journal, 20*(2), 519–525.

Gebauer, S. K., Psota, T. L., Harris, W. S., & Kris-Etherton, P. M. (2006). n−3 fatty acid dietary recommendations and food sources to achieve essentiality and cardiovascular benefits. *The American Journal of Clinical Nutrition, 83*(6), 1526S–1535S. https://doi.org/10.1093/AJCN/83.6.1526S

Givens, D. I. (2018). Review: Dairy foods, red meat and processed meat in the diet: Implications for health at key life stages. *Animal, 12*(8), 1709–1721.

Goh, K. K. T., Ye, A., & Dale, N. (2006). Characterization of ice cream containing flaxseed oil. *International Journal of Food Science and Technology, 41*(8), 946–953. https://doi.org/10.1111/j.1365-2621.2006.01151.x

Goyal, A., Sharma, V., Upadhyay, N., Gill, S., & Sihag, M. (2014). Flax and flaxseed oil: An ancient medicine & modern functional food. *Journal of Food Science and Technology, 51*(9), 1633–1653. https://doi.org/10.1007/S13197-013-1247-9/TABLES/10

Hall, C., Tulbek, M. C., & Yingying, X. (2006). Flaxseed. *Advances in Food and Nutrition Research, 51*, 1–97.

Herchi, W., et al. (2014). Flaxseed Hull: Chemical composition and antioxidant activity during development. *Journal of Oleo Science, 63*(7), 681–689.

Huang, G., Wang, J., Liu, K., Wang, F., Zheng, N., Zhao, S., Qu, X., Yu, J., Zhang, Y., & Wang, J. (2022). Effect of flaxseed supplementation on Milk and plasma fatty acid composition and plasma parameters of Holstein dairy cows. *Animals (Basel), 12*(15), 1898. https://doi.org/10.3390/ani12151898

Hussain, S., Anjum, F. M., Butt, M. S., & Sheikh, M. A. (2008). Chemical compositions and functional properties of flaxseed flour. *Sarhad Journal of Agriculture, 24*(4), 649–653.

Hyvärinen, H. K., Pihlava, J.-M., Hiidenhovi, J. A., Hietaniemi, V., Korhonen, H. J. T., & Ryhänen, E.-L. (2006). Effect of processing and storage on the stability of flaxseed Lignan added to dairy products. *Journal of Agricultural and Food Chemistry, 54*(23), 8788–8792. https://doi.org/10.1021/jf061285n

ICMR-NIN Expert Group on Nutrient Requirement for Indians. (2020). *Recommended dietary allowances (RDA) and estimated average requirement (EAR)*. ICMR-National Institute of Nutrition. ISBN: 978-81-949175-1-9.

Ivanov, S., Rashevskaya, T., & Makhonina, M. (2011). Flaxseed additive application in dairy products production. *Procedia Food Science, 1*, 275–280. https://doi.org/10.1016/j.profoo.2011.09.04

Javidi, A., Mozaffari-khosravi, H., Nadjarzadeh, A., Dehghani, A., & Eftekhari, M. H. (2016). The effect of flaxseed powder on insulin resistance indices and blood pressure in prediabetic individuals: A randomized controlled clinical trial. *Journal of Research in Medical Sciences: The Official Journal of Isfahan University of Medical Sciences, 21*, 70. https://doi.org/10.4103/1735-1995.189660

Kajla, P., Sharma, A., & Sood, D. R. (2015). Flaxseed—A potential functional food source. *Journal of Food Science and Technology, 52*(4), 1857–1871.

Kalra, A., Jose, A. P., Prabhakaran, P., Kumar, A., Agrawal, A., Roy, A., Bhargava, B., Tandon, N., & Prabhakaran, D. (2023). The burgeoning cardiovascular disease epidemic in Indians—Perspectives on contextual factors and potential solutions. *The Lancet Regional Health – Southeast Asia, 12*, 100156. https://doi.org/10.1016/J.LANSEA.2023.100156

Kaushik, P., Dowling, K., McKnight, S., Barrow, C. J., Wang, B., & B. & Adhikari, B. (2016). Preparation, characterization and functional properties of flaxseed protein isolate. *Food Chemistry, 197*, 212–220.

Khandouzi, N., Zahedmehr, A., Mohammadzadeh, A., Sanati, H. R., & Nasrollahzadeh, J. (2018). Effect of flaxseed consumption on flow-mediated dilation and inflammatory biomarkers in patients with coronary artery disease: A randomized controlled trial. *European Journal of Clinical Nutrition, 73*(2), 258–265. https://doi.org/10.1038/s41430-018-0268-x

Koca, A. F., & Anil, M. (2007). Effect of flaxseed and wheat flour blends on dough rheology and bread quality. *Journal of the Science of Food and Agriculture, 87*(6), 1172–1175. https://doi.org/10.1002/jsfa.2739

Kris-Etherton, P. M., Harris, W. S., & Appel, L. J. (2002). Fish consumption, fish oil, Omega-3 fatty acids, and cardiovascular disease. *Circulation, 106*(21), 2747–2757.

Kris-Etherton, P. M., Harris, W. S., & Appel, L. J. (2003). Omega-3 fatty acids and cardiovascular disease. *Arteriosclerosis, Thrombosis, and Vascular Biology, 23*(2), 151–152. https://doi.org/10.1161/01.ATV.0000057393.97337.AE

Kristensen, M., et al. (2012). Flaxseed dietary fibers lower cholesterol and increase fecal fat excretion, but magnitude of effect depend on food type. *Nutrition and Metabolism, 9*, 8.

Kuang, X., Li, K., Shi, Y., Shao, X., Li, H., & Li, D. (2023). Gene-diet interaction in response to defatted flaxseed flour supplementation on obesity-related traits in Chinese overweight and obese adults: A randomized controlled trial. *Nutrition, 105*, 111870. https://doi.org/10.1016/j.nut.2022.111870

Kumar, F., Tyagi, P. K., Mir, N. A., Dev, K., Begum, J., Biswas, A., Sheikh, S. A., Tyagi, P. K., et al. (2019). Dietary flaxseed and turmeric is a novel strategy to enrich chicken meat with long chain ω-3 polyunsaturated fatty acids with better oxidative stability and functional properties. *Food Chemistry, 305*, 125458. https://doi.org/10.1016/j.foodchem.2019.125458

Kumari, N., & Khetarpaul, N. (2019). Value Added Egg Muffins Incorporating Full Fat Rice Bran (10 and 20%) and Flax Seeds (10%). *Journal of Pharmacognosy and Phytochemistry, 8*(5), 2374–2377.

Kumari, J., & Morya, S. (2021). Celiac disease: An epidemiological condition: Insight on gluten free diet, significance and regulatory recommendations. *The Pharma Innovation, 6*(7), 641–654.

Lan, Y., Ohm, J. B., Chen, B., & Rao, J. (2020). Physicochemical properties and aroma profiles of flaxseed proteins extracted from whole flaxseed and flaxseed meal. *Food Hydrocolloids, 104*, 105731. https://doi.org/10.1016/j.foodhyd.2020.105731

Lange, O., Proczko-Stepaniak, M., & Mika, A. (2023). Short-chain fatty acids—A product of the microbiome and its participation in two-way communication on the microbiome-host mammal line. *Current Obesity Reports, 12*(2), 108–126. https://doi.org/10.1007/S13679-023-00503-6/TABLES/6

Lemay, A., et al. (2002). Flaxseed dietary supplement versus hormone replacement therapy in Hypercholesterolemic menopausal women. *Obstetrics and Gynecology, 100*(3), 495–504.

Lim, C. W., Norziah, M. H., & Lu, H. F. S. (2010). Effect of flaxseed oil towards physicochemical and sensory characteristic of reduced fat ice creams and its stability in ice creams upon storage. *International Food Research Journal, 17*(2), 393–403.

Lipilina, E., & Ganji, V. (2009). Incorporation of ground flaxseed into bakery products and its effect on sensory and nutritional characteristics – a pilot study. *Journal of Foodservice, 20*(1), 52–59. https://doi.org/10.1111/j.1748

Liu, J., Shim, Y. Y., Tse, T. J., Wang, Y., & Reaney, M. J. T. (2018). Flaxseed gum a versatile natural hydrocolloid for food and non-food applications. *Trends in Food Science & Technology, 75*, 146–157. https://doi.org/10.1016/j.tifs.2018.01.011

Livingston, D. B. H., Sweet, A., Rodrigue, A., Kishore, L., Loftus, J., Ghali, F., Mahmoodianfard, S., Celton, C., Hosseinian, F., & Power, K. A. (2023). Dietary flaxseed and flaxseed oil differentially modulate aspects of the microbiota gut–brain axis following an acute Lipopolysaccharide challenge in male C57Bl/6 mice. *Nutrients, 15*(16), 3542. https://doi.org/10.3390/nu15163542

Luo, J., Qi, J., Wang, W., Luo, Z., Liu, L., Zhang, G., et al. (2019). Antiobesity effect of flaxseed polysaccharide via inducing satiety due to leptin resistance removal and promoting lipid metabolism through the AMPK signaling pathway. *Journal of Agricultural and Food Chemistry., 67*(25), 7040–7049. https://doi.org/10.1021/acs.jafc.9b0243

Mahdavi, A., Bagherniya, M., Mirenayat, M. S., Atkin, S. L., & Sahebkar, A. (2021). Medicinal plants and phytochemicals regulating insulin resistance and glucose homeostasis in type 2 diabetic patients: A clinical review. In G. E. Barreto & A. Sahebkar (Eds.), *Pharmacological properties of plant-derived natural products and implications for human health* (pp. 161–183). Springer. https://doi.org/10.1007/978-3-030-64872-5_13

Man, S. M., Stan, L., Păucean, A., Chiş, M. S., Mureşan, V., Socaci, S. A., et al. (2021). Nutritional, sensory, texture properties and volatile compounds profile of biscuits with roasted flaxseed flour partially substituting for wheat flour. *Applied Sciences, 11*(11), 4791. https://doi.org/10.3390/app11114791

Manderson, L., & Jewett, S. (2023). Risk, lifestyle and non-communicable diseases of poverty. *Globalization and Health, 19*(1), 1–9. https://doi.org/10.1186/S12992-023-00914-Z/TABLES/2

Martínez, E., García-Martínez, R., Álvarez-Ortí, M., Rabadán, A., Pardo-Giménez, A., & Pardo, J. E. (2021). Elaboration of gluten-free cookies with defatted seed flours: Effects on technological, nutritional, and consumer aspects. *Food, 10*(6), 1213. https://doi.org/10.3390/foods10061213

Mazza, G., & Biliaderis, C. (1989). Functional properties of flax seed mucilage. *Journal of Food Science, 54*(5), 1302–1305.

Menendez, C., Dueñas, M., Galindo, P., González-Manzano, S., Jimenez, R., Moreno, L., Zarzuelo, M. J., Rodríguez-Gómez, I., Duarte, J., Santos-Buelga, C., & Perez-Vizcaino, F. (2011). Vascular deconjugation of quercetin glucuronide: The flavonoid paradox revealed? *Molecular Nutrition & Food Research, 55*(12), 1780–1790. https://doi.org/10.1002/MNFR.201100378

Mishra, A., & Poonia, A. (2021). Flaxseed: An underrated superfood with functional properties. In *Handbook of Cereals, Pulses, Roots, and Tubers* (pp. 491–514). CRC Press. https://doi.org/10.1201/9781003155508-33

Morris, D. H. (2007). *Flax—A health and nutrition primer* (4th ed., pp. 49–51). Flax Council of Canada. Available from: www.flaxcouncil.ca

Mousavi, M., et al. (2019). Texture and sensory characterization of functional yogurt supplemented with flaxseed during cold storage. *Food Science and Nutrition, 7*(3), 907–917.

Mridula, D., Singh, K. K., & Barnwal, P. (2011). Development of omega-3 rich energy bar with flaxseed. *Journal of Food Science and Technology, 50*(5), 950–957. https://doi.org/10.1007/s13197-011-0425-x

Mueed, A., et al. (2022). Flaxseed bioactive compounds: Chemical composition, functional properties, food applications and health benefits-related gut microbes. *Food, 11*(20), 3307.

Nassef, S., Hafez, H., & Aly, A. (2023). Maximizing the use of flaxseed in the production of vegan bakery products free of gluten, eggs, Milk and low carbohydrates. *Assiut Journal of Agricultural Sciences, 54*(1), 102–115.

National Institute of Health (NIH) Office of Dietary Supplements. Omega-3 Fatty Acids. Fact Sheet for Consumers. https://ods.od.nih.gov/factsheets/Omega3FattyAcids-Consumer/ Updated on July 18, 2022.

Ndou, S. P., et al. (2018). Dietary supplementation with flaxseed meal and oat hulls modulates intestinal Histomorphometric characteristics, Digesta- and mucosa-associated microbiota in pigs. *Scientific Reports, 8*(1), 5880.

Nestel, P. J., Pomeroy, S. E., Sasahara, T., Yamashita, T., Liang, Y. L., Dart, A. M., Jennings, G. L., Abbey, M., & Cameron, J. D. (1997). Arterial compliance in obese subjects is improved with dietary plant n-3 fatty acid from flaxseed oil despite increased LDL Oxidizability.

Arteriosclerosis, Thrombosis, and Vascular Biology, 17(6), 1163–1170. https://doi.org/10.1161/01.ATV.17.6.1163
Nijssen, K. M. R., Mensink, R. P., Plat, J., & Joris, P. J. (2023). Longer-term mixed nut consumption improves brain vascular function and memory: A randomized, controlled crossover trial in older adults. *Clinical Nutrition, 42*(7), 1067–1075. https://doi.org/10.1016/j.clnu.2023.05.025
Noreen, S., Tufail, T., Bader, U., Ain, H., Ali, A., Aadil, R. M., Nemat, A., et al. (2023). Antioxidant activity and phytochemical analysis of fennel seeds and flaxseed. *Food Science & Nutrition, 11*(3), 1309–1317.
Nowak, W., & Jeziorek, M. (2023). The role of flaxseed in improving human health. *Healthcare, 11*(3), 395. https://doi.org/10.3390/HEALTHCARE11030395
Okinyo-Owiti, D. P., Dong, Q., Ling, B., Jadhav, P. D., Bauer, R., Maley, J. M., Reaney, M. J. T., Yang, J., & Sammynaiken, R. (2015). Evaluating the cytotoxicity of flaxseed orbitides for potential cancer treatment. *Toxicology Reports, 2*, 1014–1018. https://doi.org/10.1016/J.TOXREP.2015.06.011
Oomah, B., Dave, G. M., & Cui, W. (1994). Optimization of protein extraction from flaxseed meal. *Food Research International, 27*(4), 355–361.
Pan, A., et al. (2009). Meta-analysis of the effects of flaxseed interventions on blood lipids. *American Journal of Clinical Nutrition, 90*(2), 288–297.
Parikh, M., Netticadan, T., & Pierce, G. N. (2018). Flaxseed: Its bioactive components and their cardiovascular benefits. *American Journal of Physiology-Heart and Circulatory Physiology, 314*(2), H146–H159. 10.1152/ajpheart.00400.2017.
Parikh, M., Maddaford, T. G., Austria, J. A., Aliani, M., Netticadan, T., & Pierce, G. N. (2019). Dietary flaxseed as a strategy for improving human health. *Nutrients, 11*(5), 1171. https://doi.org/10.3390/nu11051171
Pohjanheimo, T. A., Hakala, M. A., Tahvonen, R. L., Salminen, S. J., & Kallio, H. P. (2006). Flaxseed in bread making: Effects on sensory quality, aging, and composition of bakery products. *Journal of Food Science, 71*(4), S343–S348. https://doi.org/10.1111/j.1750-3841.2006.00005.x
Prasad, K. (2000a). Antioxidant activity of secoisolariciresinol diglucoside-derived metabolites, secoisolariciresinol, Enterodiol, and enterolactone. *International Journal of Angiology, 9*(04), 220–225. https://doi.org/10.1007/BF01623898
Prasad, K. (2000b). Flaxseed: A source of Hypocholesterolemic and Antiatherogenic agents. *Drug News and Perspectives, 13*(2), 99–104.
Prasad, K. (2009). Flaxseed and cardiovascular health. *Journal of Cardiovascular Pharmacology, 54*(5), 369–377.
Punia, S., Sandhu, K. S., Dhull, S. B., Kaur, M., & Siroha, A. K. (2020). Kinetic, rheological and thermal studies of flaxseed (Linum usitatissiumum L.) oil and its utilization. *Journal of Food Science and Technology., 57, 11*, 4014–4021. https://doi.org/10.1007/s13197-020-04434-1
Ramcharitar, A., Badrie, N., Mattfeldt-Beman, M., Matsuo, H., & Ridley, C. (2005). Consumer acceptability of muffins with flaxseed (Linum usitatissimum). *Journal of Food Science, 70*(7), s504–s507. https://doi.org/10.1111/j.1365-2621.2005.tb11499.x
Rangrej, V., Shah, V., Patel, J., & Ganorkar, P. M. (2015). Effect of shortening replacement with flaxseed oil on physical, sensory, fatty acid and storage characteristics of cookies. *Journal of Food Science and Technology., 52, 6*, 3694–3700. https://doi.org/10.1007/s13197-014-1430-7
Rodriguez-Leyva, D., Bassett, C. M. C., McCullough, R., & Pierce, G. N. (2010). The cardiovascular effects of flaxseed and its omega-3 fatty acid, alpha-linolenic acid. *Canadian Journal of Cardiology, 26*(9), 489–496. https://doi.org/10.1016/S0828-282X(10)70455-4

Ros, E., & Hu, F. B. (2013). Consumption of plant seeds and cardiovascular health: Epidemiological and clinical trial evidence. *Circulation, 128*, 553–565. https://doi.org/10.1161/circulationaha.112.001119

Rowland, I., Faughnan, M., Hoey, L., Wähälä, K., Williamson, G., & Cassidy, A. (2003). Bioavailability of phyto-oestrogens. *British Journal of Nutrition, 89*(S1), S45–S58. https://doi.org/10.1079/BJN2002796

Rubilar, M., et al. (2010). Flaxseed as a source of functional ingredients. *Journal of Soil Science and Plant Nutrition, 10*(3), 373–377.

Saka, İ., Baumgartner, B., & Özkaya, B. (2022). Usability of microfluidized flaxseed as a functional additive in bread. *Journal of the Science of Food and Agriculture, 102*(2), 505–513.

Sanmartin, C., Taglieri, I., Venturi, F., Macaluso, M., Zinnai, A., Tavarini, S., et al. (2020). Flaxseed cake as a tool for the improvement of nutraceutical and sensorial features of sourdough bread. *Food, 9*(2), 204. https://doi.org/10.3390/foods9020204

Santiago, A., Ryland, D., Cui, S., Blewett, H., & Aliani, M. (2019). Effect of milled flaxseed and storage conditions on sensory properties and selected bioactive compounds in Banana and cinnamon muffins used in a clinical trial. *Journal of the Science of Food and Agriculture., 99*(2), 831–843. https://doi.org/10.1002/jsfa.9253

Schön, A.-M., & Böhringer, M. (2023). Land consumption for current diets compared with that for the planetary health diet—How many people can our land feed? *Sustainability, 15*(11), 8675. https://doi.org/10.3390/su15118675

Schumann, B. E., Squires, E. J., & Leeson, S. (2000). Effect of dietary flaxseed, flax oil and n-3 fatty acid supplement on hepatic and plasma characteristics relevant to fatty liver Haemorrhagic syndrome in laying hens. *British Poultry Science, 41*(4), 465–472.

Shahada, C., Morya, S., & Awuchi, C. G. (2024). A narrative review on nutraceutical, food and industrial applications of flaxseed (Linum usitatissimum. L). *Cogent Food & Agriculture, 10*(1), 2306017. https://doi.org/10.1080/23311932.2024.2306017

Sharma, S., Cheng, S.-F., Bhattacharya, B., & Chakkaravarthi, S. (2019). Efficacy of free and encapsulated natural antioxidants in oxidative stability of edible oil: Special emphasis on nanoemulsion-based encapsulation. *Trends in Food Science & Technology., 91*, 305–318. https://doi.org/10.1016/j.tifs.2019.07.030

Shearer, A. E. H., & Davies, C. G. A. (2005). Physicochemical properties of freshly baked and stored whole-wheat muffins with and without flaxseed meal. *Journal of Food Quality, 28*(2), 137–153.

Singh, K. K., Mridula, D., Rehal, J., & Barnwal, P. (2011). Flaxseed: A potential source of food, feed and fiber. *Critical Reviews in Food Science and Nutrition, 51*(3), 210–222.

Sirotkin, A. V. (2023). Influence of flaxseed (Linum usitatissimum) on female reproduction. *Planta Medica, 89*(06), 608–615. https://doi.org/10.1055/A-2013-2966

Sung, N. Y., Jeong, D., Shim, Y. Y., Ratan, Z. A., Jang, Y. J., Reaney, M. J. T., Lee, S., Lee, B. H., Kim, J. H., Yi, Y. S., & Cho, J. Y. (2020). The anti-cancer effect of Linusorb B3 from flaxseed oil through the promotion of apoptosis, inhibition of actin polymerization, and suppression of Src activity in glioblastoma cells. *Molecules, 25*(24), 5881. https://doi.org/10.3390/MOLECULES25245881

Sungatullina, A., Petrova, T., & Nikitina, E. (2024). Investigation on fermented Milk quality after the addition of flaxseed mucilage and the use of lactobacillus delbrueckii subsp. bulgaricus and Lactiplantibacillus plantarum AG9. *Frontiers in Bioscience, 16*(2), 11. https://doi.org/10.31083/j.fbe1602011

Sunwar, R. (2022). Effect of flaxseed on the physiochemical and sensory quality of Muffin as egg replacer. http://202.45.146.37:8080/jspui/handle/123456789/250.

Taglieri, I., et al. (2020). Effect of the leavening agent on the compositional and sensorial characteristics of bread fortified with flaxseed cake. *Applied Sciences (Switzerland), 10*(15), 5235.

Tarpila, A., Wennberg, T., & Tarpila, S. (2005). Flaxseed as a functional food. *Current Topics. Nutraceutical Research., 3*, 167–188.

Tekin, Z. H., & Karasu, S. (2020). Cold-pressed flaxseed oil by-product as a new source of fat replacers in low-fat salad dressing formulation: Steady, dynamic and 3-ITT rheological properties. *Journal of Food Processing and Preservation, 44*(9), e14650. https://doi.org/10.1111/jfpp.14650

Thomasset, S. C., Berry, D. P., Garcea, G., Marczylo, T., Steward, W. P., & Gescher, A. J. (2007). Dietary polyphenolic phytochemicals—Promising cancer chemopreventive agents in humans? A review of their clinical properties. *International Journal of Cancer, 120*(3), 451–458. https://doi.org/10.1002/IJC.22419

Thompson, L. U., et al. (2006). Phytoestrogen content of foods consumed in Canada, including Isoflavones, Lignans, and Coumestan. *Nutrition and Cancer, 54*(2), 184–201.

Thumann, T. A., Pferschy-Wenzig, E.-M., Moissl-Eichinger, C., & Bauer, R. (2019). The role of gut microbiota for the activity of medicinal plants traditionally used in the European Union for gastrointestinal disorders. *Journal of Ethnopharmacology, 245*, 112153. https://doi.org/10.1016/j.jep.2019.112153

Tonial, I. B., Matsushita, M., Furuya, W. M., de Souza, N. E., & Visentainer, J. V. (2012). Fatty acid contents in fractions of neutral lipids and phospholipids of fillets of tilapia treated with flaxseed oil. *Journal of the American Oil Chemists' Society, 89*(8), 1495–1500. https://doi.org/10.1007/s11746-012-2039-5

Vassel, B., & Nesbitt, L. L. (1945). The nitrogenous constituents of flaxseed: II. The isolation of a purified protein fraction. *Journal of Biological Chemistry, 159*(3), 571–584. https://doi.org/10.1016/S0021-9258(17)41562-6

Viana, A., Ethur, E. M., de Freitas, E. M., & Hoehne, L. (2023). Chicken eggs substitute using vegetable origin – A review. *Food and Bioprocess Technology, 16*(8), 1652–1667.

Villarreal-Renteria, A. I., Herrera-Echauri, D. D., Rodríguez-Rocha, N. P., Zuñiga, L. Y., Muñoz-Valle, J. F., García-Arellano, S., Bernal-Orozco, M. F., & Macedo-Ojeda, G. (2022). Effect of flaxseed (*Linum usitatissimum*) supplementation on glycemic control and insulin resistance in prediabetes and type 2 diabetes: A systematic review and meta-analysis of randomized controlled trials. *Complementary Therapies in Medicine, 70*, 102852. https://doi.org/10.1016/j.ctim.2022.102852

Vp, R., Rs, A., & Ka, M. (2019). Flaxseed as a functional food: A review. *Journal of Pharmacognosy and Phytochemistry, 8*(3), 352–354.

Waghmode, M., Gunjal, A., & Patil, N. (2020). Probiotic sugar confectionery fortified with flax seeds (Linum usitatissimum L.). *Journal of Food Science and Technology, 57*(5), 1964–1970. https://doi.org/10.1007/s13197-020-04276-x

Wang, H., Song, Y., Ma, J., Ma, S., Shen, L., Huang, Y., Thangaraju, P., Basharat, Z., Hu, Y., Lin, Y., Peden, A. E., Sawyer, S. M., Zhang, H., & Zou, Z. (2023). Burden of non-communicable diseases among adolescents and young adults aged 10–24 years in the South-East Asia and Western Pacific regions, 1990–2019: A systematic analysis for the global burden of disease study 2019. *The Lancet Child and Adolescent Health, 7*(9), 621–635. https://doi.org/10.1016/S2352-4642(23)00148-7

Whelan, J., & Rust, C. (2006). Innovative dietary sources of n-3 fatty acids. *Annual Review of Nutrition, 26*, 75–103. https://doi.org/10.1146/ANNUREV.NUTR.25.050304.092605/CITE/REFWORKS

Williams, C. M., & Burdge, G. (2006). Long-chain n−3 PUFA: Plant v. marine sources. *Proceedings of the Nutrition Society, 65*(1), 42–50. https://doi.org/10.1079/PNS2005473

Wirkijowska, A., et al. (2020). The possibility of using by-products from the flaxseed industry for functional bread production. *Lwt, 118*, 108860.

Xi, H., Zhou, W., Sohaib, M., Niu, Y., Zhu, R., Guo, Y., Wang, S., Mao, J., Wang, X., & Guo, L. (2023). Flaxseed supplementation significantly reduces hemoglobin A1C in patients with type 2 diabetes mellitus: A systematic review and meta-analysis. *Nutrition Research, 110*, 23–32. https://doi.org/10.1016/j.nutres.2022.12.008

Xu, Y., Hall, C., & Wolf-Hall, C. (2019). Antifungal activity of flaxseed (*Linum usitatissimum* L.) hydrolysates. *Food Control, 95*, 83–88. https://doi.org/10.1016/j.foodcont.2018.07.040

Xu, J., Zhou, X., Chen, C., Deng, Q., Huang, Q., Yang, J., Yang, N., & Huang, F. (2012). Laxative effects of partially defatted flaxseed meal on normal and experimental constipated mice. *BMC Complementary and Alternative Medicine, 12*(1), 1–5. https://doi.org/10.1186/1472-6882-12-14/FIGURES/3

Yang, C., Xu, Z., Deng, Q., Huang, Q., Wang, X., & Huang, F. (2020). Beneficial effects of flaxseed polysaccharides on metabolic syndrome via gut microbiota in high-fat diet fed mice. *Food Research International, 131*, 108994. https://doi.org/10.1016/j.foodres.2020.108994

Yang, J., Wen, C., Duan, Y., Deng, Q., Peng, D., Zhang, H., & Ma, H. (2021). The composition, extraction, analysis, bioactivities, bioavailability and applications in food system of flaxseed (*Linum usitatissimum* L.) oil: A review. *Trends in Food Science and Technology, 118*, 252–260. https://doi.org/10.1016/j.tifs.2021.09.025

Yari, Z., Cheraghpour, M., Alavian, S. M., Hedayati, M., Eini-Zinab, H., & Hekmatdoost, A. (2020a). The efficacy of flaxseed and hesperidin on non-alcoholic fatty liver disease: An open-labeled randomized controlled trial. *European Journal of Clinical Nutrition, 75*, 99–111. https://doi.org/10.1038/s41430-020-0679

Yari, Z., Cheraghpour, M., & Hekmatdoost, A. (2020b). Flaxseed and/or hesperidin supplementation in metabolic syndrome: An open-labeled randomized controlled trial. *European Journal of Nutrition, 60*, 287–298. https://doi.org/10.1007/s00394-020-02246-9

Yawale, P., Upadhyay, N., Ganguly, S., & Kumar, S. (2022). A comprehensive review on recent novel food and industrial applications of flaxseed: 2014 onwards. *Food and Feed Research, 49*(1), 67–95.

Ye, X. P., Xu, M. F., Tang, Z. X., Chen, H. J., Wu, D. T., Wang, Z. Y., et al. (2022). Flaxseed protein: Extraction, functionalities and applications. *Food Science and Technology, 42*, e22021. https://doi.org/10.1590/fst.22021

Yuan, J. P., Li, X., Xu, S. P., Wang, J. H., & Liu, X. (2008). Hydrolysis kinetics of secoisolariciresinol diglucoside oligomers from flaxseed. *Journal of Agricultural and Food Chemistry, 56*(21), 10041–10047. https://doi.org/10.1021/JF8020656/ASSET/IMAGES/LARGE/JF-2008-020656_0001.JPEG

Zarzycki, P., Sykut-Domańska, E., Sobota, A., Teterycz, D., Krawęcka, A., Blicharz-Kania, A., et al. (2020). Flaxseed enriched pasta—Chemical composition and cooking quality. *Food, 9*(4), 404. https://doi.org/10.3390/foods9040404

Zhubi-Bakija, F., Bajraktari, G., Bytyçi, I., Mikhailidis, D. P., Henein, M. Y., Latkovskis, G., Rexhaj, Z., Zhubi, E., & Banach, M. (2021). International lipid expert panel (ILEP). The impact of type of dietary protein, animal versus vegetable, in modifying cardio metabolic risk factors: A position paper from the international lipid expert panel (ILEP). *Clinical Nutrition, 40*(1), 255–276. https://doi.org/10.1016/j.clnu.2020.05.017

Zou, X. G., Hu, J. N., Li, J., Yang, J. Y., Du, Y. X., Yu, Y. F., & Deng, Z. Y. (2018). iCellular uptake of [1–9-NαC]-linusorb B2 and [1–9-NαC]-linusorb B3 isolated from flaxseed, and their anti-tumor activities in human gastric SGC-7901 cells. *Journal of Functional Foods, 48*, 692–703. https://doi.org/10.1016/J.JFF.2018.08.008

Extraction of Linseed Oil: Conventional and Novel Methods

Monika Chand, Sheetal Mane, and Anupama Singh

Abstract

Linseed oil is a valuable source of omega-3 fatty acids (particularly alpha-linolenic acid), omega-6 fatty acids, vitamin E, and phytonutrients, offering numerous health benefits due to its high polyunsaturated fatty acid (PUFA) content. However, its fatty acid profile affects its oxidative stability, leading to rancidity and reduced shelf life. Traditional extraction methods, such as mechanical pressing, yield good-quality oil but with lower yields and impurities, while solvent extraction increases yields but reduces PUFA content and poses environmental hazards. Advanced extraction techniques like supercritical, ultrasound, and microwave methods are being explored to meet the rising demand for edible oils. These methods aim to enhance extraction efficiency and oil quality while reducing environmental risks, although they present practical challenges at larger scale and may increase carbon footprints if not managed efficiently.

Keywords

Conventional extraction · Nonconventional extraction · Omega-3 fatty acids · Extraction efficiency

M. Chand
Department of Food Science and Technology, National Institute of Food Technology Entrepreneurship and Management, Kundli, Haryana, India

S. Mane · A. Singh (✉)
Department of Food Engineering, National Institute of Food Technology Entrepreneurship and Management, Kundli, Haryana, India

© The Author(s), under exclusive license to Springer Nature Singapore Pte Ltd. 2025

R. Chopra et al. (eds.), *Dynamics of Linseed and its Valorization*,
https://doi.org/10.1007/978-981-96-8927-9_4

1 Introduction

Linseed oil is an excellent source of omega-3 fatty acids, particularly alpha-linolenic acid (ALA), as well as omega-6 fatty acids, vitamin E, and phytonutrients (Pointner et al., 2024). Linseed oil is one of the richest sources of PUFA (polyunsaturated fatty acids) with tremendous health benefits and therapeutic properties (Chand et al., 2024). However, due to its fatty acid profile, it has an undesirable effect on the oxidative stability of linseed oil. One of the most common causes of deterioration in lipid-based foods is oxidation. This process occurs when fats and oils react with molecular oxygen, leading to rancidity, off-flavors, and a reduced shelf life (Szterk et al., 2010). Extraction is crucial in separating and identifying useful components from various plants.

Linseed oil has been conventionally extracted using a variety of methods, including screw presses (expellers), hydraulic presses, power-driven rotary ghanis, and bullock-driven ghani (Cakaloglu et al., 2018). However, these mechanically pressing methods often resulted in good-quality oil but lower yields and impurities. The other conventional method broadly used was using polar solvents like hexane, which has led to a significant increase in oil yield but the loss in PUFA content due to heating and environmental hazard, which were the major drawbacks of solvent extraction (Sabadin Piva et al., 2018). Over time, the demand for edible vegetable oils has consistently risen, from 87.8 million in 2000 to 186.5 million tons in 2016 and vegetable oil sales are in future expected to grow by 6.8%, with a compound annual growth rate (CAGR) of 6.5% from the year 2018 to 2028 (Sarpong, 2024; Khater et al., 2023; Nawade et al., 2018). So, to overcome this increasing demand, new underutilized sources of edible oil like linseed have been explored recently along with new novel technologies. These nonconventional methods include supercritical, ultrasound, and microwave, which aim to reduce quality issues and environmental risks and increase oil yield. These advanced extraction methods, while promising in enhancing extraction efficiency and oil quality, have certain large-scale practical challenges and require high energy and cost, potentially leading to higher carbon footprints if not managed efficiently.

In this chapter, extraction methods, the nutritional significance, and challenges associated with linseed oil production will be reviewed. Both traditional and novel extraction methodologies will be studied, highlighting their advantages and limitations. Moreover, the potential of sustainable nonconventional methods to improve yield and promote sustainability while addressing practical challenges will be explored. Figure 1 shows a diagrammatic representation of conventional and novel extraction methods.

2 Conventional Extraction Methods

Conventional extraction methods refer to well-established, traditional techniques for obtaining oil from seeds, nuts, or other plant materials. These methods generally rely on mechanical and chemical processes that have been extensively utilized in the

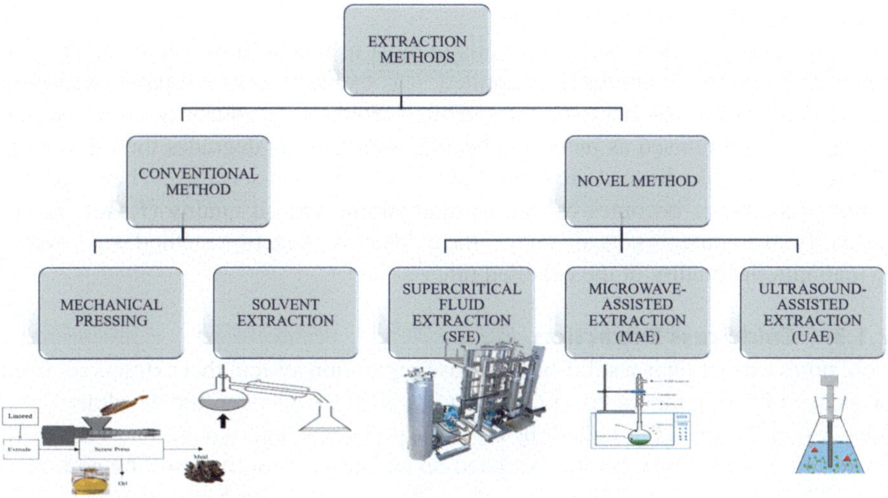

Fig. 1 Diagrammatic representation of conventional and novel extraction methods

industry for many years (Prado et al., 2021). The mechanical pressing of linseed oil has a long and rich history, progressing from basic manual techniques to advanced modern technologies. Over time, the use of mechanical expellers has increased due to their growing popularity (Singh et al., 2012). The primary goal has consistently been to extract high-quality linseed oil efficiently for diverse applications through changes and improvements in extraction methods.

2.1 Mechanical Pressing

2.1.1 Hydraulic Pressing

J. Bramah invented the hydraulic press in 1785 to extract oil from oilseeds. Afterward, in the 1800s, hydraulic presses utilized 16 press boxes and 400 tons of pressure force (Kirschenbauer, 1944). The principle of the hydraulic press is that oil is obtained by pressing the seeds filled in filter cloth inside the press boxes. The press cake remains in the filter cloth, which is manually removed. Temperature and pressure are the two most crucial factors in hydraulic pressing. While hydraulic press cages without filter cloth were common in the 1900s, they were later replaced by techniques like solvent extraction and cold extractors. These newer methods could be applied to continuous systems, maintained high efficiency, worked more quickly, required less labor, and left behind relatively small amounts of oil (Lanoiselle & Bouvier, 1994). Hydraulic pressing, on the other hand, was time-consuming and had lower oil yield, higher processing time, higher cost, and degraded oil quality (Gros et al., 2003).

2.1.2 Hot Pressing Extraction

Pressure is used in the separation of oils in most instances; however, depending on whether or not the temperature is applied, it is called hot or cold press extraction (Kiritsakis, 2002). The hot extraction method yields a high quantity of oil, but the quality is compromised as increased heating significantly degrades the oil quality. PUFA-rich oils like linseed are quite light-, air-, and heat-sensitive. Therefore, the temperature factor becomes crucial to maintaining the oil quality (Kasote et al., 2013). To overcome this disadvantage, the cold press extraction method was devised to maintain the quality of the expelled oil.

2.1.3 Cold Press Extraction

Cold press extraction is a solid-liquid phase separation system that extracts oil from oilseeds at lower temperatures (Zuorro et al., 2014). Anderson first developed cold press expellers in 1902, including the cold press machine having one inlet with seeds and two exits: one for the extracted oil and another for the resulting non-oiled cake. The oil is separated from the cake and removed through slots between regularly spaced metal bars, facilitated by the rotating screw (Uitterhaegen & Evon, 2017). Among all the techniques for linseed oil extraction, cold pressing is a simple, rapid, cost-effective, safe, and eco-friendly method. The oil is not subjected to chemicals, heating, and refining processes and thus does not degrade major sensitive phenolics and antioxidant compounds (Bhargavi et al., 2018; Szydłowska-Czerniak et al., 2020). However, merely removing heating leads to lowered yield and high residual oil (Kasote et al., 2013). It extracts less than 70% of the oil content from the seeds (Pradhant et al., 2010b). Due to this incompetency of the process, the seeds are mostly doubly or triply pressed, although no significant effect is seen with triply pressed, and it is not an economically viable process (Kasote et al., 2013). Furthermore, oil quality decreases, such as altered color, decreased saponification value, and increased free fatty acids, but few compounds like phenolics and flavonoids tend to increase with double pressing.

2.2 Solvent Extraction

Solvent extraction (or liquid extraction) involves using an organic solvent. It involves using a solvent, typically hexane, acetone, petroleum ether, methanol, and n-hexane dichloromethane to dissolve the oil from the linseed. It can also utilize an aqueous medium to obtain desired compounds by selectively separating the component from the aqueous mixture (Kumar et al., 2017). The linseeds are cleaned and dried to remove impurities and maintain moisture, or size reduction might be given and then placed in an extraction unit where it is mixed with solvent, forming a mix known as miscella. The oil seeps into the organic solvent. The miscella is then processed to recover the solvent through a distillation process where the solvent is distilled for reuse. Further, this oil can undergo refining or processing to obtain a solvent-free final oil product (Serrato, 1981). Hexane is commonly used as a solvent due to its advantageous properties, including easy recovery, nonpolar nature, low latent heat of vaporization (330 kJ/kg), and high selectivity for solvents (Liu & Mamidipally, 2005). Figure 2 shows diagrammatic linseed oil using solvent extraction.

Solvent extraction is preferred for its high efficiency and oil recovery compared to cold press extraction. However, solvent extraction faces several challenges, including quality, food safety, and environmental concerns. The main issue is that solvent emissions and residues pose environmental risks, as they can react with pollutants to form ozone and other compounds (Hanmoungjai et al., 2000). To address these disadvantages, several alternative solutions have been explored to improve this process's efficiency and sustainability, including using alternative green solvents, aqueous-assisted enzyme extraction, and process optimization.

Green solvents like terpenes and ionic liquids are viable alternatives for eco-friendly oil extraction due to their lower energy requirements, nontoxic nature, and environmentally friendly properties (Wan et al., 1995). These natural solvents have good solubilizing abilities. Ionic liquids are another option, as they are nonflammable and have a wide temperature range, making them versatile. They are suitable solvents with specific conductivity, polarity, hydrophobicity, and solubility properties, which can facilitate efficient compound recovery depending on the nature of the solute (Cooney et al., 2009).

Adjusting process parameters like pressure, temperature, and solvent can improve oil yield and quality. Pressurized liquid extraction uses solvents at temperatures above their boiling points under increased pressure. This higher pressure

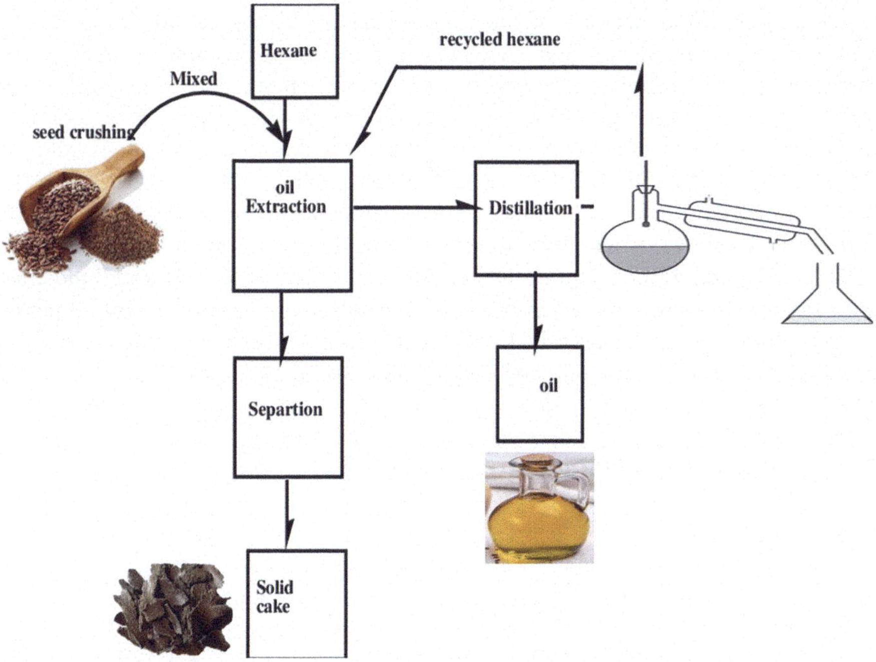

Fig. 2 Diagrammatic representation of linseed oil using solvent extraction

reduces the solvent's surface tension, enhancing its ability to penetrate the matrix pores. This leads to better disruption and mass transfer, ultimately increasing the extraction efficiency (Jesus et al., 2013).

A different alternative for solvent extraction is enzyme-assisted extraction (EAA), an eco-friendly method that offers higher yield and does not damage the by-products. Enzymes hydrolyze the structural cell wall by breaking the polysaccharides and proteins, thus easily releasing oils from the cell (Long et al., 2011). In this process, water serves as a medium to extract oil from oilseeds. Lipid molecules have an amphipathic character, and the water-soluble constituents eventually diffuse into the water to create emulsions. Enzymes can de-emulsify the oil emulsified in water, efficiently separating the desired extracted ingredient (Gros et al., 2003; Li et al., 2013). Although the enzyme-assisted extraction (EAE) process is safer, healthier, and more environmentally friendly, it has some drawbacks, such as high costs for downstream processing and enzyme production and a lengthy incubation period.

3 Novel Extraction Methods (Nonconventional)

Several novel or green extraction methods have been proposed for extracting oil from linseed, including supercritical/subcritical fluid extraction, microwave-assisted extraction, and ultrasonic-assisted extraction. The composition and quantity of unsaturated fatty acids and other bioactive compounds extracted through different methods quite differ because of the complex nature of linseed oil. Linseed oil is traditionally obtained through mechanical pressing. Mechanical methods for extracting linseed oil offer advantages such as cost-effectiveness, minimal equipment requirements, acceptable quality, unchanged oil taste, and no use of chemicals in the extraction process (Bhargavi et al., 2018). Although mechanical pressing has these advantages, few studies documented its disadvantages. Kasote (2013) reported that the quality of linseed oil and its ALA content was maintained using cold press extraction. However, it has drawbacks including low yield, high residual oil, and notable decreases in concentrations of vitamins, phytosterols, phospholipids, and antioxidants. Recently, there has been significant interest in modern oil extraction techniques such as supercritical CO_2 extraction, subcritical fluid extraction, microwave-assisted extraction, and ultrasound-assisted extraction.

3.1 Supercritical Fluid Extraction (SFE)

Supercritical fluid extraction (SFE) utilizes supercritical fluids to isolate components from the matrix. It is also known as supercritical carbon extraction. Various solvents, including compressed gases like ethane, ethylene, propane, dinitrogen oxide, and carbon dioxide, are utilized in this method (Yoswathana, 2013). CO_2 is commonly preferred due to its low critical temperature (31.1 °C), lack of toxicity and flammability, good solvent properties, high diffusivity, low viscosity, easy removal without leaving residues, and cost-effectiveness (Ara & Raofie, 2016). The key benefits of SFE are rapid extraction time, excellent selectivity, high diffusivity, low viscosity, lower extraction temperatures, and high solvent power (Hasanov et al., 2023). The supercritical fluid extraction (SFE) process has three phases. Initially, the supercritical solvent permeates the linseed material, reducing mass transfer resistance. Then, soluble compounds dissolve into the supercritical fluid (SCF), diffusing first onto the solid surface and then into the fluid phase. Finally, the solute and bulk fluid phases are transported and removed from the extractor, completing the oil extraction process (Ibanez et al., 2016).

The modern approach for extracting linseed oil includes supercritical CO_2 fluid extraction, known for its environmental friendliness. In a comparative study of extraction methods such as supercritical fluid extraction (SFE), accelerated solvent extraction (ASE), and solvent extraction (SE) in terms of oil yield, SFE was found to yield less oil than ASE and SE. However, SFE yields high-quality oil and retains high concentrations of omega-3 fatty acids, lignans, and phenolic compounds. Therefore, it could be used in various food products (Khattab & Zeitoun, 2013). Moreover, its production efficiency surpasses mechanical methods (Soxhlet and screw press) by approximately 25% (Pradhan et al., 2010a). Similarly, Chauhan found that supercritical fluid extraction (SFE) had a lower oil yield (32.16%) compared to solvent (35.73%), Soxhlet (36.26%), and ultrasonic (US) (33.05%) extraction methods. However, the oil obtained through SFE was rich in n-3 fatty acids and exhibited significant antioxidant activity compared to the other methods (Chauhan et al., 2015). Various factors affect SFE, including cosolvents, raw materials, solvent-to-feed ratio, and solubility. Rombaut's study optimized key SFE parameters—CO_2 pressure, flow rate, and temperature—to improve oil yield and product quality. They found that at optimal conditions of 42.5 MPa pressure, 120 °C temperature, 12.5 kg/h CO_2 flow rate, and a solvent-to-feed ratio of 125 g/g, around 60% oil yield was achieved (Rombaut et al., 2017).

3.2 Microwave-Assisted Extraction (MAE)

Microwave-assisted extraction (MAE) represents a modern and compelling alternative to traditional pressing extraction methods for oil extraction (Hasene et al., 2017). Microwave-induced rapid cell heating efficiently extracts oil in a short time with minimal solvent use and maintains high quality. Another significant benefit is that low energy needs result in lower environmental consequences and financial expenses (Fathi-Achachlouei et al., 2019; Yu et al., 2016). The MAE mechanism involves ionic conduction and dipole rotation within the material due to microwave energy. This leads to electrophoretic migration and realignment of ions under an electromagnetic field, increasing the temperature of the extraction medium, and facilitating the extraction of compounds (Nde & Foncha, 2020). Figure 3 represents the mechanism of extraction. MAE, parameters such as power, extraction time, and temperature play pivotal roles in the extraction process. Most studies reported on the impact of process parameters on oil yield and quality. For instance, Suri et al.

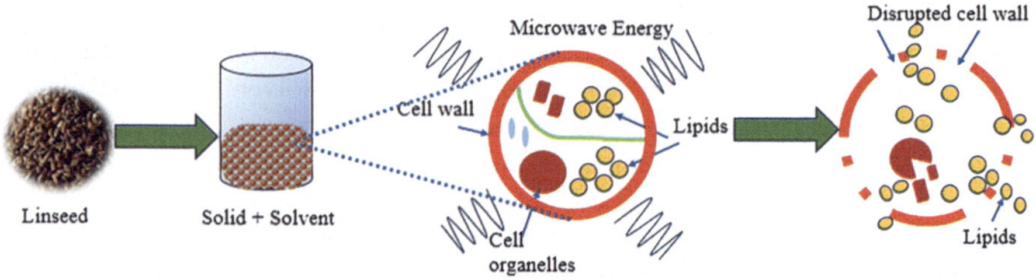

Fig. 3 Mechanism of microwave-assisted extraction

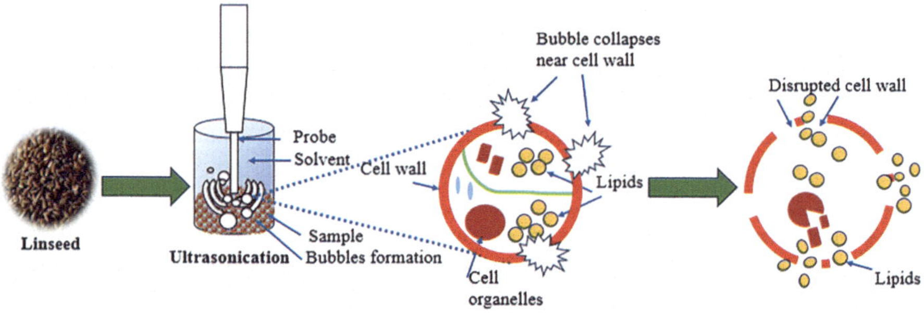

Fig. 4 Mechanism of ultrasound-assisted extraction

(2020) discovered that subjecting linseeds to microwave roasting at 540 W for 10 min increased linseed oil yield and enhanced the oils' oxidative stability and antioxidant activity. Likewise, Szydlowska-Czerniak et al. (2020) optimized microwave process parameters for linseed oil extraction, revealing that MAE-treated oil exhibited superior oxidative stability and antioxidant activity compared to untreated oil. Also, Lv et al. (2020) further explored optimal microwave process conditions, noting that employing a microwave power of 65 W and an extraction duration of 3 min resulted in a 46.60% oil yield, an increase of 14.9% in polyphenol content, and a subsequent delay in oil oxidation, ultimately enhancing its oxidative stability.

3.3 Ultrasound-Assisted Extraction (UAE)

Ultrasound is a sound wave with a frequency range of 20–100 MHz. UAE is primarily driven by cavitation, leading to bubble formation, growth, and collapse. This collapse causes physicochemical and mechanical effects that disrupt the material matrix, facilitating extractable compounds release and aiding solvent movement into the sample, thereby enhancing the release of target compounds from the matrix into the solvent (Nde & Foncha, 2020). Figure 4 Depicts mechanism of ultrasound assisted extraction. UAE offers several advantages, including cost-effectiveness, enhanced mass transfer, improved solvent diffusion, reduced solvent dependency leading to lower consumption, extraction at lower temperatures, quicker and shorter extraction times, higher purity of extracts, increased and more consistent extraction efficiency, reduced fossil energy usage, expanded solvent options for selective extraction, use of compact equipment, safety and health benefits, and environmental friendliness (Marhamati et al., 2020).

Furthermore, ultrasonic power has also been employed for linseed oil extraction. Similar to other extraction methods in UAE extraction oils, factors like solvent type, ultrasound power (amplitude), extraction time, extraction temperature, and solid-to-solvent ratio are crucial parameters (Xu et al., 2017). Zhang et al. (2007) investigated the impact of operating parameters on linseed oil recovery. They found that increasing ultrasonic power led to higher oil yield, while extraction temperature elevation resulted in decreased yield. The maximum recovery rate achieved was 84.9%. Gutte et al. (2015) investigated the effect of ultrasound parameters on linseed oil yield and quality, and results showed significantly highest recovery with α-Linolenic acid (ω-3) acid obtained at optimal conditions of ultrasonic frequency of 40 kHz, temperature of 30 °C, extraction time of 40 min, and solid to solvent ratio: 1:10. Long et al. (2011) also investigated ultrasound-assisted extraction using immobilized enzymes, achieving a 68.1% oil recovery with increased unsaturated fatty acid content.

4 Factors Affecting Oil Yield and Quality

There are various physical parameters of raw material as well as process parameters that affect the linseed oil yield and quality. Physical parameters such as seed variety (genotypes), cultivating conditions, growing locations, harvesting time, picking operations, seed storage conditions, seed drying temperature, and storage all play a significant role (Kasote et al., 2013). Another important factor is the sample preparation of the oilseeds, which includes dehulling, flaking, size reduction, and thickness reduction. It has proven to facilitate oil extraction as it provides greater interfacial area (Zhang et al., 2007). In case of cold press extraction, other process parameters affecting extraction are the moisture content, temperature, feed rate, diameter of restriction dye, and rotation speed.

Temperature plays a significant role in oil quality and yields with an increase in temperature up to 350 °C, oil yield increased as reported by Moknatjou et al. (2015). However, increasing temperature for a longer duration might affect oil quality characteristics, as there is a change in the fatty acid values of linseed oil due to roasting temperature. In addition to the previously mentioned process parameters solvent type (polar or nonpolar, green solvents), solvent quantity, the use of a single solvent (polar or nonpolar) or a mixture of polar and nonpolar solvents, and the particle size of raw material are also important factors for enhancing oil yield and quality. Piva et al. (2018) showed that the linseed oil yield obtained using subcritical propane was 28.39%, higher than pressurized ethanol (8.05%) under comparable conditions.

Meanwhile, in soxhlet extraction (using hexane), it was 36.12%. To facilitate the release of oil from cells in oil-bearing material, it is essential to increase the surface area of contact between the material and the solvent. This enhancement allows for

Table 1 Effect of different extraction parameters on oil yield and quality of linseed oil

	Extraction method	Extraction conditions	Oil yield (%)	Antioxidants	Quality assessment		References
Conventional					DPPH	Fatty acid composition	
	Cold press				1.25 to 1.42 mM of Trolox kg^{-1} oil,	45–65% of α linolenic acid	(Symoniuk et al. (2017)
			22.34–23.84%	Vit. E = 400 mg/kg		51.01 g/100 g	(Wang et al. 2022)
	Hot press	Temperature: 160–180 °C	24.36–30.00%	Vit. E = 330.30–424.90 mg/kg.		50.77 g/100 g	(Wang et al. 2022)
		Temperature: −50 to +150 °C)	Whole: 39.91% Dehulled: 52.14%			α-linolenic acid content: 53.34% to 54.21%	(Mridula et al. 2015)
	Soxhlet extraction	Solvent: petroleum ether, Time: 8 h Temperature: 70 °C.	31.88–34.50%	Vit. E- ~380.00 mg/kg.		48.14 g/100 g	(Wang et al. 2022)
		Solvent: petroleum ether, Time: 13 h Temperature: 60 to 80 °C	41.53%		19.37%		(Kulkarni et al. 2017)
		Solvent/solid ratio- 20:1 Temperature: 60 °C Time: 8 h	100%	□- and α tocopherols- 56.37 mg/100 g			(Omar et al. 2014)

Nonconventional	Supercritical fluid extraction (SFE)	CO_2, pressure-10–65 MPa, Temperature- 40–120 °C, Flow Rate-5 to 20 kg/h	~60%	γ-tocopherol or Polyphenols- 100 mg FAE/kg oil)			(Rombaut et al. 2017)
		CO_2, DET 36–60 min, Temperature- ambient −120 °C, Pressure 45.57–62.05 MPa (6000–9000 psi). Extraction flow rate, 0–3 L/min	40%			α-linolenic acid (C18:3n-3) is approximately 4% higher than Soxhlet extracts	(Ivanov et al. 2012)
		CO_2, pressure—200 to 400 bar, Time- 60 to 180 min Temperature −40 to 60 °C	30.03%		19.94%		(Kulkarni et al. 2017)
	Microwave extraction	Treatment time-1 to 3 min, MP-450 to 800 W,	–	–	209.9–315.1 μmol TE/100 g)		(Szydłowska-Czerniak et al. 2020)
		MW radiation intensities-12, 18, and 24 W/g, pretreatment time-90, 150, and 210	78.11%	–	–	No significant effect on FAs by MW treatment	(Ren et al. 2015)
	Microwave-assisted screw press oil expeller (below 60 °C.)	MP-180,360, and 540 W Roasting time-5 and 10 min	34.9%	–	–	C18:3n3c (α-Linolenic)- 53.61 to 54.30	(Suri et al. 2020)

(continued)

Table 1 (continued)

	Extraction method	Extraction conditions	Oil yield (%)	Antioxidants	Quality assessment		References
	Ultrasound extraction	Temperature-25–40 °C, Amplitude-20–80 kHz, Solid to solvent ratio-1:5, 1:10, and 1:15 Sonication time-20–80 min S	~35%	–	–	No significant effects on α-Linolenic acid (ω-3)	(Gutte et al. 2015)
		Solvent/solid ratio-10:1, 10:1, 15:1 Extraction time: 30, 30, 20 min, Extraction temperature: 30, 20, 30 °C, and	80.05%	□- and α-tocopherols- 40.39 mg/100 g	–	No significant differences in fatty acids	(Omar et al. 2014)
	Ultrasound pretreated three-phase partitioning	Power- 30, 50, and 70 W, duty cycle (30, 50, and 70%) and time (5, 10, and 15 min)	27.05%	–	16.20%	–	(Kulkarni et al. 2017)

faster and easier infiltration of the transfer medium. Reducing the size of the material leads to greater disruption of the cell wall and shortens the diffusion path for cellular components (Passos & Ribeiro, 2016). Agitation also plays a vital role in improving oil yield by disrupting the mechanical barriers and causing uniform constituents to mix, enabling mass transfer and decreasing process time. Moisture content is another factor affecting the oil yield, lower moisture content offers enhanced oil yield, the oil yield increases from 76% to 82.5% with a decrease in moisture from 6% to 3.5%. Additional processes like drying, peeling, and applying pressure can improve the oil yield and bioactive components of linseed oil (Bargale & Patil, 2007). Table 1 depicts the effect of different extraction parameters on oil yield and quality of linseed oil (Table 1).

5 Challenges and Future Directions

Linseed oil is a PUFA-rich oil that is highly sensitive to light, air, and heat. Extraction is a crucial step that significantly impacts the oil's yield and quality, affecting its nutritional value and economic parameters. Conventional cold pressing methods produce higher quality oil but lower yields. Solvent extraction can increase yields but compromises quality and poses environmental risks. Emerging nonconventional techniques aim to maintain quality and enhance yields but are not yet cost-effective or scalable. Therefore, there is an urgent need to develop extraction methods that are safe, environmentally friendly, scalable, and cost-effective to meet the demand for linseed oil while reducing the burden on the environment.

References

Ara, K. M., & Raofie, F. (2016). Application of response surface methodology for the optimization of supercritical fluid extraction of essential oil from pomegranate (Punica granatum L.) peel. *Journal of Food Science and Technology, 53*, 3113–3121.

Bargale, P. C., & Patil, R. T. (2007). *Effect of pretreatments on oil recovery and oil-point pressure of soybean under uniaxial pressing*.

Bhargavi, G., Nageswara Rao, P., & Renganathan, S. (2018). Review on the extraction methods of crude oil from all generation biofuels in last few decades. *IOP Conference Series: Materials Science and Engineering, 330*(March), 012024. https://doi.org/10.1088/1757-899X/330/1/012024

Cakaloglu, B., Ozyurt, V. H., & Otles, S. (2018). Cold press in oil extraction. A review. Ukrainian food journal, (7, Issue 4), 640–654.

Chand, M., Chopra, R., Talwar, B., Homroy, S., Singh, P. K., Dhiman, A., & Payyunni, A. W. (2024). Unveiling the potential of linseed mucilage, its health benefits, and applications in food packaging. *Frontiers in Nutrition, 11*, 1334247.

Chauhan, R., Chester, K., Khan, Y., Tamboli, E. T., & Ahmad, S. (2015). Characterization of Linum usitatissimum L. oil obtained from different extraction technique and in vitro antioxidant potential of supercritical fluid extract. *Journal of Pharmacy and Bioallied Sciences, 7*(4), 284–288.

Cooney, M., Young, G., & Nagle, N. (2009). Extraction of bio-oils from microalgae. *Separation & Purification Reviews, 38*(4), 291–325. https://doi.org/10.1080/15422110903327919

Fathi-Achachlouei, B., Azadmard-Damirchi, S., Zahedi, Y., & Shaddel, R. (2019). Microwave pretreatment as a promising strategy for increment of nutraceutical content and extraction yield of oil from milk thistle seed. *Industrial Crops and Products, 128*, 527–533.

Gros, C., Lanoisellé, J.-L., & Vorobiev, E. (2003). Towards an alternative extraction process for linseed oil. *Chemical Engineering Research and Design, 81*(9), 1059–1065. https://doi.org/10.1205/026387603770866182

Gutte, K. B., Sahoo, A. K., & Ranveer, R. C. (2015). Effect of ultrasonic treatment on extraction and fatty acid profile of linseed oil. *OCL, 22*(6), D606.

Hanmoungjai, P., Pyle, L., & Niranjan, K. (2000). Extraction of rice bran oil using aqueous media. *Journal of Chemical Technology & Biotechnology, 75*(5), 348–352. https://doi.org/10.1002/(SICI)1097-4660(200005)75:5<348::AID-JCTB233>3.0.CO;2-P

Hasanov, J., Salikhov, S., & Oshchepkova, Y. (2023). Techno-economic evaluation of supercritical fluid extraction of linseed oil. *The Journal of Supercritical Fluids, 194*, 105839.

Hasene, K. Ç., Derya, K. Y., Ugur, G., & Fahrett, G. (2017). Optimization of microwave-assisted extraction of pomegranate (Punicagranatum L.) seed oil and evaluation of its physicochemical and bioactive properties. *Food Technology and Biotechnology, 55*, 86–94.

Ibanez, E., Mendiola, J. A., & Castro-Puyana, M. (2016). *Supercritical fluid extraction*. Institute of Food Science Research (CIAL-CSIC).

Ivanov, D. S., Čolović, R. R., Lević, J. D., & Sredanović, S. A. (2012). Optimization of supercritical fluid extraction of linseed oil using RSM. *European Journal of Lipid Science and Technology, 114*(7), 807–815.

Jesus, A. A., Almeida, L. C., Silva, E. A., Filho, L. C., Egues, S. M. S., Franceschi, E., Fortuny, M., et al. (2013). Extraction of palm oil using propane, ethanol and its mixtures as compressed solvent. *The Journal of Supercritical Fluids, 81*(September), 245–253. https://doi.org/10.1016/j.supflu.2013.06.011

Kasote, D. M., Badhe, Y. S., & Hegde, M. V. (2013). Effect of mechanical press oil extraction processing on quality of linseed oil. *Industrial Crops and Products, 42*, 10–13. https://doi.org/10.1016/j.indcrop.2012.05.015

Khattab, R. Y., & Zeitoun, M. A. (2013). Quality evaluation of linseed oil obtained by different extraction techniques. *LWT-Food Science and Technology, 53*(1), 338–345.

Khater, S. I., Shalabi, M., Alammash, B. B., Alrais, A. I., Al-Ahmadi, D. S., Alqahtani, L. S., & El-Dawy, K. (2023). Evaluation of flaxseed lignan-enriched extract targeting autophagy, apoptosis, and hedgehog pathways against experimentally induced obesity. *Journal of Advanced Veterinary and Animal Research, 10*(2), 321.

Kiritsakis A.K. (2002). Virgin olive oil composition and its effect on human health, Inform., 13, pp. 237–241.

Kirschenbauer, H. G. (1944). *Fats and oils* (pp. 122–123). Reinhold Publishing.

Kulkarni, N. G., Kar, J. R., & Singhal, R. S. (2017). Extraction of linseed oil: A comparative study of three-phase partitioning and supercritical carbon dioxide using response surface methodology. *Food and Bioprocess Technology, 10*, 940–948.

Kumar, S. P., Jeevan, S. R., Prasad, R. B., Agarwal, D. K., Kulkarni, K. S., & Ramesh, K. V. (2017). Green solvents and technologies for oil extraction from oilseeds. *Chemistry Central Journal, 11*(1), 9. https://doi.org/10.1186/s13065-017-0238-8

Lanoiselle, J. L., & Bouvier, J. M. (1994). *Le pressage hydraulique des oleagineux* (p. 41). Revue française des corps gras.

Li, Y., Fine, F., Fabiano-Tixier, A.-S., Abert-Vian, M., Carre, P., Pages, X., & Chemat, F. (2013). Evaluation of alternative solvents for improvement of oil extraction from rapeseeds. *Comptes Rendus. Chimie, 17*(3), 242–251. https://doi.org/10.1016/j.crci.2013.09.002

Liu, S. X., & Mamidipally, P. K. (2005). Quality comparison of rice bran oil extracted with d-limonene and hexane. *Cereal Chemistry, 82*(2), 209–215. https://doi.org/10.1094/CC-82-0209

Long, J.-j., Yu-jie, F., Yuan-gang, Z., Li, J., Wang, W., Cheng-bo, G., & Luo, M. (2011). Ultrasound-assisted extraction of linseed oil using immobilized enzymes. *Bioresource Technology, 102*(21), 9991–9996. https://doi.org/10.1016/j.biortech.2011.07.104

Marhamati, M., Kakhaki, Z. K., & Rezaie, M. (2020). Advance in ultrasound-assisted extraction of edible oils: A review. *Journal of Nutrition, Fasting & Health, 8*(4).

Moknatjou, R., Hajimahmoodi, M., Toliyat, T., Moghaddam, G., Sadeghpour, O., Monsef-Esfahani, H., & Shams-Ardekani, M. (2015). Effect of roasting on fatty acid profile of brown and yellow varieties of linseed (Linum Usitatissimum L). *Tropical Journal of Pharmaceutical Research, 14*(1), 117. https://doi.org/10.4314/tjpr.v14i1.17

Mridula, D., Barnwal, P., & Singh, K. K. (2015). Screw pressing performance of whole and dehulled linseed and some physico-chemical characteristics of linseed oil. *Journal of Food Science and Technology, 52*, 1498–1506.

Nawade, B., Mishra, G. P., Radhakrishnan, T., Dodia, S. M., Ahmad, S., Kumar, A., Kundu, R. (2018). High oleic peanut breeding: Achievements, perspectives, and prospects. *Trends in Food Science & Technology, 78*, 107–119.

Nde, D. B., & Foncha, A. C. (2020). Optimization methods for the extraction of vegetable oils: A review. *Processes, 8*(2), 209.

Omar, K. A., Liu, R., & Wang, X. (2014). Effects of ultrasound-assisted extraction on yield of linseed oil, β-and γ-tocopherols optimized by orthogonal array design. *European Journal of Lipid Science and Technology, 116*(10), 1412–1420.

Passos, M. L., & Ribeiro, C. P. (2016). Innovation in food engineering: new techniques and products. CRC Press.

Piva, G. S., Weschenfelder, T. A., Franceschi, E., Cansian, R. L., Paroul, N., & Steffens, C. (2018). Linseed (Linum usitatissimum) oil extraction using different solvents. *Food Technology and Biotechnology, 56*(3), 366–372.

Pointner, T., Rauh, K., Auñon-Lopez, A., Veličkovska, S. K., Mitrev, S., Arsov, E., & Pignitter, M. (2024). Comprehensive analysis of oxidative stability and nutritional values of germinated linseed and sunflower seed oil. *Food Chemistry, 454*(October), 139790. https://doi.org/10.1016/j.foodchem.2024.139790

Pradhan, R. C., et al. (2010a). Supercritical CO2 extraction of fatty oil from linseed and comparison with screw press expression and solvent extraction processes. *Journal of Food Engineering., 98*(4), 393–397.

Pradhan, R. C., Meda, V., Naik, S. N., & Tabil, L. (2010b). Physical properties of Canadian grown linseed in relation to its processing. *International Journal of Food Properties, 13*(4), 732–743. https://doi.org/10.1080/10942910902818137

Prado, J. M., Vardanega, R., Debien, I. C., Meireles, M. A. A., Gerschenson, L. N., Sowbhagya, H. B., & Chemat, S. (2021). Conventional extraction. In *Food waste recovery* (pp. 109–127). Academic Press.

Ren, G., Zhang, W., Sun, S., Duan, X., & Zhang, Z. (2015). Enhanced extraction of oil from linseed (Linum usitatissimum L.) using microwave pre-treatment. *Journal of Oleo Science, 64*(10), 1043–1047.

Rombaut, N., Savoire, R., Van Hecke, E., & Thomasset, B. (2017). Supercritical CO2 extraction of linseed: Optimization by experimental design with regards to oil yield and composition. *European Journal of Lipid Science and Technology, 119*(9), 1600078.

Sarpong, P. (2024, May 1). Emerging trends in vegetable oil market: Healthier oils, safety challenges, and sustainability. *Safety Challenges, and Sustainability.*

Serrato, A. G. (1981). Extraction of oil from soybeans. *Journal of the American Oil Chemists' Society, 58*(3Part1), 157–159. https://doi.org/10.1007/BF02582327

Singh, K. K., Jhamb, S. A., & Kumar, R. (2012). Effect of pretreatments on performance of screw pressing for flaxseed. *Journal of Food Process Engineering, 35*(4), 543–556.

Suri, K., Singh, B., Kaur, A., Yadav, M. P., & Singh, N. (2020). Influence of microwave roasting on chemical composition, oxidative stability and fatty acid composition of linseed (Linum usitatissimum L.) oil. *Food Chemistry, 326*, 126974.

Symoniuk, E., Ratusz, K., & Krygier, K. (2017). Oxidative stability 441 and the chemical composition of market cold-pressed linseed oil. *European Journal of Lipid Science and Technology, 119*, 1700055.

Szydłowska-Czerniak, A., Tymczewska, A., Momot, M., & Włodarczyk, K. (2020). Optimization of the microwave treatment of linseed for cold-pressing linseed oil – changes in its chemical and sensory qualities. *LWT, 126*(May), 109317. https://doi.org/10.1016/j.lwt.2020.109317

Uitterhaegen, E., & Evon, P. (2017). Twin-screw extrusion technology for vegetable oil extraction: A review. *Journal of Food Engineering, 212*(November), 190–200. https://doi.org/10.1016/j.jfoodeng.2017.06.006

Wan, P. J., Hron, R. J., Dowd, M. K., Kuk, M. S., & Conkerton, E. J. (1995). Alternative hydrocarbon solvents for cottonseed extraction: Plant trials. *Journal of the American Oil Chemists' Society, 72*(6), 661–664. https://doi.org/10.1007/BF02635651

Wang, S., Wang, J., Dong, G., Chen, X., Wang, S., Lei, F., et al. (2022). Effect of different extraction methods on quality characteristics of rapeseed and linseed oils. *Journal of Food Quality, 2022*, 8296212.

Xu, D. P., Zheng, J., Zhou, Y., Li, Y., Li, S., & Bin, L. H. (2017). Ultrasound-assisted extraction of natural antioxidants from the flower of Limonium sinuatum: Optimization and comparison with conventional methods. *Food Chemistry, 217*, 552–559.

Yoswathana, N. (2013). Optimization of ScCO2 extraction of rambutan seed oil using response surface methodology. *International Journal of Chemical Engineering and Applications, 4*(4), 187.

Yu, S., Hongkun, X., Chenghai, L., Chai, L., Xiaolin, S., & Xianzhe, Z. (2016). Comparison of microwave-assisted extraction with hot reflux extraction in acquirement and degradation of anthocyanin from powdered blueberry. *International Journal of Agricultural and Biological Engineering, 9*(6), 186–199.

Zhang, S. B., Wang, Z., & Shi Ying, X. (2007). Optimization of the aqueous enzymatic extraction of rapeseed oil and protein hydrolysates. *Journal of the American Oil Chemists' Society, 84*(1), 97–105. https://doi.org/10.1007/s11746-006-1004-6

Zuorro, A., Lavecchia, R., Medici, F., & Piga, L. (2014). Use of cell wall degrading enzymes for the production of high-quality functional products from tomato processing waste. *Chemical Engineering Transactions, 38*, 355–360. https://doi.org/10.3303/CET1438060

Refining Linseed Oil: Recent Trends, Advancements, and Sustainability Indicators

Sayani Mavai, Lalit Goswami, Gaurav Singh, Neelam Lohiya, Praveen Kumar Singh Yadav, and Seungdae Oh

Abstract

Refining linseed oil is a critical process that ensures its quality, stability, and suitability for industrial applications, particularly in the food sector. Linseed oil, known for its high α-linolenic acid content (34.1–63%), is widely used in food industries. However, its high polyunsaturated fatty acid content makes it prone to rancidity, necessitating effective refining methods to retain its quality. The refining processes, including degumming, neutralization, bleaching, winterization, and deodorization, are addressed in this chapter, highlighting their role in maintaining oil stability and extending its shelf life. The potential of green technologies such as electrical field treatments, ultrasound, microwave, and ion exchange has been discussed as promising alternatives to conventional refining methods. These green technologies offer enhanced refining efficiency, reduced energy consumption, and improved sustainability in linseed oil production. The challenges faced during linseed oil processing and novel pretreatment technologies aimed at improving oil quality and sustainability are also discussed in this chapter.

S. Mavai
Department of Food Science and Technology, National Institute of Food Technology Entrepreneurship and Management, Kundli, Haryana, India

L. Goswami · S. Oh
Department of Civil Engineering, College of Engineering, Kyung Hee University, Yongin, Republic of Korea

G. Singh · P. K. S. Yadav
Department of Oil Technology, Harcourt Butler Technical University, Kanpur, Uttar Pradesh, India

N. Lohiya (✉)
Global Active Clay LLP, Ahmedabad, Gujarat, India

© The Author(s), under exclusive license to Springer Nature Singapore Pte Ltd. 2025
R. Chopra et al. (eds.), *Dynamics of Linseed and its Valorization*,
https://doi.org/10.1007/978-981-96-8927-9_5

Keywords

Linseed oil · α-linolenic acid · Conventional refining methods · Novel refining methods · Green technology

1 Introduction

Linseed, also known as flax (*Linum usitatissimum*), is one of the world's oldest cultivated crops grown in 47 countries for its versatile seed oil and valuable fiber. While regions like Southwest Asia and Canada primarily cultivate linseed for their oil, countries such as Russia, Egypt, and Northwestern Europe emphasize its superior fiber for linen production (Payasi et al., 2024; Suri & Singh, 2024). Globally, linseed spans 32.23 lakh hectares, yielding 30.68 lakh tonnes at an average productivity of 952 kg/ha. India, ranking fifth in area and sixth in production, faces challenges like marginal soils, low seed replacement rates, and limited market support, resulting in lower yields compared to leading nations like Canada and China (Kaur et al., 2024). Flaxseed, available in brown and yellow varieties, is a multi-component system rich in bioactive compounds, including oil, dietary fiber, lignans, vitamins (B and E), and minerals like phosphorus, magnesium, and zinc (Chand et al., 2024; Yu et al., 2024). Linseed oil, extracted from seeds, comprises 73% polyunsaturated fatty acids (linolenic and linoleic acids), 18% monounsaturated fatty acids (oleic acid), and 9% saturated fatty acids (stearic acid). It also contains minor components like arachidic and palmitoleic acids (Fernandes et al., 2024).

Crude linseed oil contains various natural impurities, including phosphatides, gums, and waxes, which must be removed to ensure the oil meets quality standards (Kong et al., 2024). During storage, up to 1% of impurities in crude oil naturally separate and settle at the bottom of the tank. When the settled crude oil is rapidly heated to approximately 110 °C, the heat causes the crude oil to destabilize, enhancing the separation process and promoting the deposition of up to 0.5% of polysaccharide-based impurities (Abdulhussein et al., 2023). Additionally, chilling the oil may cause some waxes to crystallize and separate, necessitating further refinement to achieve the desired clarity and stability (H. Wang et al., 2023). The bleaching process is crucial for enhancing the color and quality of the oil. Typically, up to 3% of highly acid-activated bleaching clay removes pigments such as chlorophylls and carotenoids, which influence appearance and oxidative stability (Chen & Sun, 2023; Ferfuia et al., 2023). Deodorization, another key refining step, eliminates volatile compounds responsible for unpleasant odors and flavors, ensuring a neutral sensory profile (Kong et al., 2024). To improve stability, trace metals like iron and copper, which act as oxidation catalysts, are removed using adsorbents. Moisture content is also reduced during refining to prevent hydrolytic rancidity (Langyan et al., 2023). Oxidation products, such as peroxides, are eliminated to extend the shelf life, while soap residues from neutralization are thoroughly washed out to ensure purity. Harmful contaminants, including polycyclic aromatic hydrocarbons (PAHs) and residual solvents, are effectively removed during deodorization, further enhancing the quality of oil. These refining steps work collectively to produce linseed oil that meets industry standards, ensuring its suitability for various applications while maintaining its stability, clarity, and sensory attributes (Chand et al. 2024; Orlova et al., 2021). This chapter provides a detailed overview of the traditional and advanced refining techniques employed in linseed oil processing, with a focus on enhancing oil quality and stability. It highlights innovations in refining technologies that improve efficiency while addressing challenges related to impurities, oxidation, and sensory attributes. Additionally, the chapter explores sustainability considerations in refining processes, emphasizing the importance of minimizing environmental impact and aligning production practices with global sustainability goals.

2 Conventional Refining Process

2.1 Degumming

Degumming is a crucial step in the refining of linseed oil, aims at removing phospholipids, trace metals, and mucilaginous substances, which can adversely affect the quality, clarity, and stability of oil (Fig. 1) (Khamies et al., 2024; Selge et al., 2024). Removing these impurities is essential to prevent undesirable chemical reactions, such as oxidation and hydrolysis, that could compromise the oil's shelf life and sensory attributes. Several techniques are employed to achieve degumming, including chemical, enzymatic, and membrane-based methods, each offering unique benefits and challenges (Une et al., 2024).

The traditional hydration degumming method is widely utilized for linseed oil (Liu et al., 2024a). This method relies on the addition of water to hydrate phospholipids, causing them to swell and form a colloidal phase (Khamies et al., 2024). The

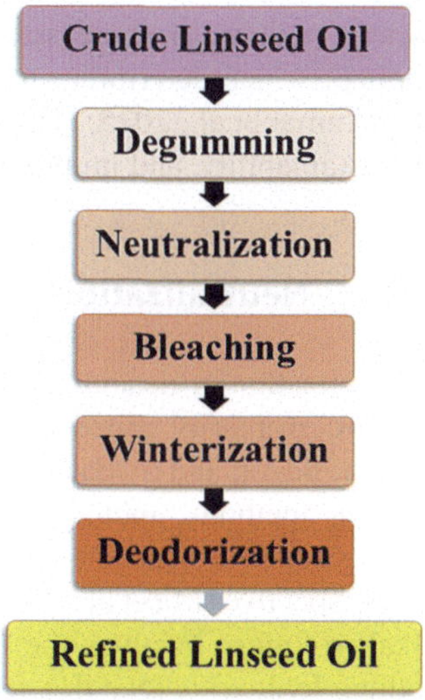

Fig. 1 Flowchart depicting the conventional refining process of linseed oil

intermolecular forces between the hydrophilic head groups of the phospholipids and water molecules facilitate this process. However, this technique is limited in its ability to eliminate nonhydrated phospholipids (Pan et al., 2024). To overcome this, acids such as phosphoric or citric acid are introduced, thus altering the non-hydrated phospholipids by protonating the polar groups, thereby converting them into hydrated forms. These hydrated phospholipids can then be separated through centrifugation. However, one of the drawbacks of acid degumming is the potential loss of oil due to the emulsification of triglycerides during the process, which affects the overall yield during large-scale processing (Khamies et al., 2024; Wu et al., 2024).

Alternatively, enzymatic degumming involves the use of phospholipase enzymes, which catalyze the hydrolysis of the ester bonds in the fatty acid chains of phospholipids (Pan et al., 2024). This enzymatic conversion produces hydrophilic lysophospholipids more easily separated from the oil. The biocatalytic specificity of enzymes ensures minimal disruption to the triglyceride matrix, preserving the quality of the oil. Enzymatic degumming operates under mild temperatures (35–60 °C) and pH (4.5–6.5) conditions compared to chemical methods, offering higher efficiency and being more environmentally friendly (Kong et al., 2024). However, the higher cost of enzymes remains a significant challenge, hindering its widespread adoption in industrial-scale production (Hou et al., 2023; Khamies et al., 2024).

Furthermore, membrane filtration technology has emerged as an innovative approach for degumming linseed oil (Liu et al., 2024b). It employs membranes with pore sizes in the nanofiltration or ultrafiltration range, with pore diameters ranging from 0.001 to 0.1 μ. This process utilizes the selective permeability of membranes to separate phospholipids from triglycerides (Hudaib et al., 2024; Kong et al., 2024). Phospholipids form reverse micelles due to their amphiphilic nature, where the hydrophilic heads orient inward, encapsulating water molecules, and the hydrophobic tails interact with the oil phase (Wang et al., 2024). These reverse micelles, with their larger molecular weight compared to triglycerides, are retained during membrane filtration (Zhang et al., 2024b). The separation efficiency is influenced by factors such as the pore size of the membrane and the transmembrane pressure applied, which determines the rate of filtration and the retention of phospholipids (Jayakumar et al., 2025). This technique is preferred for its simplicity, environmental sustainability, and minimal use of chemicals.

2.2 Neutralization

Neutralization or deacidification plays a critical role in the refining process of linseed oil, primarily aimed at reducing the free fatty acid content, which impacts the quality, flavor, and oxidative stability of the oil (Kong et al., 2024). Several deacidification methods, including chemical, physical, and biological techniques, are employed, each with distinct advantages and limitations from a chemical and practical perspective (Ma et al., 2024). Chemical deacidification, commonly referred to as alkali refining, involves the reaction of free fatty acids with an alkali, typically sodium hydroxide (NaOH), to form soap stocks (sodium salts of fatty acids), which are separated through centrifugation. This neutralization reaction follows the equation:

$$R - COOH + NaOH \rightarrow R - COONa + H_2O$$

Conversely, the deacidification also uses vacuum steam distillation to evaporate free fatty acids and other volatile compounds, such as aldehydes and ketones, at elevated temperatures under reduced pressure (Elaine & Nyam, 2025; Seifollahi et al., 2024). The process relies on the differences in boiling points between triglycerides and free fatty acids. However, high temperatures (>200 °C) pose a risk of thermal degradation of heat-sensitive bioactive compounds like omega-3 fatty acids, containing multiple double bonds, which are subjected to oxidative cleavage (Dai et al., 2024). The reaction mechanism for degradation involves the formation of lipid radicals, which can initiate chain reactions, emphasizing the need for precise temperature and pressure control during this process (Panasenko et al., 2024). Additionally, biological deacidification uses enzymes such as lipases to target the free fatty acids. Lipases catalyze the esterification of free fatty acids with glycerol, converting them into acylglycerols, effectively reincorporating them into the oil structure:

$$\text{Free fatty acids} + \text{Glycerol} \rightarrow \text{Monoglycerides / Diglycerides} + \text{Water}$$

This method preserves the bioactive properties of oil, such as tocopherols and phenolics, which act as natural antioxidants. However, the biochemical pathways in enzymatic processes are influenced by factors like pH, temperature, and substrate specificity, requiring careful consideration for optimal efficiency (Albayati et al., 2024).

Thus, each deacidification method plays a distinct role in removing free fatty acids from linseed oil. Chemical methods are valued for their simplicity and cost-effectiveness, though they may result in minor oil loss. While offering a solvent-free approach, physical methods carry the risk of thermal degradation of sensitive compounds. While biological methods hold promise for sustainability and nutrient preservation they pose challenges related to scalability and cost-effectiveness.

2.3 Bleaching of Linseed Oil

Bleaching is a critical step in refining linseed oil, aimed at removing pigments such as carotenoids and chlorophyll to produce a lighter-colored oil, often appearing light yellow when sufficient bleaching clay is employed (Kong et al., 2024). The process commonly uses acid-activated bentonite clay, chemically treated with acids like sulfuric or hydrochloric acid and thermally activated (Tyagi, 2024). This treatment enhances the clay's adsorption capacity by increasing its surface area and introducing active sites for binding impurities. The clay functions through physical adsorption and ionic interactions, effectively capturing pigments, residual soaps from alkali refining, trace metals, and other contaminants (Zhao et al., 2024).

Carotenoids and chlorophyll, being conjugated systems with multiple double bonds, interact strongly with the active sites on the clay surface via van der Waals forces and π-π interactions (Griep et al., 2024). Trace metals are often adsorbed onto the clay through cation exchange mechanisms, further improving oil stability (Xie et al., 2024). However, linseed oil derived from solin varieties (marketed under the trademark Linola™) demonstrates better stability even after bleaching, making it an exception to this limitation (Dabour et al., 2024; Suri & Singh, 2024). The improved stability of solin oil allows for bleaching without significantly impacting its quality. Nevertheless, the production of solin linseed oil has declined in recent years. In Australia, cultivation ceased after a decrease in demand, and in Canada, solin varieties were deregistered in 2013 following several years of inactivity in production. Consequently, the practice of bleaching linseed oil is now selective, determined largely by the specific characteristics of the oil and its intended use (Langyan et al., 2024).

Despite its effectiveness, bleaching is not commonly used for linseed oil because it removes oil-soluble antioxidants, such as tocopherols, which are crucial in delaying lipid oxidation. The reduction in antioxidant content compromises the oxidative stability of linseed oil, making it more prone to rancidity and reducing its shelf life. Careful optimization of bleaching conditions, including quantity of clay, contact time, and temperature, is essential to minimize these adverse effects while achieving the desired pigment removal.

2.4 Winterization of Linseed Oil

Winterization is a methodology used to address cloudiness in linseed oil, which is often caused by trace amounts of wax that impact the clarity and quality of oil (Dubrovskaya et al., 2023). This involves chilling the oil to encourage the crystallization of waxes composed of long-chain esters. The crystallized waxes can then be removed through filtration, resulting in a clearer oil. Linseed oil usually does not undergo winterization because it typically does not form significant waxy deposits even during storage at lower temperatures (Jing et al., 2024). Instead, the oil is allowed to rest for extended periods, enabling suspended impurities to naturally settle out (Khan et al., 2021). These impurities, which include fine solids and colloidal particles, gradually precipitate due to differences in density and weak intermolecular forces, such as van der Waals attractions. The molecular interactions between the waxes, particulates, and the triglycerides in the oil play a crucial role during these processes (Bray et al., 2020). The cooling process alters the physical properties of the wax molecules, causing them to aggregate and separate from the liquid phase (Cao et al., 2022). While these treatments improve the clarity of the oil, some wax content and minor components may be lost, underscoring the importance of optimizing processing methods to preserve the chemical integrity and functional properties of the oil.

2.5 Deodorization of Linseed Oil

Deodorization is the final stage in the refining process of linseed oil, designed to remove volatile substances that cause undesirable odors and flavors (Kong et al., 2024). This step uses steam distillation under vacuum to effectively remove compounds such as aldehydes, ketones, and free fatty acids, which are by-products of fatty acid oxidation (Gharby, 2022). By targeting these molecules, deodorization enhances the sensory qualities and overall acceptability of the oil. This process involves the reduction of partial pressure of volatile compounds, breaking their intermolecular bonds, and allowing their evaporation in the presence of steam. Despite its effectiveness, deodorization has a drawback, as it can result in the loss of tocopherol, a naturally occurring antioxidant in the oil (Tzompa-Sosa et al., 2021). Tocopherols stabilize the oil by neutralizing free radicals, which prevents oxidation and prolongs shelf life. In most cases, linseed oil is not deodorized to preserve these valuable antioxidants, which contribute to its natural stability and health benefits (Jesus et al., 2023). While deodorization can improve purity and extend shelf life, it can reduce the antioxidant content of linseed oil, highlighting a trade-off between refining and maintaining nutritional value.

3 Challenges and Considerations in Conventional Linseed Oil Refining

Conventional processing of linseed oil involves several steps that present challenges, which can significantly influence both the yield and quality of the final product (Yang et al., 2021). A primary concern in linseed oil processing is the presence of various impurities, including phospholipids, free fatty acids, pigments, and trace metals (Yang et al., 2021). These impurities can negatively impact the color, stability, and nutritional profile of oil. Degumming and deacidification are crucial stages that help remove phospholipids and free fatty acids (Selvamuthukumaran, 2020). However, these methods, particularly when chemical treatments are employed, often lead to some oil loss and do not always preserve the valuable bioactive components of linseed oil. Additionally, the high content of polyunsaturated fatty acids, such as alpha-linolenic acid (ALA), makes linseed oil highly susceptible to oxidation, contributing to its inherent instability. Moreover, bleaching and deodorization are important steps in removing undesirable compounds, including pigments and volatile impurities, to enhance the appearance and sensory qualities of oil (Abdelbasir et al., 2023; Karim et al., 2022). However, these processes also remove antioxidants, such as tocopherols, which are essential for preventing oxidative degradation and extending the shelf life (Fig. 2). As a result, bleaching and deodorization are not commonly used in linseed oil processing, as these treatments can reduce the oxidative stability of oil.

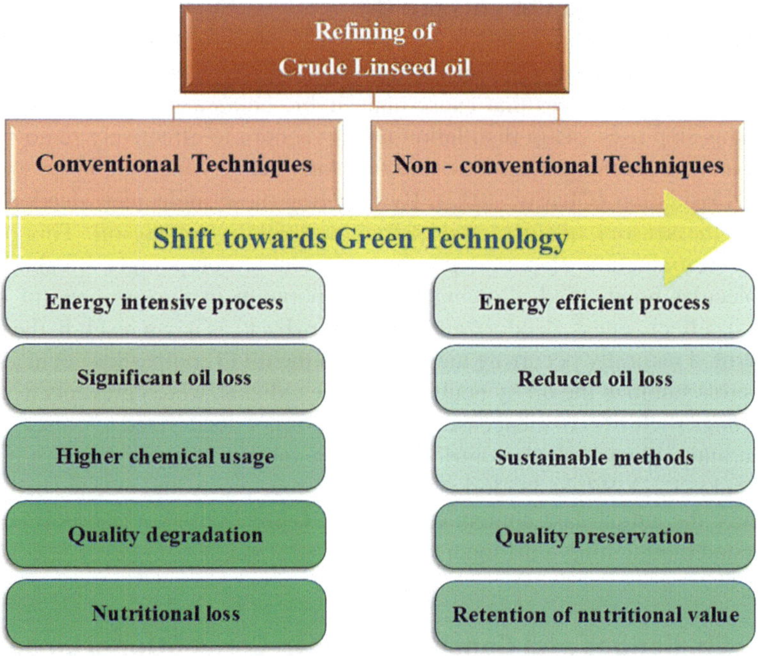

Fig. 2 Comparative analysis of traditional and novel refining techniques

4 Novel Methods and Pretreatment in Refining

4.1 Electrostatic Field Treatment

The use of electrostatic field technology in linseed oil refining provides an innovative, precise, and efficient method for separating polar and nonpolar compounds (Li et al., 2024a). This technique capitalizes on the dielectric differences between these molecules to remove impurities while preserving the nutritional quality of the oil. In this method, polar substances such as phospholipids, free fatty acids (FFAs), and peroxides respond to a high-voltage electrostatic field, typically in the range of 10–30 kV. These impurities are attracted to a charged electrode due to their high permittivity. On the other hand, nonpolar compounds like tocopherols, phytosterols, and polyphenols remain unaffected and are retained (Drozd-Rzoska et al., 2024; Razola-Díaz et al., 2024).

The refining process involves subjecting crude linseed oil to the electrostatic field for a specific period, usually ranging between 30 min and 90 min, depending on the oil composition and impurity load (Fan et al., 2024). A pleated cellulose collector is strategically placed near the electrode to trap the polar compounds as they migrate under the influence of the field. The pleated design enhances the surface area of the collector, improving the efficiency of capturing the ability of impurities. This selective removal ensures the elimination of polar impurities while preserving the nonpolar bioactive compounds. Moreover, the electrostatic field method is operated typically below 50 °C, which minimizes thermal degradation and oxidative damage (Mangang et al., 2024; Shen et al., 2024). This is crucial for maintaining the integrity and maximizing the health benefits of linseed oil.

By refining linseed oil through electrostatic separation, the final product achieves improved purity, stability, and shelf life without the need for chemical treatments or excessive heating. This sustainable approach aligns with modern demands for eco-friendly and high-quality processing technologies, enabling the production of premium-grade linseed oil for food industrial applications.

4.2 Ultrasound-Assisted Refining

Recent advancements in sustainable processing techniques have highlighted ultrasound-assisted refining as an innovative and efficient method for oil refining, particularly for linseed oil (Chew & Ali, 2021). High-intensity ultrasound waves, with frequencies exceeding 20 kHz, induce a phenomenon known as cavitation. This process involves the rapid formation, expansion, and disintegration of microscopic gas bubbles in the liquid medium, which generates localized high temperatures and pressures, creating intense shear forces. These physical effects facilitate the separation of impurities from the oil, while avoiding the need for excessive external heat or chemical exposure (Dengaev et al., 2023; Thilakarathna et al., 2023).

Furthermore, the ultrasound waves accelerate molecular interactions by increasing the surface area and promoting the dispersion of reagents, which leads to faster and more effective reactions (Das et al., 2024). During degumming, the cavitation effect disrupts the molecular bonds between phospholipids and the oil, facilitating their separation and removal (Sankarappa et al., 2005). In the neutralization process, ultrasound increases the effectiveness of alkali treatments by enhancing the dispersion of the alkali in the oil, allowing for the complete removal of free fatty acids (Yan et al., 2019). In the bleaching process, ultrasound helps disperse the bleaching agents more uniformly, resulting in better adsorption and removal of pigments, peroxides, and oxidation products. These processes reduce the need for excess chemicals and energy, making the process more sustainable and efficient (Wen et al., 2023). Moreover, ultrasonic baths during the refining process offer a controlled environment that minimizes the oxidative effects associated with cavitation. Cavitation-induced heat can lead to undesirable oxidation reactions in the oil, but this risk can be minimized by controlling the temperature and cavitation intensity. This is particularly important for linseed oil, as it is highly sensitive to oxidation (Xin et al., 2022). Mild conditions preserve bioactive compounds, such as tocopherols and polyphenols, which are valuable antioxidants.

Hence, ultrasound-assisted refining offers a cost-effective, environmentally friendly, and chemical-free alternative to traditional refining methods. It improves the purity of linseed oil while retaining its essential bioactive properties. As this technology continues to evolve, it is poised to meet the growing demand for high-quality, sustainably produced edible oils, offering an innovative solution to modern refining challenges.

4.3 Microwave-Assisted Refining

Microwave-assisted refining of linseed oil represents an efficient approach to oil processing, with the principle of dielectric heating (Tajik et al., 2024). This technique utilizes microwave energy, typically at a frequency of 2.45 GHz, to induce rapid heating within the seed material through molecular interactions. Polar molecules such as water and phospholipids absorb microwave energy, undergoing rapid vibration and friction, which results in uniform and efficient heat generation. This controlled heating process is particularly beneficial for refining linseed oil, as it minimizes thermal degradation and preserves key nutritional properties. During microwave treatment, the reduction of seed moisture and the softening of cellular structures facilitate the disruption of cell walls, promoting efficient release of oil fraction. Additionally, the heat generated inactivates enzymatic activity of lipases and peroxidases (Chetima et al., 2024; Li et al., 2024a). This enzymatic control ensures greater stability of the oil both during extraction and in storage. Moreover, microwave pretreatment contributes to the retention of beneficial bioactive compounds, such as tocopherols and phenolics (Porch et al., 2012). These compounds play a crucial role in maintaining the oxidative stability of linseed oil and protecting its polyunsaturated fatty acids, particularly alpha-linolenic acid, from degradation. The uniform heating provided by microwaves also limits the formation of oxidative by-products, such as peroxides (Farmonov et al., 2024).

Moreover, microwave-assisted refining enhances oil extraction efficiency, whether through mechanical pressing or solvent extraction. Softening the seed matrix and improving oil diffusion led to higher yields while preserving the bioactive components. Compared to conventional thermal processing, microwave-assisted refining is not only more energy-efficient but also more environmentally sustainable, aligning with modern industrial goals for cleaner and greener production methods.

4.4 Ion Exchange

The application of ion exchange resins in the refining of linseed oil offers a sustainable and efficient solution for impurity removal, aligning with modern industrial needs for environmentally friendly processes (Esquerre Verastegui et al., 2024). These resins, composed of polymeric matrices embedded with functional groups, operate on the principle of ion exchange to selectively remove contaminants such as phospholipids, metallic ions, and other charged impurities from the oil. This method provides a precise and controlled purification process while preserving the nutritional quality of the oil (Selimi et al., 2024; Susik & Ptasznik, 2023).

Primarily, the raw linseed oil is passed through a packed bed of ion exchange resin contained within a purification reactor (Thomas et al., 2024). As the oil flows through the resin, the charged impurities interact with the functional groups on the resin and get bound to its matrix. The ion exchange mechanism is driven by electrostatic interactions and chemical affinities between the resin's active sites and the contaminants. This allows the oil to be purified without requiring additional solvents or extensive processing steps. Depending on the type of resin, specific impurities can be targeted, with acidic resins effectively binding positively charged species, basic resins removing negatively charged contaminants, and mixed-bed resins offering broader purification capabilities (Mhadmhan et al., 2023; Ngouangna et al., 2022).

A notable advantage of ion exchange resins lies in their regenerative capability (Abusultan et al., 2023). Once the resin becomes saturated with impurities, it can be restored to its active state by treating it with a small quantity of regenerant, such as a diluted acid or base. This regeneration process not only enhances the reusability of the resin but also minimizes waste generation, significantly reducing the environmental footprint of the refining process (Osazuwa & Abidin, 2020). Compared to conventional wet washing methods, ion exchange resin purification eliminates the need for solvents, avoids liquid-liquid separation steps, and requires less energy, thereby lowering operational costs and enhancing sustainability.

Hence, the use of ion exchange resins in linseed oil refining aligns closely with the principles of green chemistry by reducing waste, conserving energy, and promoting environmentally conscious production. By eliminating excessive chemical usage and energy-intensive processes, this method represents a sustainable advancement in oil refining. Though it is still a relatively new approach, its potential to transform lipid purification is significant.

5 Challenges of Emerging Technologies and Future Solutions

Emerging technologies, including electrostatic field treatment, ultrasound, microwave-assisted refining, and ion exchange resins, offer substantial promises in enhancing the efficiency and sustainability of linseed oil refining (Ao et al., 2023; Oyekunle et al., 2024). However, each of these methods presents distinct challenges that must be addressed before they can be fully integrated into large-scale industrial applications (Table 1).

Electrostatic field treatment, which is employed to remove charged impurities from oils, faces difficulties related to consistency and scalability (Ferraz & Silva, 2025; Ranjha et al., 2021). The efficiency of this process is influenced by factors such as oil composition, viscosity, and the presence of natural polar compounds (Aneed & Najim, 2024). Furthermore, the process requires precise control over operational parameters, such as the strength and configuration of the electric field, which adds to the complexity. The energy consumption associated with scaling up this technology also raises concerns, as it may reduce its overall cost-effectiveness in large-scale operations (Huang et al., 2024). While ultrasound-assisted refining shows promise, one of the main challenges is achieving uniform treatment across large batches (Walayat et al., 2024; Zhang et al., 2024a). The energy required for cavitation can be inconsistent, resulting in uneven processing and potentially affecting the quality and efficiency of the refining process (Chew & Ali, 2021). As a

Table 1 Comparison of parameters between conventional and nonconventional refining of crude linseed oil

Parameter	Conventional refining	Nonconventional refining	References
Chemical usage	High chemical dependency	Minimal chemical usage	Cárdenas et al. (2021)
		Rely on enzymes, membranes, and bio-adsorbents	
Energy consumption	High due to thermal processes	Low energy consumption	Ishfaq et al. (2024), Yang et al. (2020)
Environmental impact	High environmental impact	Low environmental impact; eco-friendly and sustainable processes	Chen and Sun (2023), Wen et al. (2023)
Oil quality	Quality degradation due to high temperatures and chemical interactions	Superior oil quality, nutrients, antioxidants, and flavor are preserved	Hashempour-Baltork et al. (2022), Hernandez-Centeno et al. (2020)
Processing time	Relatively longer processing time	Faster processing due to efficient techniques	Kong et al. (2024), Selge et al. (2024)
Cost	Lower initial setup cost; higher operational costs due to energy and chemicals	Higher initial setup cost	Akhtaruzzaman and Rahman (2024), Saleem et al. (2024)
		Lower operational costs	
Adoption	Highly scalable for large-scale production	Limited scalability for industrial production	Yatimi et al. (2024)
		Still under development	

result, the energy efficiency of ultrasound-assisted refining can be a limiting factor, especially in industrial applications where large volumes of oil need to be processed (Chemat et al., 2004). Moreover, microwave-assisted refining also poses challenges, particularly in ensuring uniform heating of the oil. This lack of consistency can negatively affect the quality of the refined oil and lead to the formation of undesirable by-products (Tajik et al., 2024; Zhang et al., 2018). Optimizing microwave power, treatment duration, and oil flow rate is essential to mitigate these issues but achieving uniform and controlled heating across large-scale operations remains a significant hurdle. Notably, the performance of ion exchange resins can degrade over time as they become saturated with impurities, necessitating periodic regeneration. While this process is generally low in energy consumption and waste production, it still adds complexity and cost to the operation. Furthermore, ion exchange resins may not be effective at removing nonionic impurities, such as certain polyphenols, which are commonly found in linseed oil. As a result, further research is required to develop more efficient resin materials and to optimize regeneration processes to ensure that ion exchange can be applied effectively in oil refining (Fu et al., 2016; Nir et al., 2024).

Despite these challenges, the potential of these technologies to revolutionize the linseed oil refining process remains substantial. Overcoming the limitations will require ongoing research and development focused on optimizing operational parameters, enhancing energy efficiency, and improving the scalability of these methods. Innovations in precise control systems, advanced resin formulations, and improved heat distribution technologies will be key to making these emerging techniques more effective and commercially viable. As the food sector moves toward more sustainable and environmentally friendly practices, these technologies hold the potential to transform the linseed oil refining process, offering more efficient, cost-effective, and eco-conscious solutions for the future.

6 Environmental Indicators for Sustainability Assessment in Linseed Oil Processing Industry

Sustainable development is vital for the linseed oil processing industry, especially regarding environmental impact. To ensure sustainability and remain competitive in the market, sustainability assessments play a key role. These assessments use various indicators and methodologies to evaluate sustainability, often presenting findings through qualitative reports that highlight relevant indicators. They are becoming increasingly important as they guide decision-making on sustainability, provide accurate data for policy analysis and monitoring, serve as key resources for environmental reporting, and raise awareness of sustainability issues (Guo et al., 2020).

6.1 Sustainability Indicators and Characteristics

A Sustainability indicator (SI) refers to any metric that offers insight or characterizes a process, system, or activity in the context of sustainability (Shukor & Ng, 2022). These indicators are crucial tools for providing an overarching view of a nation's progress toward sustainability, focusing on the economic, social, and environmental pillars. They also play a vital role in informing decision-making processes. Specifically, environmental indicators, a subset of SIs, are instrumental in tracking environmental progress, supporting policy evaluation, and keeping the public informed. Table 2 represents the indicators used for sustainability assessment and their key characteristics (Shukor & Ng, 2022).

Building on these attributes and earlier research on environmental sustainability metrics within the food processing sector, it introduces a suite of metrics specifically designed for the linseed oil processing industry. The chosen metrics are guided by benchmarks from comparable industries, including the Roundtable on Sustainable Palm Oil (RSPO) (Shukor & Ng, 2022)

6.2 Sustainability Assessment

The international standard methods such as the Food and Agriculture Sustainability Assessment (SAFA) (Zarba et al., 2025), Environmental Performance Indicators (EPIs) for ISO 14001 (Shukor & Ng, 2022), and the Traffic Light Assessment by

Table 2 The indicators utilized for sustainability assessment and their respective key characteristics

Indicators	Characteristics
Comparability	Metrics must be analogous, capturing shifts in ecological outcomes and assisting stakeholders in making informed decisions
Target-orientation	Metrics must track advancement toward the organization's objectives and precisely mirror the processes or functions they signify
Balance and clarity	Metrics should depict environmental performance trends in an even-handed way, emphasizing both challenges and advantages. They must also be straightforward, dependable, and readily accessible
Consistency and practicality	It should remain stable over time, employing matching units and timelines to facilitate comparisons. They should also be practical, whether in qualitative or quantitative terms
Frequency	Indicators must be updated frequently enough to prompt timely actions by firms, such as monthly, quarterly, or annually
Comprehensibility	Indicators should be understandable to users and align with their information needs

DEFRA are often too broad or general for application in the food processing industry. Additionally, current evaluation methods like Corporate Sustainability Performance (SCP) often fall short due to insufficient integration of sustainability dimensions and the reliance on varied indicators (Shukor & Ng, 2022). Although Life Cycle Sustainability Assessment (LCSA) provides a more holistic approach, its complexity demands expert guidance. Techniques such as the Cobble Nest Graph and Cylindrical Sustainability are easier to understand and interpret, yet they struggle with data collection and presentation validity.

Previous research has shown that existing methods and evaluations fall short in effectively assessing sustainability and are often unsuitable for the food processing sector. There is a lack of standardized indicators tailored to this industry, with many current indicators not comprehensively addressing environmental factors. The existing indicators tend to be overly broad and do not align with the specific needs of the edible oil processing industry. Some indicators focus solely on specific aspects, such as waste treatment or cost analysis, rather than providing a complete environmental overview. Additionally, many approaches have been oriented toward internal assessments based on individual organizational needs, failing to encompass all environmental aspects.

7 Conclusions

In summary, refining linseed oil for food-based applications requires a careful approach that prioritizes both optimizing production efficiency and maintaining its nutritional value and quality. Conventional refining techniques, when integrated with advanced methods, offer an effective strategy for producing high-quality linseed oil that meets the stringent standards required by the food industry. These processes, such as degumming, neutralization, bleaching, and deodorization, are essential for removing impurities, improving sensory attributes, and extending shelf life while ensuring compliance with food safety regulations. However, maintaining the inherent nutritional properties, particularly its rich α-linolenic acid content, and ensuring long-term oxidative stability are critical considerations during processing. Emerging green technologies, including ultrasound-assisted extraction, microwave treatments, and enzymatic methods, present an opportunity to enhance the efficiency and sustainability of the refining process without compromising quality. Despite these advancements, conventional refining methods continue to play a pivotal role in retaining the quality of linseed oil throughout the refining stages, ensuring its suitability for diverse food applications.

References

Abdelbasir, S. M., Shehab, A. I., & Khalek, M. A. A. (2023). Spent bleaching earth; recycling and utilization techniques: A review. *Resources, Conservation & Recycling Advances, 17*(200124), 200124. https://doi.org/10.1016/j.rcradv.2022.200124

Abdulhussein, Z., Al-sharify, Z., Alzuraiji, M., & Onyeaka, H. (2023). Environmental significance of fouling on the crude oil flow. A comprehensive review. *Journal of Engineering and Sustainable Development, 27*(3), 317–338. https://doi.org/10.31272/jeasd.27.3.3

Abusultan, A. A. M., Wood, J. A., Sainio, T., Kemperman, A. J. B., & van der Meer, W. G. J. (2023). Ion exchange resin – Bipolar membrane electrodialysis hybrid process for reverse osmosis permeate remineralization: Cation exchange resins equilibria and kinetics. *Separation and Purification Technology, 317*(123798), 123798. https://doi.org/10.1016/j.seppur.2023.123798

Akhtaruzzaman, M., & Rahman, M. R. (2024). Commonality in systemic risk from green and conventional energy. *Energy Economics, 107404*, 107404. https://doi.org/10.1016/j.eneco.2024.107404

Albayati, S. H., Nezhad, N. G., Taki, A. G., & Rahman, R. N. Z. R. A. (2024). Efficient and easible biocatalysts: Strategies for enzyme improvement. A review. *International Journal of Biological Macromolecules, 276*(Pt 2), 133978. https://doi.org/10.1016/j.ijbiomac.2024.133978

Aneed, T. S., & Najim, S. T. (2024). Review of electrical methods for enhancing crude oil viscosity and flowability. *BIO Web of Conferences, 97*, 00033. https://doi.org/10.1051/bioconf/20249700033

Ao, S., Chhandama, M. V. L., Li, H., & Lalthazuala Rokhum, S. (2023). Microwave-assisted sustainable production of biodiesel: A comprehensive review. *Current Microwave Chemistry, 10*(1), 3–25. https://doi.org/10.2174/2213335610666230223100707

Bray, D. J., Anderson, R. L., Warren, P. B., & Lewtas, K. (2020). Wax formation in linear and branched alkanes with dissipative particle dynamics. *Journal of Chemical Theory and Computation, 16*(11), 7109–7122. https://doi.org/10.1021/acs.jctc.0c00605

Cao, H., Cao, X., Zhao, X., Guo, D., Liu, Y., & Bian, J. (2022). Molecular dynamics simulation of wax molecules aggregational crystallization behavior during cooling of crude oil mixture. *Case Studies in Thermal Engineering, 37*(102298), 102298. https://doi.org/10.1016/j.csite.2022.102298

Cárdenas, J., Orjuela, A., Sánchez, D. L., Narváez, P. C., Katryniok, B., & Clark, J. (2021). Pretreatment of used cooking oils for the production of green chemicals: A review. *Journal of Cleaner Production, 289*(125129), 125129. https://doi.org/10.1016/j.jclepro.2020.125129

Chand, M., Chopra, R., Talwar, B., Homroy, S., Singh, P. K., Dhiman, A., & Payyunni, A. W. (2024). Unveiling the potential of linseed mucilage, its health benefits, and applications in food packaging. *Frontiers in Nutrition, 11*, 1334247. https://doi.org/10.3389/fnut.2024.1334247

Chemat, F., Grondin, I., Costes, P., Moutoussamy, L., Sing, A. S. C., & Smadja, J. (2004). High power ultrasound effects on lipid oxidation of refined sunflower oil. *Ultrasonics Sonochemistry, 11*(5), 281–285. https://doi.org/10.1016/j.ultsonch.2003.07.004

Chen, X., & Sun, S. (2023). Color reversion of refined vegetable oils: A review. *Molecules (Basel, Switzerland), 28*(13), 5177. https://doi.org/10.3390/molecules28135177

Chetima, A., Nde Bup, D., Kewir, F., & Wahaboua, A. (2024). Activated carbons from open air and microwave-assisted impregnation of cotton and neem husks efficiently decolorize neutral cotton oil. *Heliyon, 10*(1), e24060. https://doi.org/10.1016/j.heliyon.2024.e24060

Chew, S. C., & Ali, M. A. (2021). Recent advances in ultrasound technology applications of vegetable oil refining. *Trends in Food Science & Technology, 116*, 468–479. https://doi.org/10.1016/j.tifs.2021.08.001

Dabour, S. A., Abozid, M., & Abdelgwad, S. M. (2024). A comparative study between sunflower oil and flaxseed oil as oils with high nutritional value. *Menoufia Journal of Agricultural Biotechnology, 9*(8), 115–123. https://doi.org/10.21608/mjab.2024.299746.1020

Dai, M., Niu, Q., Wu, S., Lin, Y., Biswas, J. K., & Yang, C. (2024). Hydroxyl radicals in ozone-based advanced oxidation of organic contaminants: A review. *Environmental Chemistry Letters, 22*(6), 3059–3106. https://doi.org/10.1007/s10311-024-01772-w

Das, N., Kumar Praharaj, M., & Panda, S. (2024). Exploring ultrasonic wave transmission in liquids and liquid mixtures: A comprehensive overview. *Journal of Molecular Liquids, 403*(124841), 124841. https://doi.org/10.1016/j.molliq.2024.124841

Dengaev, A. V., Khelkhal, M. A., Getalov, A. A., Baimukhametov, G. F., Kayumov, A. A., Vakhin, A. V., & Gafurov, M. R. (2023). Innovations in oil processing: Chemical transformation of oil components through ultrasound assistance. *Fluids, 8*(4), 108. https://doi.org/10.3390/fluids8040108

do Espírito Santo de Jesus, F., de Jesus Freitas, T., Bispo, A. M., de Matos Santos, L., Braga Alves, A. S., Aparecida Souza Machado, B., & Ferreira Ribeiro, C. D. (2023). Edible oils and development of new products: Sensory, microbiological, and cytotoxic aspects. *Current Organic Chemistry, 27*(22), 1917–1945. https://doi.org/10.2174/0113852728267166231123111707

Drozd-Rzoska, A., Rzoska, S. J., & Łoś, J. (2024). Supercriticality, glassy dynamics, and the new insight into melting/freezing discontinuous transition in linseed oil. *Biophysica, 4*(1), 34–57. https://doi.org/10.3390/biophysica4010003

Dubrovskaya, I. A., Butina, E. A., Slobodyanik, M. V., & Kopytova, N. S. (2023). Method for the identification and quantification of waxes in vegetable oils. *AIP Conference Proceedings, 2777*, 020077. https://doi.org/10.1063/5.0140399

Elaine, E., & Nyam, K. L. (2025). Application of distillation in edible oil deodorization. In *Mass transfer operations in the food industry* (pp. 283–305). Elsevier. https://doi.org/10.1016/b978-0-12-819536-9.00009-6

Esquerre Verastegui, J. E., López López, A., González Domínguez, R. A., Zamora Antuñano, M. A., Dávila Ignacio, C. V., & García García, R. (2024). Production of coconut oil bioturbosine without water by using ultrasound as a source of energy and ion exchange for its purification. *Energies, 17*(3), 614. https://doi.org/10.3390/en17030614

Fan, J.-N., Yang, Y., Wang, Y., Chen, H., & Qian, B. (2024). Intense field dielectric purification of oil droplets in machining buildings. *Journal of Building Engineering, 84*(108543), 108543. https://doi.org/10.1016/j.jobe.2024.108543

Farmonov, J., Hunupolagama, D., Dissanayake, K., Boynazarova, Y., Serkaev, K., Samadiy, M., & Rifky, M. (2024). Application of microwave technology to extract pure sesame oil. *E3S Web of Conferences, 494*, 04025. https://doi.org/10.1051/e3sconf/202449404025

Ferfuia, C., Zuliani, F., Piani, B., Costa, L. D., Corazzin, M., Turi, M., & Baldini, M. (2023). Bleaching techniques impact on some quality parameters in two different cold-pressed oils obtained at farm scale. *Journal of Food Process Engineering, 46*(7). https://doi.org/10.1111/jfpe.14357

Fernandes, C. D. P., Pott, A., Hiane, P. A., do Nascimento, V. A., Filiú, W. F. D. O., de Oliveira, L. C. S., Sanjinez-Argandoña, E. J., Cavalheiro, L. F., Nazário, C. E. D., Caires, A. R. L., Michels, F. S., Freitas, K. D. C., Asato, M. A., Donadon, J. R., Bogo, D., & Guimarães,

R. D. C. A. (2024). Comparative analysis of grape seed oil, linseed oil, and a blend: In vivo effects of supplementation. *Foods (Basel, Switzerland), 13*(14), 2283. https://doi.org/10.3390/foods13142283

Ferraz, L. P., & Silva, E. K. (2025). Pulsed electric field-assisted extraction techniques for obtaining vegetable oils and essential oils: Recent progress and opportunities for the food industry. *Separation and Purification Technology, 354*(128833), 128833. https://doi.org/10.1016/j.seppur.2024.128833

Fu, J., Li, Z., Xing, S., Wang, Z., Miao, C., Lv, P., & Yuan, Z. (2016). Cation exchange resin catalysed biodiesel production from used cooking oil (UCO): Investigation of impurities effect. *Fuel (London, England), 181*, 1058–1065. https://doi.org/10.1016/j.fuel.2016.04.131

Gharby, S. (2022). Refining vegetable oils: Chemical and physical refining. *TheScientificWorldJOURNAL, 2022*, 6627013. https://doi.org/10.1155/2022/6627013

Griep, P., Gayeski, L., Colet, R., Zeni, J., & Valduga, E. (2024). Recent updates of carotenoid encapsulation by spray-drying technique. *Journal of Microencapsulation, 1–21*, 26. https://doi.org/10.1080/02652048.2024.2430643

Guo, Z., Ge, S., Yao, X., Li, H., & Li, X. (2020). Life cycle sustainability assessment of pumped hydro energy storage. *International Journal of Energy Research, 44*(1), 192–204. https://doi.org/10.1002/er.4890

Hashempour-Baltork, F., Farshi, P., Alizadeh, A. M., Azadmard-Damirchi, S., & Torbati, M. (2022). Nutritional aspects of vegetable oils: Refined or unrefined? *European Journal of Lipid Science and Technology: EJLST, 124*(12), 2100149. https://doi.org/10.1002/ejlt.202100149

Hernandez-Centeno, F., Universidad Autónoma Agraria Antonio Narro, Hernández-González, M., López-De la Peña, H. Y., López-Trujillo, R., Zamudio-Flores, P. B., Ochoa-Reyes, E., Tirado-Gallegos, J. M., & Martínez-Vázquez, D. G. (2020). Changes in oxidative stability, composition and physical characteristics of oil from a non-conventional source before and after processing. *Revista Mexicana de Ingenieria Quimica, 19*(3), 1389–1400. https://doi.org/10.24275/rmiq/alim937

Hou, Z., Jiang, S., Cao, X., Cao, L., Pang, M., Yang, P., & Jiang, S. (2023). Performances of phospholipids and changes of antioxidant capacity from rapeseed oil during enzymatic degumming. *Lebensmittel-Wissenschaft Und Technologie [Food Science and Technology], 173*(114222), 114222. https://doi.org/10.1016/j.lwt.2022.114222

Huang, L., Huang, S., Chen, L., Ren, B., OuYang, P., & Li, Y. (2024). Molecular dynamics promotes study of droplet electrocoalescence: A mini-review. *Journal of Electrostatics, 129*(103929), 103929. https://doi.org/10.1016/j.elstat.2024.103929

Hudaib, B., Al-Qodah, Z., Abu-Zurayk, R., Waleed, H., & Omar, W. (2024). Fabrication of blended cellulose acetate/poly-pyrrole ultrafiltration membranes for crude oil wastewater separation. *Case Studies in Chemical and Environmental Engineering, 9*(100692), 100692. https://doi.org/10.1016/j.cscee.2024.100692

Ishfaq, K., Sana, M., Waseem, M. U., Anwar, S., & Zia, A. W. (2024). Circular usage of waste cooking oil towards green electrical discharge machining process with lower carbon emissions. *The International Journal of Advanced Manufacturing Technology., 131*, 5133. https://doi.org/10.1007/s00170-024-13322-3

Jayakumar, S., Trens, P., Barboiu, M., & Cerneaux, S. (2025). Hydrophobic cordierite-based capillary membranes applied to desalination. *Separation and Purification Technology, 359*(130679), 130679. https://doi.org/10.1016/j.seppur.2024.130679

Jing, J., Cao, L., Shan, Y., Sun, J., & Tan, J. (2024). Optimizing the low-temperature performance of high-wax-content crude oil with emulsion-based wax inhibitors: Mechanisms and efficacy. *Annals of the New York Academy of Sciences, 1541*(1), 255–265. https://doi.org/10.1111/nyas.15248

Karim, N. A. A., Othman, N. H., & Yusoff, M. M. (2022). Vegetable oil refining. In *Recent advances in edible fats and oils technology* (pp. 101–140). Springer Singapore. https://doi.org/10.1007/978-981-16-5113-7_4

Kaur, V., Gomashe, S. S., Yadav, S. K., Singh, D., Sheela, Chauhan, S. S., Kumar, V., Jat, B., Tayade, N. R., Langyan, S., Kaushik, N., Singh, M., Kheralia, M., Wankhede, D. P., Aravind,

J., Srivastava, V., Gupta, K., Kumar, A., & Singh, G. P. (2024). Leveraging genetic resource diversity and identification of trait-enriched superior genotypes for accelerated improvement in linseed (Linum usitatissimum L.). *Scientific Reports, 14*(1), 20266. https://doi.org/10.1038/s41598-024-71044-8

Khamies, M., Hagar, M., Kassem, T. S. E., & Moustafa, A. H. E. (2024). Case study of chemical and enzymatic degumming processes in soybean oil production at an industrial plant. *Scientific Reports, 14*(1), 4064. https://doi.org/10.1038/s41598-024-53865-9

Khan, A., Nadeem, M., Imran, M., & Khalique, A. (2021). Impact of winterization on fatty acids' composition, isomers, and oxidative stability of conjugated linoleic acids produced from selected vegetable oils. *Journal of Food Processing and Preservation, 45*(3). https://doi.org/10.1111/jfpp.15254

Kong, M., Du, Y., Chen, X., Cai, R., Xie, J., & Shen, M. (2024). Investigation into the effects of the refining steps before deodorization on the formation of trans fatty acids in linseed oils. *Journal of Food Composition and Analysis: An Official Publication of the United Nations University, International Network of Food Data Systems, 134*(106549), 106549. https://doi.org/10.1016/j.jfca.2024.106549

Langyan, S., Yadava, P., Khan, F. N., Sharma, S., Singh, R., Bana, R. S., Singh, N., Kaur, V., Kalia, S., & Kumar, A. (2023). Trends and advances in pre- and post-harvest processing of linseed oil for quality food and health products. *Critical Reviews in Food Science and Nutrition, 1–24*, 746. https://doi.org/10.1080/10408398.2023.2280768

Langyan, S., Kaur, V., & Kumar, A. (2024). Overview of linseed as multipurpose-multisector crop. In *Linseed* (pp. 1–18). Elsevier. https://doi.org/10.1016/b978-0-443-15439-3.00019-9

Li, J., Lin, L., Ju, T., Meng, F., Han, S., Chen, K., & Jiang, J. (2024a). Microwave-assisted pyrolysis of solid waste for production of high-value liquid oil, syngas, and carbon solids: A review. *Renewable and Sustainable Energy Reviews, 189*(113979), 113979. https://doi.org/10.1016/j.rser.2023.113979

Li, Q., Song, T., Yu, Y., Ren, Y., & Qian, J.-Y. (2024b). Electric fields and transglutaminase in preparing adzuki bean protein emulsion gel for plant-based steamed egg custard. *Innovative Food Science & Emerging Technologies: IFSET: The Official Scientific Journal of the European Federation of Food Science and Technology, 98*(103871), 103871. https://doi.org/10.1016/j.ifset.2024.103871

Liu, L., Cai, H., Zhang, Y., Jin, Q., Wang, X., & Jin, J. (2024a). Chemical compositions and oxidative stabilities of cold-pressed walnut oils (Juglans regia L.): Effects of chemical refining, water degumming, and molecular distillation. *Journal of Food Science, 89*(11), 7589–7598. https://doi.org/10.1111/1750-3841.17402

Liu, X., Huang, C., Lan, D., Wang, W., & Wang, Y. (2024b). Combining phospholipase A1 with monoacylglycerol lipase for crude vegetable oil degumming through improved oil-water separation. *Food Chemistry, 467*, 142366. https://doi.org/10.1016/j.foodchem.2024.142366

Ma, R., Jia, L., Zhang, H., Cao, F., Shao, J., Zhang, J., Yan, S., & Xu, J. (2024). Structural analysis of petroleum acids in highly acidic crude oil and deacidification using organic amines. *Fuel (London, England), 360*(130117), 130117. https://doi.org/10.1016/j.fuel.2023.130117

Mangang, I. B., Nongmaithem, R., Sasikumar, R., Mohan, R. J., & Manickam, L. (2024). Influence of high-voltage electrical discharges on oil extraction and its quality. In *Emerging methods for oil extraction from food processing waste* (pp. 107–116). CRC Press. https://doi.org/10.1201/9781003408567-6

Mhadmhan, S., Yoosuk, B., Chareonteraboon, B., Janetaisong, P., Pitakjakpipop, P., Henpraserttae, S., & Udomsap, P. (2023). Elimination of free fatty acid from palm oil by adsorption process using a strong base anion exchange resin. *Separation and Purification Technology, 310*(123211), 123211. https://doi.org/10.1016/j.seppur.2023.123211

Ngouangna, E. N., Zaidi Jaafar, M., Norddin, M., Agi, A., Oseh, J. O., & Mamah, S. (2022). Surface modification of nanoparticles to improve oil recovery mechanisms: A critical review of the methods, influencing parameters, advances and prospects. *Journal of Molecular Liquids, 360*(119502), 119502. https://doi.org/10.1016/j.molliq.2022.119502

Nir, S. Z., Salem, A., & Salem, S. (2024). Application of clay-based waste collected in landfill of vegetable oil refinery for immobilization of heavy metal ions from wastewater of zinc industry through fabrication of zeolite LTA and hydroxysodalite. *Sustainable Chemistry and Pharmacy, 39*(101618), 101618. https://doi.org/10.1016/j.scp.2024.101618

Orlova, Y., Harmon, R. E., Broadbelt, L. J., & Iedema, P. D. (2021). Review of the kinetics and simulations of linseed oil autoxidation. *Progress in Organic Coatings, 151*(106041), 106041. https://doi.org/10.1016/j.porgcoat.2020.106041

Osazuwa, O. U., & Abidin, S. Z. (2020). The functionality of ion exchange resins for esterification, transesterification and hydrogenation reactions. *ChemistrySelect, 5*(25), 7658–7670. https://doi.org/10.1002/slct.202001381

Oyekunle, D. T., Gendy, E. A., Barasa, M., Oyekunle, D. O., Oni, B., & Tiong, S. K. (2024). Review on utilization of rubber seed oil for biodiesel production: Oil extraction, biodiesel conversion, merits, and challenges. *Cleaner Engineering and Technology, 21*(100773), 100773. https://doi.org/10.1016/j.clet.2024.100773

Pan, F. G., Liu, J., Yang, J. X., Ren, J. R., Sun, Y. Y., Li, P. Z., Yang, E. Q., Chen, X. M., & Liu, B. Q. (2024). Research progress on the genesis and removal methods of non-hydratable phospholipids from vegetable oils. *Grasas y Aceites, 75*(1), e543. https://doi.org/10.3989/gya.0325231

Panasenko, O. M., Vladimirov, Y. A., & Sergienko, V. I. (2024). Free radical lipid peroxidation induced by reactive halogen species. *Biochemistry. Biokhimiia, 89*(Suppl 1), S148–S179. https://doi.org/10.1134/S0006297924140098

Payasi, D. K., Garg, D., Payasi, S., & Yogranjan. (2024). Preharvesting processing of linseed crop. In *Linseed* (pp. 21–45). Elsevier. https://doi.org/10.1016/b978-0-443-15439-3.00018-7

Porch, A., Slocombe, D., Beutler, J., Edwards, P., Aldawsari, A., Xiao, T., Kuznetsov, V., Almegren, H., Aldrees, S., & Almaqati, N. (2012). Microwave treatment in oil refining. *Applied Petrochemical Research, 2*(1–2), 37–44. https://doi.org/10.1007/s13203-012-0016-4

Ranjha, M. M. A. N., Kanwal, R., Shafique, B., Arshad, R. N., Irfan, S., Kieliszek, M., Kowalczewski, P. Ł., Irfan, M., Khalid, M. Z., Roobab, U., & Aadil, R. M. (2021). A critical review on pulsed electric field: A novel technology for the extraction of phytoconstituents. *Molecules (Basel, Switzerland), 26*(16), 4893. https://doi.org/10.3390/molecules26164893

Razola-Díaz, M. D. C., Genovese, J., Tylewicz, U., Guerra-Hernández, E. J., Rocculi, P., & Verardo, V. (2024). Enhanced extraction of procyanidins from avocado processing residues by pulsed electric fields pre-treatment. *Lebensmittel-Wissenschaft Und Technologie [Food Science and Technology], 212*(116952), 116952. https://doi.org/10.1016/j.lwt.2024.116952

Saleem, M., Ali, M., & Saeed, A. (2024). Current trends in extraction, purification, and refining of oils from various biological sources using a biochemical method. In *Recent advances in industrial biochemistry* (pp. 29–47). Springer International Publishing. https://doi.org/10.1007/978-3-031-50989-6_3

Sankarappa, T., Prashant Kumar, M., & Ahmad, A. (2005). Ultrasound velocity and density studies in some refined and unrefined edible oils. *Physics and Chemistry of Liquids, 43*(6), 507–514. https://doi.org/10.1080/00319100500192889

Seifollahi, F., Eikani, M. H., & Khandan, N. (2024). Optimization of operating conditions for lampante olive oil deacidification by short path molecular distillation: Waste valorization approach. *Journal of Cleaner Production, 454*(142304), 142304. https://doi.org/10.1016/j.jclepro.2024.142304

Selge, B., Gusovius, H.-J., & Ouagne, P. (2024). Processing of linseed straw: State-of-the-art and further perspectives. *Industrial Crops and Products, 222*(119518), 119518. https://doi.org/10.1016/j.indcrop.2024.119518

Selimi, J., Langschwager, F., Tunå, P., Hulteberg, C. P., & Abdelaziz, O. Y. (2024). Purification of lipid oil using ion exchange resins. *Biomass Conversion and Biorefinery, 15*, 5523. https://doi.org/10.1007/s13399-024-05388-6

Selvamuthukumaran, M. (2020). Membrane technology for degumming, dewaxing and decolorization of crude oil. In *Applications of membrane Technology for Food Processing Industries* (pp. 201–210). CRC Press. https://doi.org/10.1201/9780429276408-8

Shen, L., Li, F., Jiang, C., Cao, X., Jin, J., Wang, X., Wei, W. (2024). Comparative analysis of DHA positional distribution and triacylglycerol molecular species in algal oil (Schizochytrium sp.) from different oil processing. Food Bioscience 58103634. https://doi.org/10.1016/j.fbio.2024.103634

Suri, S., & Singh, S. (2024). Global linseed food market and recent technological advances. In *Linseed* (pp. 119–137). Elsevier. https://doi.org/10.1016/b978-0-443-15439-3.00021-7

Susik, J., & Ptasznik, S. (2023). The first stage of refining of post-fermentation corn oil with a high content of free fatty acids and phytosterols – comparison of neutralisation by an ion-exchange resin without solvent and base neutralisation. *Food Research International (Ottawa, Ont.), 164*(112302), 112302. https://doi.org/10.1016/j.foodres.2022.112302

Shukor, S. A., & Ng, G. K. (2022). Environmental indicators for sustainability assessment in edible oil processing industry based on Delphi Method. *Cleaner Engineering and Technology* 10100558. https://doi.org/10.1016/j.clet.2022.100558

Tajik, A., Vakhin, A. V., Nazimov, N. A., Mirzayev, O., Latypov, R. R., & Gafurov, M. R. (2024). Investigating the effect of microwave radiation at different frequencies on improving the quality of heavy oil. *Fuel (London, England), 375*(132547), 132547. https://doi.org/10.1016/j.fuel.2024.132547

Thilakarathna, R. C. N., Siow, L. F., Tang, T.-K., & Lee, Y. Y. (2023). A review on application of ultrasound and ultrasound assisted technology for seed oil extraction. *Journal of Food Science and Technology, 60*(4), 1222–1236. https://doi.org/10.1007/s13197-022-05359-7

Thomas, E., Panjagari, N. R., Ganguly, S., Kapila, S., & Singh, A. K. (2024). Flaxseed lignan: Metabolism, extraction and isolation techniques, potential health benefits and food applications. *Indian Journal of Dairy Science, 77*(5) https://epubs.icar.org.in/index.php/IJDS/article/view/134613

Tyagi, S. (2024). Linseed market dynamics: Demand and supply. In *Linseed* (pp. 139–148). Elsevier. https://doi.org/10.1016/b978-0-443-15439-3.00001-1

Tzompa-Sosa, D. A., Dewettinck, K., Gellynck, X., & Schouteten, J. J. (2021). Replacing vegetable oil by insect oil in food products: Effect of deodorization on the sensory evaluation. *Food Research International (Ottawa, Ont.), 141*(110140), 110140. https://doi.org/10.1016/j.foodres.2021.110140

Une, S., Sutardi, Hastuti, P., & Susanto, H. (2024). Effect of micelle concentration on degumming of sesame oil (Sesamum indicum L) with ultrafiltration membrane. *IOP Conference Series. Earth and Environmental Science, 1379*(1), 012032. https://doi.org/10.1088/1755-1315/1379/1/012032

Walayat, N., Yurdunuseven-Yıldız, A., Kumar, M., Goksen, G., Öztekin, S., & Lorenzo, J. M. (2024). Oxidative stability, quality, and bioactive compounds of oils obtained by ultrasound and microwave-assisted oil extraction. *Critical Reviews in Food Science and Nutrition, 64*(27), 9974–9991. https://doi.org/10.1080/10408398.2023.2219452

Wang, H., Boyer, S. A. E., Bellet, M., & Dalle, F. (2023). Effects of wax components and the cooling rate on crystal morphology and mechanical properties of wax–oil mixtures. *Crystal Growth & Design, 23*(3), 1422–1433. https://doi.org/10.1021/acs.cgd.2c00941

Wang, X., Chen, Y., McClements, D. J., Meng, C., Zhang, M., Chen, H., & Deng, Q. (2024). Recent advances in understanding the interfacial activity of antioxidants in association colloids in bulk oil. *Advances in Colloid and Interface Science, 325*(103117), 103117. https://doi.org/10.1016/j.cis.2024.103117

Wen, C., Shen, M., Liu, G., Liu, X., Liang, L., Li, Y., Zhang, J., & Xu, X. (2023). Edible vegetable oils from oil crops: Preparation, refining, authenticity identification and application. *Process Biochemistry (Barking, London, England), 124*, 168–179. https://doi.org/10.1016/j.procbio.2022.11.017

Wu, X., Gao, T., Shang, B., Geng, M., Li, L., Feng, X., Wang, X., & Teng, F. (2024). Effect of ultrasonic treatment on soybean oil: Focus on degumming of soybean crude oil and the quality of degummed oil. *European Journal of Lipid Science and Technology: EJLST, 126*(12). https://doi.org/10.1002/ejlt.202400115

Xie, S., Huang, L., Su, C., Yan, J., Chen, Z., Li, M., Du, M., & Zhang, H. (2024). Application of clay minerals as adsorbents for removing heavy metals from the environment. *Green and Smart Mining Engineering, 1*(3), 249–261. https://doi.org/10.1016/j.gsme.2024.07.002

Xin, L., Guo, L., Edirs, S., Zhang, Z., Cai, C., Yang, Y., Lian, Y., & Yang, H. (2022). An efficient deacidification process for safflower seed oil with high nutritional property through optimized ultrasonic-assisted technology. *Molecules (Basel, Switzerland), 27*(7), 2305. https://doi.org/10.3390/molecules27072305

Yan, J., Wright, W. M. D., O'Mahony, J. A., Roos, Y., Cuijpers, E., & van Ruth, S. M. (2019). A sound approach: Exploring a rapid and non-destructive ultrasonic pulse echo system for vegetable oils characterization. *Food Research International (Ottawa, Ont.), 125*(108552), 108552. https://doi.org/10.1016/j.foodres.2019.108552

Yang, K., Liu, S., He, C., Zhang, B., Chen, Q., & Pan, M. (2020). Improving energy saving of crude oil distillation units with optimal operations. *Journal of Cleaner Production, 263*(121340), 121340. https://doi.org/10.1016/j.jclepro.2020.121340

Yang, J., Wen, C., Duan, Y., Deng, Q., Peng, D., Zhang, H., & Ma, H. (2021). The composition, extraction, analysis, bioactivities, bioavailability and applications in food system of flaxseed (Linum usitatissimum L.) oil: A review. *Trends in Food Science & Technology, 118*, 252–260. https://doi.org/10.1016/j.tifs.2021.09.025

Yatimi, Y., Mendil, J., Marafi, M., Alalou, A., & Al-Dahhan, M. H. (2024). Advancement in heavy oil upgrading and sustainable exploration emerging technologies. *Arabian Journal of Chemistry, 17*(3), 105610. https://doi.org/10.1016/j.arabjc.2024.105610

Yu, X., Qin, X., Yang, F., Sun, H., Deng, Q., Tang, X., Chen, Y., & Zhu, Y. (2024). The physicochemical stability and in vivo gastrointestinal fates of flaxseed oil bodies with the introduction of soluble flaxseed gum polysaccharides. *Food Hydrocolloids, 156*(110287), 110287. https://doi.org/10.1016/j.foodhyd.2024.110287

Zarbà, C., Gravagno, R.M., Chinnici, G., Scuderi, A. (2025). A systematic review of the SAFA framework in the literature: An approach to assess sustainability in agri-food systems. *Cleaner Environmental Systems*, 16100267. https://doi.org/10.1016/j.cesys.2025.100267

Zhang, Y., Adam, M., Hart, A., Wood, J., Rigby, S. P., & Robinson, J. P. (2018). Impact of oil composition on microwave heating behavior of heavy oils. *Energy & Fuels: An American Chemical Society Journal, 32*(2), 1592–1599. https://doi.org/10.1021/acs.energyfuels.7b03675

Zhang, H., Gao, C., Zhang, H., Song, N., & Cao, Q. (2024a). Revisiting the application of ultrasonic technology for enhanced oil recovery: Mechanisms and recent advancements. *Energies, 17*(14), 3517. https://doi.org/10.3390/en17143517

Zhang, M., Wang, C., Xie, Z., Gao, B., & Yu, L. (2024b). Chemical structures, analytical approaches and toxicological effects of oxidative derivatives of triglycerides as potential hazards in lipid thermal processing: A review. *Grain & Oil Science and Technology., 7*, 270. https://doi.org/10.1016/j.gaost.2024.07.001

Zhao, C., Zhang, W., Zhang, Y., Yang, Y., Guo, D., Liu, W., & Liu, L. (2024). Influence of multivalent background ions competition adsorption on the adsorption behavior of azo dye molecules and removal mechanism: Based on machine learning, DFT and experiments. *Separation and Purification Technology, 341*(126810), 126810. https://doi.org/10.1016/j.seppur.2024.126810

Composition of Linseed Oil: Major and Minor Components

Himanshi Madan, Rajni Chopra, and Monika Chand

Abstract

Linseed oil, derived from the *Linum usitatissimum* plant of the *Linaceae* family, is renowned for its extraordinary composition, earning it a distinguished place among superfoods. It is a plant-based source rich in polyunsaturated fatty acids (PUFA), especially α-linolenic acid (ALA), which is an indispensable nutrient for maintaining optimal health. The unique fatty acid profile of linseed oil supports cardiovascular and brain health and contributes to cellular structure and function. Beyond its fatty acids, linseed oil is also a reservoir of minor phytonutrients such as vitamin E, phospholipids, phytosterols, polyphenols, lignin, and squalene, collectively referred to as concomitant substances. These compounds not only promulgate the health benefits of linseed oil but also contribute to its stability and functional properties. The composition and stability of linseed oil are influenced by various geographical and genetic factors, which directly or indirectly influence its yield and fatty acid composition, particularly the ALA content. In contrast, other minor constituents are less affected by environmental factors. Understanding the major and minor constituents of linseed oil provides valuable insights into the oil's potential to promote general health and well-being and pave the way to explore its diverse applications in food industries.

Keywords

Linseed oil · Phospholipids · Phytosterols · Squalene · Functional properties · Oil stability · Shelf life of oil

H. Madan · R. Chopra (✉) · M. Chand
Department of Food Science and Technology, National Institute of Food Technology Entrepreneurship and Management, Kundli, Haryana, India

© The Author(s), under exclusive license to Springer Nature Singapore Pte Ltd. 2025

R. Chopra et al. (eds.), *Dynamics of Linseed and its Valorization*,
https://doi.org/10.1007/978-981-96-8927-9_6

1 Introduction

Linseed, commonly known as flaxseed, an annual herbaceous plant botanically known as *Linum usitatissimum*, holds significant importance and versatility in the social and economic development of human civilizations. It is one of the earliest domesticated plants, having been cultivated for 8000–10,000 years for the purpose of oil and fiber, and shows remarkable versatility in its utility (Franke et al., 2010). Linseed is classified into three categories based on its functionality: the first is the oilseed variety that yields linseed oil and is popularly used in paints and varnishes, wood treatment, and linoleum flooring; the second variety is the fiber-flax, which is an integral part of the textile industry for producing linen; and the third variety is the dual-purpose type, distinguished by its ability to produce both seed and fiber (Goyal et al., 2014).

Global linseed production is dominated by a few key countries; Russia is the largest producer, with approximately 1.77 million tonnes, followed by Kazakhstan and Canada. These three countries collectively account for 71% of the world's linseed production. Other notable producers include China, India, the United States, Ethiopia, and France, which together contribute an additional 21% to the global output production of linseed (Saleem et al., 2020). In India, linseed is cultivated across an area of 3.420 lakh hectares, producing 1.537 lakh tonnes, popularly grown in the states of Madhya Pradesh, Uttar Pradesh, and Rajasthan. Madhya Pradesh and Uttar Pradesh together provide around 70% of the country's linseed production (Shakya et al., 2023).

Linseed has been widely used in industrial applications for the longest period in history, but its potential as a food crop has not been explored much despite its astonishing nutritional value. It is highly nutritious, having valuable components such as fats, proteins, vitamins, minerals, and phytochemicals; it contains oil (41%), protein content (20%), dietary fiber (28%), and ash (3.3%) (Piironen et al., 2000). It contains up to 75% polyunsaturated fatty acids (PUFA), 57% α- linolenic acid (ALA, n-3), and 16% linoleic acid (LA, n-6). Linseed also boasts a favorable proportion of amino acids, including asparagine, glutamic acid, leucine, and arginine, making it a good source of these nutrients. However, it is a poor source of sulfur-containing amino acids, such as methionine and cysteine, and branched-chain amino acids, with lysine, threonine, and tyrosine being the limiting amino acids. Linseed is low in carbohydrate content and encompasses 1 g /100 g (Beema et al., 2022). Several factors, including lack of awareness, low oil yield, the vulnerability of crops to pests, disease, adverse weather conditions, susceptibility to oxidation, and poor miscibility in hydrophilic matrices, influence its limited use in food applications and the food industry. Additionally, competition from other oilseed crops, soybeans, groundnuts, and sunflowers, along with limited infrastructure and facilities for processing and storage, further affects the commercial viability of the crop. (Al-Madhagy et al., 2023).

In India, the consumption of linseed has been growing due to increased awareness of its health benefits and its emergence as a dietary supplement and nutraceutical supplement. The demand for linseed oil in both global and Indian markets is also rising, spurred by its applications in health foods and natural products (Zeng et al., 2022).

Linseed oil is extracted from the mature and dried seeds of *Linum usitatissimum*, a species belonging to the Linaceae family. It is esteemed for its abundant phytoconstituents, including fatty acids, pigments, peptides, and vitamins, making it a noteworthy inclusion in trophology and the food industry (Gandova et al., 2023). It is a potent source of ALA, an omega-3 PUFA, pivotal for sustaining human health, supporting cardiovascular health, reducing inflammation, and aiding cognitive functions. The oil also contains a spectrum of bioactive compounds like polyphenols, phytosterols, and tocopherols, which impart significant anti-inflammatory and antioxidant effects (Mueed et al., 2022). These components enhance the development of linseed-based functional foods, nutraceuticals, and therapeutic agents, highlighting the oil's potential to promote health and well-being through innovative dietary and therapeutic applications (Gutte et al., 2015; Sharma et al., 2019).

2 Linseed Oil Composition

The oil content in linseeds typically varies from 35% to 45% (w/w). Linseed oil is renowned for its diverse health benefits, mainly due to its exceptional chemical configuration. Linseed oil is among the richest plant-based sources of unsaturated fatty acid, typically comprising 83.78–89.97% of oil (Pali & Mehta, 2014). This fatty acid content in total oil varied from 10.2% to 16.22%. The oil contains a significant concentration of α-linolenic acid (ALA; 18:3n-3), which accounts for 53.01–50.49%, and linoleic acid (LA; 18:2n-6), which ranges from 15.88% to 17.83% (Dixit et al., 2012). The oil content in linseed is primarily stored in the seed coat and the embryo, with approximately 22% in the seed coat and 4% in the embryo as triacylglycerols in oil bodies having an average diameter of 0.5–0.2 micrometers. These oil bodies are essential for storing the oil within the seed, contributing to the efficient encapsulation and stability of the triacylglycerols (Bai et al., 2021).

Natural fats derived from linseeds are intricate mixtures of various lipids, with triacylglycerols being the primary component. Additionally, linseed oil contains lipophilic constituents, including phospholipids, cyclolinopeptides (CLs), phytosterols, tocopherol, polyphenols, and squalene, collectively called concomitant substances. These lipid concomitants, also known as fat or oil concomitants, are natural phytochemicals present in oil in trace amounts, with concentrations less than 1% (Bekhit et al., 2018). These oleophilic adjuncts not only enhance the quality of linseed oil but also impact the biochemical functions, synergistically improving the functionality of oil with ALA. The proportion of these components varies depending on factors like seed maturity, extraction methods, and storage conditions (Mueed et al., 2022) (Fig. 1).

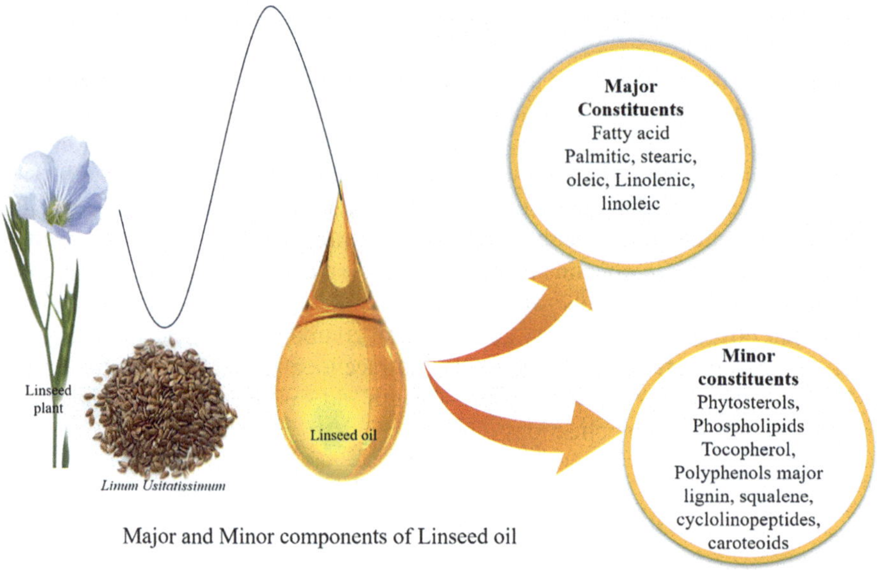

Fig. 1 Depiction of the major and minor components of linseed oil

2.1 Major Components of Linseed Oil

Linseed oil primarily comprises three triglycerides: linolein, linolenin, and olein. Its main triglycerides feature five major fatty acids: α-linolenic, linoleic, oleic, palmitic, and stearic acid (Farag et al., 2021) depicted in Table 4.1. These fatty acids include both saturated and unsaturated types. Saturated fatty acids (SFAs) in linseed oil include myristic acid (14:0) at concentrations of ≤0.1%, palmitic acid (16:0) ranging from 5.1% to 5.3%, stearic acid (18:0) constituting about 3.8% to 6.2%, arachidic acid (20:0) ranging from 0.1% to 0.65%, lignoceric acid (24:0) and behenic acid (22:0) both at concentration ≤ 0.1%. These SFAs are present in amounts ranging from 12.61% to 19.99% of the oil. Specifically, palmitic and stearic acids contribute approximately 9–11% of the oil (Bozan & Temelli, 2008; Lewinska et al., 2015).

Unsaturated fatty acids (USFAs) are present in abundance in linseed oil exceeding 75–90%. It includes monounsaturated fatty acids (MUFAs), in particular, hexadecenoic acid (16:1), oleic acid (18:1), and eicosenoic acid (20:1), which together make up 22.88% to 29.61% (Yang et al., 2021). Linseed oil also consists of 50–55% α-linolenic acid (ALA; 18:3n-3), an omega-3 tri-unsaturated fatty acid. It also includes approximately 20% linolein, the triglyceride formed by esterifying three linoleic acid molecules (LA; 18:2n-6) to a glycerol backbone with the chemical formula $C_{57}H_{98}O_6$. These fatty acids are crucial in defining the oil's nutritional and health benefits and are responsible for the inherent physiochemical and functional characteristics of linseed oil (Kostik et al., 2013).

Table 1 Major fatty acid composition of linseed oil

S. No.	Fatty acids	Percentage (%)				
1	Palmitic acid	4.5–4.8	6.86	7.68	5.17	4.9–5.2
2	Stearic acids	2.24–3.92	4.59	4.1	3.07	3.2–2.7
3	Oleic acid	13.44–22.21	15.07	16.1	16.04	16.5–17.2
4	Linoleic acid	15.17–17.44	13.96	14.4	15.86	14.1-`5.1
5	Alpha-Linolenic acid	51.0–60.42	58.31	50.0	59.85	53.2–53.7
References		Beema et al. (2022)	Bozan and Temelli (2008)	Gandova et al. (2023)	Farag et al. (2021)	Long et al. (2011)

However, ALA bioavailability is higher in linseed oil compared to ground or whole linseeds, making linseed oil a suitable source of this essential fatty acid (Katoch & Bhatia, 2021). The unique fatty acid composition of linseed oil, particularly its high ALA content, contributes significantly to its nutritional value and health-promoting qualities. It is known for its cardiovascular protective and anti-inflammatory effects; it also enhances brain function and promotes healthy skin (Al-Madhagy et al., 2023). Regular consumption of linseed oil can reduce the risk of heart disease, manage obesity, improve insulin resistance, and protect against diabetic retinopathy (Kaur et al., 2023). Additionally, it can benefit individuals with hypertension and hyperlipidemia. The hypocholesterolemia effect of linseed oil is primarily due to its presence of ALA, which helps lower low-density lipoprotein (LDL) levels and total plasma cholesterol (Tripathi et al., 2013) (Table 1).

2.2 Minor Components of Linseed Oil

Linseed oil is not solely defined by these primary components. An extensive spectrum of bioactive compounds, although present in smaller quantities, also contribute to the oil's functional characteristics. These minor constituents, including phytosterols, polyphenols, lignans, and various antioxidants, contribute to the oil's functional characteristics. Understanding these bioactive compounds provides a more comprehensive view of linseed oil's composition and its diverse applications (Younas et al., 2023).

Lipid concomitants, based on their composition, can be divided into three categories: simple form, complex, and derived form. Simple lipid are esters formed by the conjugation of acids and alcohols that can further be hydrolyzed into two parts, such as glycerol esters, sterol esters, and glutamates (Wu et al., 2022). On the other hand, auxiliaries, such as phospholipids (PLs), in which non-lipid molecules coexist with fatty acids and alcohols, fall under the category of complex lipid concomitant. Further, derived lipid concomitants encompass compounds related to or originating from simple and complex lipids, such as steroids and terpenes (Bozan & Temelli, 2008; Zuk et al., 2015).

Lipid concomitants are also classified in terms of hydrophilicity or molecular polarity into polar, amphiphilic, and nonpolar types. Polar lipid concomitants include polyphenolic compounds like phenolic acids and flavonoids. Nonpolar lipid concomitants encompass tocopherol, squalene, and carotenoids (Beema et al., 2022; Lewinska et al., 2015). Phytosterols and phospholipids fall under the category of amphiphilic lipid concomitants. Polar lipid concomitants have a high hydrophilic-lipophilic balance (HLB) and are particularly effective and active in less polar or nonpolar media such as bulk oils. They are predominantly located at the oil interface, where they bind readily to metal ions, thus slowing oxidation and improving the oxidative stability of edible oils. Their antioxidant activity is chiefly facilitated through the single-electron transfer (SET) mechanism (Al-Madhagy et al., 2023).

2.2.1 Phospholipids

Phospholipids are a crucial component of linseed, commonly used as emulsifiers and dietary supplements. Phospholipids have the tendency to enhance the dispersion of solid particles in the aqueous phase and ameliorate the texture of multiphase systems, thereby offering a number of advantageous processing characteristics as well as physiological actions (Wang et al., 2021). Six classes of glycerophospholipids have been identified in linseed oil, namely: phosphatidylglycerol (PG: 1–4%), phosphatidylcholine (PC: 7–18%), phosphatidic acid (PA: 1–9%), lysophosphatidylcholine (LPC: 8–21%), phosphatidylethanolamine (PE: 27–40%), and phosphatidylinositol (PI: 29–32%) (Zhang et al., 2020).

The total phospholipid content, mainly comprising phosphatidylcholine (PC) and phosphatidylinositol (PI), ranges from 1.0% to 1.5% being the major constituents, typical of plant oils, followed by phosphatidylethanolamine (PE), lysophosphatidylcholine (LPC), phosphatidic acids (PA), and phosphatidylglycerol (PG) (Ali et al., 2019). Throughout all phospholipid classes, the most prevalent fatty acid is palmitic acids (23.3–48.5%), thereafter oleic acid (14.0–39.8%) (Dumarey et al., 1975), and the prevalence of linoleic and linolenic acids is comparatively lower. Markedly, phosphatidylinositol contains the highest levels of saturated fatty acids, primarily palmitic and stearic acids (43.5–69.7%), whereas phosphatidylcholine and phosphatidylethanolamine have comparatively lower levels (39.1–59.6% and 39.7–61.1%, respectively) but higher levels of linolenic acid. Additionally, phosphatidylcholine is rich in MUFA (25.6–41.0%), while phosphatidylethanolamine is notable for its PUFA content (21.7–35.3%). Stearic acid predominantly exists in the form of PC and LPC (Xu et al., 2022).

- *Phosphatidylglycerol (PG):* Phosphatidylglycerol (PG) is a kind of glycerophospholipid, present in very small quantities, making about 1.5–4.2% of the total phospholipid content. Both PG (C16:0/C18:2) and PG (C16:0/C18:1) are the primary molecular species present in PG (Gutte et al., 2015). Phosphatidylglycerol is amphiphilic in nature, which allows it to reduce surface tension, form protective layers around droplets, provide electrostatic repulsion, and increase the viscosity of the emulsion, thereby contributing to oil stability (Teneva et al., 2014).

- *Phosphatidic Acid (PA):* PA constitutes 0.9–8.6% of the total phospholipids. PA (16:0/18:3), PA (16:0/18:2), and PA (18:1/18:2) are the most common species in phosphatidic acid. PA levels may be low due to its role as a signaling molecule and its conversion to triglycerides. Phosphatidic acid is a key intermediate in the biosynthesis of triglycerides, which can lead to its relatively low concentration in linseed oil. PA plays a critical role in various cellular signaling pathways that contribute to the dynamic metabolism of the oil's components (Zhang et al., 2020).
- *Phosphatidylethanolamine (PE):* PE makes up to 40% of all phospholipids; PE is the most widespread among all phospholipids. PE (18:2/18:2), PE (18:2/18:1), and PE (16:0/18:2) are the primary molecular species involved. Linoleic acid possesses antioxidant properties and increases the stability and shelf life of the oil; it is the most pertinent molecular in PE (Topnikova et al., 2022; Zhang et al., 2021).
- *Phosphatidylinositol (PI):* PI comprises 29–32% of the phospholipids, with the main molecular species being PI (16:0/18:2) and PI (16:0/18:1). The distribution of linolenic acid is less prevalent in PI compared to PA or PG (Wang et al., 2021).
- *Phosphatidylcholine (PC):* PC constituents 7–18% of phospholipids, with PC (C18:2/18:1) and PC (C18:1/18:1) being the two major molecular species. In vitamin and nutritional supplements, PC is an alternative to choline bitartrate and choline chloride and is essential for liver and cell activities (Yasmeen et al., 2018).
- *Lysophosphatidylcholine (LPC):* LPC accounts for 8–21% of the phospholipids, with the main molecular species being LPC (C18:1) and LPC (C18:2). LPC can arise from the hydrolysis of PC catalyzed by phospholipase A2 enhancing the overall health benefits of linseed oil (Zhang et al., 2020).

2.2.2 Phytosterols

Linseed oil encompasses about 250 mg of sterols per 100 grams. Six phytosterols were identified in linseed oil, including campesterol, stigmasterol, β-sitosterol, Δ5-avenasterol, cycloartenol, and 2,4-methylene cycloartenol (Dąbrowski et al., 2019; Zeb, 2021). Most of the sterol fraction of linseed oil predominantly consists of β-sitosterol, stigmasterol, and campesterol, which make up the majority of the unsaponifiable fraction common to most vegetable oils, followed by Δ5-avenasterol, 2,4-methylene, and cycloartenol. Brassicasterol and Δ5-avenasterol are present in smaller amounts (Teneva et al., 2014). Cholesterol is found in minimal quantities (0.2%), resulting from the biosynthetic pathway shared with phytosterols via cycloartenol (Younas et al., 2023).

The total sterol content of linseed oil is approximately 0.5%, with β-sitosterol being the predominant component. Sitosterol ranges from 54.8% to 72.9%, followed by stigmasterol and campesterol present at 13.1–26.1% and 3.4–15.0%, respectively (Zuk et al., 2015). Free sterols make up more than 75% of the total sterols, and the rest accounts for sterol esters. Sterol esters and free sterols have similar individual compositions but differ quantitatively; Campesterol and stigmasterol are more prevalent in free sterols (22.1–26.1% and 8.0–15.0%, respectively) than in sterol esters conversely, β-sitosterol is more abundant in sterol esters. There are 12 recognized fatty acids found in sterol esters, with oleic acid accounting for the most (38.0–43.5%), followed by palmitic acid (29.2–34.6%) and stearic acid (8.2–20.5%). Linolenic and linoleic acids are present in smaller amounts (0.3–1.5%) (Sharma et al., 2019) (Table 2).

2.2.3 Tocopherols

Linseed oil has the highest unsaponifiable matter among oilseeds, which correlates to its rich antioxidant profile. Tocopherols are lipid-soluble phytocompounds, present in four isomeric forms: α, β, γ, and δ, each with significant antioxidant and anticancer properties. Linseed oil is characterized by higher tocopherol content but contains relatively lower levels of tocotrienols (Al-Madhagy et al., 2023).

Linseed oil contains tocopherols and tocotrienols, together termed tocochromanols, which have both hydrophilic and hydrophobic properties. Their poly-prenyl side chain and polar moiety, which is produced from tyrosine, are the sources of this duality. Tocopherols have a phytyl-side chain, while tocotrienols have a geranyl-geranyl side chain (Lewinska et al., 2015).

Tocopherol content is substantial in Linseed oil, with approximately 37.4 mg per 100 grams of oil (Alireza et al., 2010). γ-Tocopherol is the predominant form, comprising over 65% of the total tocopherol content, ranging from 248.21 to 516.82 mg/kg. In comparison, the levels of α-tocopherol, averaging about 1–8 mg/kg, β, and

Table 2 Total content of unsaponifiable matter, sterols, and tocopherols in linseed oil

Biologically active components	Content (%)
Unsaponifiable matter % of the oil	1.4
Phospholipid	1.5
Phospholipid fraction, % of Linseed oil	
Phosphatidylglycerol (PG)	1–4
Phosphatidic acid (PA)	1–9
Phosphatidylethanolamine (PE)	27–40
Phosphatidylinositol (PI)	29–32
Phosphatidylcholine (PC)	7–18
Lysophosphatidylcholine (LPC)	8–21
Phytosterols	0.5
Phytosterols fraction (% of Linseed oil)	
Cholesterol	0.2
Brassicasterol	5.9
Campesterol	3.415.0
Stigmasterol	13.1–26.1
β-sitosterol	54.8–72.9
Δ5-avenasterol	1.1
Tocopherol mg/kg of oil	374
γ-Tocopherol mg/kg of oil	248.21 to 516.82
γ-tocotrienol mg/kg of oil	270 to 370

Source: Bayrak et al. (2010), Sharma et al. (2019), Teneva et al. (2014)

δ-tocopherol are relatively lower, making up about 30% of the total tocopherol content (Feng et al., 2022).

The tocopherol content of linseed oil also has a substantial quantity of plastochromanol-8, a functional analog of γ-tocotrienol, which ranges from 270 mg/kg to 370 mg/kg. Studies have shown that γ-tocotrienol and plastochromanol-8 levels correlate positively with temperature and the amount of sunlight received during seed ripening, whereas δ-tocopherol shows a negative correlation (Mueed et al., 2022).

Linseed oil's tocopherol composition sets it apart from other common oils with different predominant tocopherols, like sesame oil (where γ-tocopherol is also the prime component) and sunflower oil (where α-tocopherol predominates), soybean oil (where δ- and γ tocopherols are significant components), and corn oil (where γ-tocopherol is prevalent but also contains traces of δ- and α- tocopherols) (Cheng et al., 2022).

2.2.4 Phenols

Linseed contains numerous phenolic compounds, which can be divided into two groups: lignans and phenolic acids. The total phenolic acids were found to range between 790 and 1030 mg/100 g. Among these, chlorogenic acid, ferulic acid, p-hydroxybenzoic acid, coumaric acid, and vanillic acid constitute the largest portion (Herchi et al., 2014; Zeb, 2021). Linseed oil contains a wide range of phenolic compounds from various classes.

A spectrum of hydroxybenzoic acid derivatives is found in linseed oil, including syringic aldehyde present at concentrations of about 3 to 5 μg/kg, vanillic acid ranges from 0.5 mg/kg, p-hydroxybenzoic acid up to 1.2 mg/kg, protocatechuic acid 1.48 μg/100 g, and vanillin 20–60 μg/kg. Specifically, p-hydroxybenzoic acid and vanillic acid are prominent hydroxybenzoic acid derivatives, with syringic aldehyde present in the oil at 0.3 to 0.5 μg per 100 g. Studies have shown vanillic acid is found at 0.54 mg/kg and p-hydroxybenzoic acid at 1.08 mg/kg in the phenolic dry extract of linseed oil (Zuk et al., 2015).

Linseed also contains various derivatives of hydroxycinnamic acids, another critical group of phenolic compounds. These include ferulic acid, caffeic acid, and other derivatives, namely, ferulic acid methyl ester, ferulic acid 4-glucoside, p-coumaric acid 4- glucoside, and coumaroyl methyl ester, which are present in alkaline and acid hydrolysates of linseed oil (Zeb, 2021). Ferulic acid is the main fingerprinting phenolic compound in the plants of the *Linaceae* family, present in the highest amount. Ferulic acid, caffeic acid, and p-coumaric acid are found in both free form and bound form, the concentration of caffeic acid ranging from 5.18 to 8.7 mg/kg, p-coumaric acid from 9.2 to 17.8 mg/kg, ferulic acid from 3.99 to 46.4 mg/kg as observed in studies (Ma et al., 2023).

- *Ester of hydroxycinnamic acid:* Chlorogenic acid, an ester of quinic and caffeic acid, is a prominent phenolic compound, belonging to the hydroxycinnamic acid group, and is known for its potent antioxidant properties. In linseed oil, chlorogenic acid contributes to the overall phenolic content, enhancing its health benefits and stability (Shim et al., 2014).

Important flavonoids such as epicatechin, kaempferol, quercetin-3-rutinoside, and catechin are abundant in linseed oil. Linseed oils have a total bound flavonoid concentration ranging from 1317 to 2506 mg/kg, while the total free flavonoid content varies from 1026 to 2492 mg/kg, measured as catechin equivalents (Fila et al., 2018). Phenolic compounds, including these flavonoids, are well-known for their potent antioxidant properties and numerous health benefits, including antibacterial, antioxidant, anti-obesity, cardioprotective, antihyperlipidemic, antitumor, antidiabetic, neuroprotective, anti-hepatotoxic effects. Specifically, in refined linseed oil, antioxidants such as myricetin, (+)-catechin, genistein, and caffeic acid are present at concentrations of 555 μmol/kg, enhancing the oil's stability and health-promoting properties (Morya et al., 2022).

2.2.5 Lignin

Lignans are phenolic dimers having low molecular weight and base structure of 2,3-dibenzylbutane primarily located in the seed's outer coat. Plant lignans are phenolic secondary metabolites consisting of two connected phenylpropanoid units (Alireza et al., 2010). They can be classified mainly into furofuran lignans and dibenzylbutane lignans. Examples include secoisolariciresinol diglucoside (SDG) from linseed and sesamin from sesame seeds, which are primary sources of plant lignans and are notable for their antioxidant and phytoestrogenic properties, which result from their conversion into active metabolites by colon bacteria (Rudnik et al., 2001).

Secoisolariciresinol diglucoside (SDG) is the predominant lignan in linseed, matairesinol, pinoresinol, diphyllin, and secoisolariciresinol represent a smaller fraction (Wang et al., 2021). Linseed contains approximately 2653 mg of SDG per 100 g of non-defatted extract, underscoring its status as a significant lignan source; Coniferyl aldehyde is also present at the concentration of 0.5 to 3.0 μg per 100 g of oil. Lignans provide stability to the oil and water mixtures while forming emulsions and nano-emulsions (Xu et al., 2022).

Secoisolariciresinol diglucoside (SDG) consists of two connected phenylpropanoid units with a molecular weight of 686.7 Da. SDG, often referred to simply as secoisolariciresinol or SECO (its aglycone form), exists in two isomeric forms in linseed: (+)-SDG and (−)-SDG, with (+)-SDG being the predominant isomer. In addition to SDG, smaller quantities of other lignans such as matairesinol, lariciresinol, demethoxysecoisolariciresinol, isolariciresinol, and pinoresinol have been identified in linseed. About 75% of the total lignan consumption in ordinary diets comes from pinoresinol and lariciresinol, with the remaining 25% coming from secoisolariciresinol and matairesinol (Mueed et al., 2022).

The plant lignans, including SDG, are phytoestrogens and serve as precursors for mammalian lignans. The intestinal microbiota converts plant lignans into enterolactone and enterodiol, which are metabolites with enhanced antioxidant activity compared to their precursors. These metabolites also exhibit antiplatelet effects and can act as either weak estrogens or antiestrogens, depending on the body's estradiol levels (Franke et al., 2010).

2.2.6 Squalene

Squalene, a triterpene with the molecular formula $C_{30}H_{50}$ and the chemical name 2,6,10,15,19,23-hexamethyl-2,6,10,14,18,22-tetrahexaene, acts as a precursor in the biosynthesis reactions of sterols, and terpenoids including carotenoids, in plants (Dąbrowski et al., 2019). Its structure is highly unsaturated and thus unstable. Squalene is one of the minor components of linseed oil, and its content typically does not exceed 24 mg/kg. Overall, squalene, along with tocopherols and phytosterols, significantly contributes to the functional characteristics and health-promoting properties of linseed oil, making it a superior choice among edible oils (Dumarey et al., 1975).

The inclusion of squalene in the diet is advisable due to its safety and broad health benefits. Employing efficient extraction methods to concentrate squalene in oil is essential because of the limited natural sources of this compound (Sharif et al., 2017).

2.2.7 Cyclolinopeptides (CLs)

The naturally occurring cyclic hydrophobic peptides known as cyclolinopeptides (CLs) are present in linseed oil and fall under type VI peptides, classified explicitly as "Caryophyllaceae Type VI homomonocyclopeptides," and consist of eight or nine amino acid residues, with a molecular weight of approximately 1 kDa. Cyclic peptides in linseed contain proteinogenic amino acids and their oxidized derivatives. The first cyclolinopeptide (CL 1) was identified from sediments recovered from crude linseed oil (Shim et al., 2014). These peptides have been demonstrated to have immunosuppressive properties and to cause apoptosis in stomach cancer cells (SGC-7901) (Morya et al., 2022).

2.2.8 Carotenoids

Carotenoids are 40-carbon organic compounds found in several seeds and fruits, imparting yellow, orange, and red hues and serving as precursors to vitamin A (Tolkachev & Zhuchenko, 2000). β-Carotene, a significant pigment within this group, exhibits the highest pro-vitamin A activity. The carotenoid content in linseed generally ranges from 0.7 to 3.1 mg/kg; a much higher β-carotene content of 77 mg/kg in linseed oil is observed in studies. Additionally, a positive correlation exists between the amount of daylight hours during seed development and levels of tocochromanol and carotenoids in linseed. Carotenoids are crucial for protecting against photo-oxidation, which is particularly important because of the high unsaturated lipid in linseed oil (Goldstein & Reifen, 2022).

2.3 Role of Major and Minor Components of Linseed Oil

Linseed oil stands out among plant-based oils for its unique fatty acid composition, particularly its high content of alpha-linolenic acid (ALA) and a favorable n-6 to n-3 fatty acid ratio of approximately 0.3:1. This balance is advantageous for maintaining a healthy equilibrium of essential fatty acids in the diet (Ciftci et al., 2012). ALA, an essential omega-3 PUFA, naturally cannot be synthesized by the human body, necessitating dietary intake from ALA-rich sources like linseed oil to meet omega-3 requirements. ALA can be metabolized into docosahexaenoic acid (DHA) and eicosapentaenoic acid (EPA), which are crucial for growth, development, and maintaining normal physiological functions (Herchi et al., 2014). However, enzyme competition and limited enzyme efficiency restrict the conversion rate of ALA to DHA and EPA. Enzymes like delta-6 desaturase and elongases are rate-limiting factors, as they also convert linoleic acid (LA) to arachidonic acid (AA), and LA is typically more abundant in the diet. It competes with ALA for these enzymes, reducing the amount of ALA converted to EPA and DHA (Vereshchagin & Novitskaya, 1965). Omega-3 fatty acids in linseed oil have been shown to offer a wide range of health benefits, including protection against infections and the treatment of conditions such as ulcers, migraines, ADHD, eating disorders, preterm labor, emphysema, psoriasis, glaucoma, Lyme disease, lupus, and panic attacks. Linseed oil, in particular, demonstrates a notable ability to reduce the incidence of ulcers and exhibits cytoprotective effects, thereby promoting gastrointestinal health (Campos et al., 2019). The anti-inflammatory and cardioprotective properties of omega-3 fatty acids further enhance the health benefits of linseed oil, making it a valuable addition to a balanced diet.

In addition to ALA, linseed oil contains other fatty acids that contribute to its nutritional profile. Linoleic acid (LA), an omega-6 fatty acid, plays a crucial role in cellular function and metabolism (Wakjira et al., 2004). However, maintaining a balanced intake of omega-6 and omega-3 fatty acids is essential to prevent inflammatory responses associated with excessive omega-6 consumption. Oleic acid, a MUFA present in linseed oil, is known for its beneficial effects on lowering bad cholesterol levels, improving lipid profiles, and maintaining the immune system. The presence of SFA-like palmitic and stearic acids, although in smaller amounts, also contributes to the structural integrity of cell membranes and skin health (Parikh et al., 2018) (Fig. 2).

Phospholipids, phytosterols, tocopherols, and other minor constituents such as phenols, lignans, cyclolinopeptides, and carotenoids of linseed oil play crucial roles in stabilizing the oil and enhancing its functional properties. Phospholipids are essential for stabilizing oil droplets in an aqueous medium by increasing surface pressure and dilational modulus, thus preventing the coalescence of oil droplets, especially when interacting synergistically with oleosins (Beema et al., 2022; Yadav et al., 2018). Moreover, phospholipids significantly increase the solubility of bioactive compounds in oil, enhancing their bioavailability and contributing to the overall stability of oil. Natural phospholipids exhibit an exceptional ability to inhibit the oxidative damage to PUFAs in linseed oil, with higher concentrations (greater than

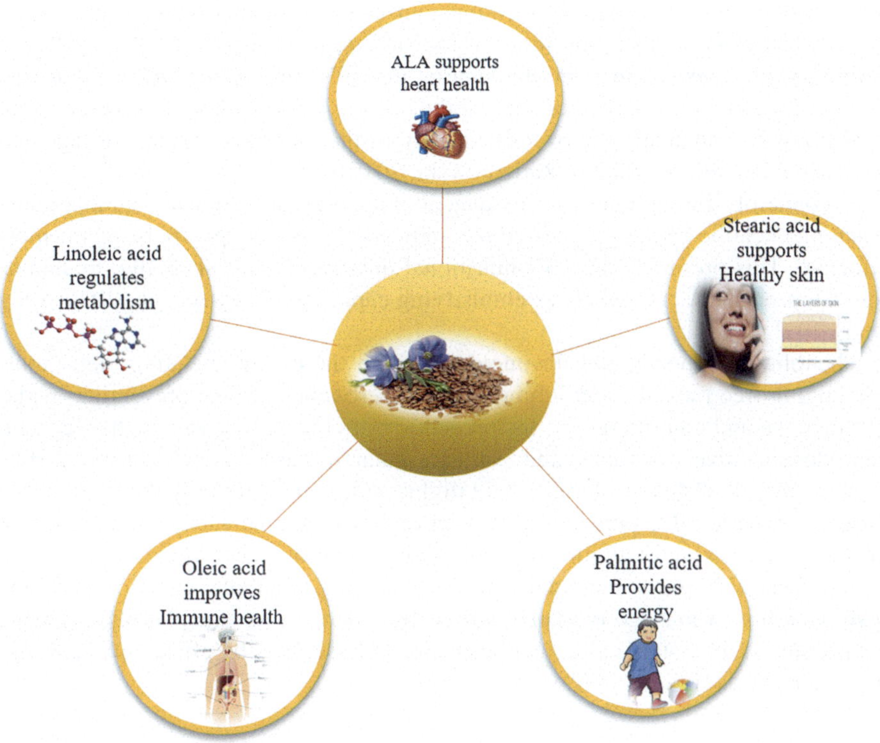

Fig. 2 Illustration of the role of major components of linseed oil

0.2%) showing a notably pronounced effect on storage stability (Bozan & Temelli, 2008). They also interact with trace metals that can catalyze oxidation reactions, thereby mitigating this effect and preserving the integrity of the oil. Additionally, nitrogen-containing phospholipids demonstrate higher hydroperoxide-decomposing activity compared to phosphatidic acids, which is crucial for breaking down initial oxidation products and preventing the propagation of oxidative degradation. By stabilizing oil bodies and preventing oxidation, phospholipids improve the functional properties of linseed oil, maintaining its nutritional quality, extending shelf life, and enhancing its performance in industrial applications (Gutte et al., 2015).

Phytosterols also significantly enhance the stability and functional characteristics of linseed oil. Acting as potent antioxidants, phytosterols such as β-sitosterol and campesterol interrupt oxidative chain reactions by donating hydrogen atoms to lipid radicals, which hinders the propagation of lipid peroxidation, the primary cause of rancidity (Bai et al., 2021). This antioxidant action extends the shelf life of linseed oil and preserves its nutritional quality over time. Furthermore, phytosterols improve the functional properties of linseed oil by enhancing its emulsifying capacity (Bayrak et al., 2010). Their amphiphilic nature allows them to align at oil–water interfaces, stabilizing emulsions crucial for incorporating linseed oil into various food products and industrial applications, ensuring consistent texture and performance. Phytosterols also contribute to the structural integrity of cell membranes within the oil matrix, aiding in maintaining the oil's consistency and resistance to thermal degradation. Their presence modulates the fluidity and phase behavior of lipid bilayers, enhancing the overall stability of the oil under varying storage and processing conditions (Piłat & Zadernowski, 2010).

Tocopherols, through their antioxidant activity, prevent oxidative degradation by donating phenolic hydrogens to lipid free radicals, with α-tocopherol being the most effective. This preserves the oil's nutritional quality, extends shelf life, maintains sensory properties, and enhances emulsifying capacity (Shadyro et al., 2020; Yang et al., 2021).

Phenolic compounds and flavonoids stabilize the oil by chelating metal ions, scavenging free radicals, and inhibiting lipid peroxidation, thus preventing oxidative damage and contributing to the prevention of chronic diseases such as cancer, neurodegenerative disorders, and cardiovascular diseases (Herchi et al., 2014). Lignans like SDG (secoisolariciresinol diglucoside), the chief polyphenol found in linseed, are believed to prevent the production of oxygen radicals, reducing the risk of atherosclerosis and exhibiting potential anticancer properties (Alireza et al., 2010).

Squalene also plays a pivotal role in enhancing metabolic functions and the body's ability to manage oxidative stress. In synergy with tocopherols, squalene contributes to the potent antioxidant capacity of linseed oil by effectively scavenging free radicals (Prasad, 2009).

2.4 Factors Affecting Major and Minor Components of Linseed Oil

Linseed oil is profoundly influenced by a multitude of environmental, genetic, and processing factors that impact its yield, composition, and quality (Bayrak et al., 2010). The oil yield is highly correlated with environmental conditions, whereas the composition of the oil shows a weaker correlation. Specifically, oil yield is closely linked to ALA content, while no significant correlation exists between oil yield and other compositional characters apart from ALA (Čeh et al., 2020).

Key weather conditions, such as pluviometry (rainfall), sunshine hours and degree days (temperature), and water shortages, directly influence oil quality and yield (Fila et al., 2018). While oil-producing linseed variants use less water than other varieties (transpiration coefficients ranging from 300 to 400), adequate rainfall and increased soil water availability (from 40% to 80%) nearly double seed yield per plant and boost oil content by approximately 2.5%. Linseed requires substantial water, about 400–550 mm, during its growth period (Langyan et al., 2023). A cool climate leads to higher oil yields and lower protein content, enhancing the proportion of omega-3 fatty acids. In contrast, a continental temperate climate increases PUFA content while reducing oleic acid levels. High temperatures can negatively affect the soil, indirectly reducing seed and oil yields (Singh et al., 2015). Soil properties significantly impact the linseed growing season. Wet and cold soils in spring can prolong the growing period, while a lack of precipitation and high temperatures in summer often lead to lower seed yields but higher oil content. These soil conditions directly influence the overall productivity and quality of linseed oil (Tomaszewska-Gras et al., 2021).

Genetic factors and seed variety also play a vital part in determining oil characteristics. The ALA content in linseed oil is particularly sensitive to both environmental and genetic factors (Teneva et al., 2014). The oil yield itself is positively associated with the content of PUFA, such as linoleic and linolenic acids, while showing a negative correlation with SFA, like palmitic and stearic acids. A weak positive relationship exists between oil yield and monounsaturated oleic acid content (Farag et al., 2021; Kaur et al., 2023).

Processing and storage facilities also significantly impact the composition and quality of linseed oil. Extraction methods, such as cold pressing and solvent extraction, affect the oil's fatty acid profile and minor component content (Yang et al., 2021). Pretreatment techniques like roasting, at temperatures ranging from 90 to 120 °C, influence the levels of bioactive compounds such as carotenoids, phenols, and flavonoids, as well as antioxidant activity. For instance, the oil content of linseeds can vary between 34.07% and 42.57%, depending on the roasting temperature. Roasting also affects the concentration of dominant phenolic compounds, including isorhamnetin, resveratrol, quercetin, catechin, apigenin-7-glucoside, and kaempferol. Enzyme treatments can enhance oil yield and modify the composition by breaking down cell walls and facilitating the release of oil and bioactive components (Zhang et al., 2020) (Fig. 3).

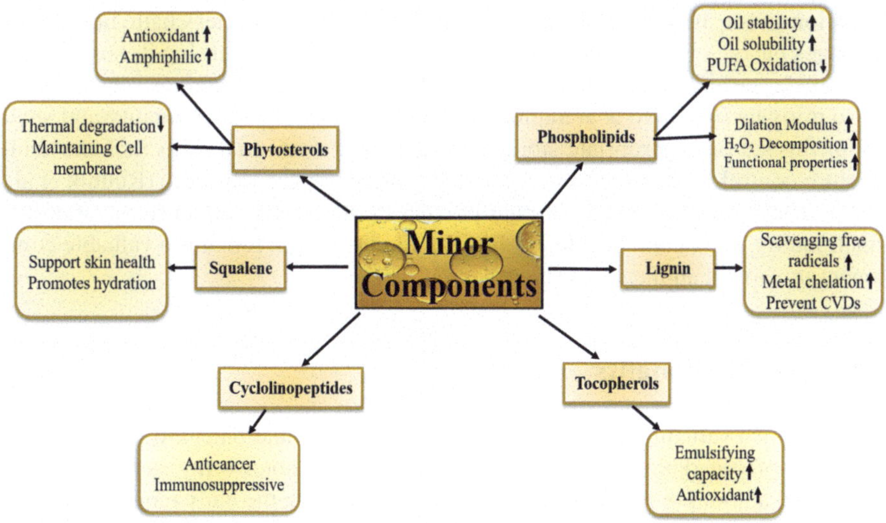

Fig. 3 Illustration of the role of minor components of linseed oil

3 Functional Properties of Linseed Oil

The functional properties of linseed oil are shaped by its fatty acid profile and the presence of bioactive substances, which are critical for its various applications and nutritional value.

3.1 Stability and Shelf Life

The stability and shelf life of linseed oil is significantly influenced by its fatty acid composition. Commercial linseed oil contains 87.33–89.17% USFAs, with linolenic acid being the predominant fatty acid (46.57–4.24%), followed by oleic acid (20.46–24.00%) and linoleic acid (14.06–18.21%) (Bayrak et al., 2010). Notably, the oxidation rate of esters from linolenic acid is 96 times higher than that of oleic acid due to the presence of two bis-allylic carbons in its molecular structure, making it highly prone to oxidation (Kaur et al., 2023).

Unsaturated fatty acids are inherently more susceptible to oxidation, leading to rancidity and a reduced shelf life. This oxidative instability necessitates meticulous handling, storage, and processing to retain the oil's quality and nutritional value (Shadyro et al., 2020). Key indicators of these properties include the saponification number and iodine value, which reflect the amount of alkali required to saponify a given quantity of oil and the degree of unsaturation in the oil, respectively (Rudnik et al., 2001). A high saponification number indicates a higher proportion of lower molecular weight fatty acids, while a high iodine value suggests a higher proportion of unsaturated fatty acids, particularly polyunsaturated fatty acids (PUFAs) like alpha-linolenic acid (ALA) (Piironen et al., 2000). These properties confirm the oxidation-prone nature of linseed oil; the presence of shorter-chain fatty acids enhances the oil's fluidity and decreases its melting point, increasing its susceptibility to oxidation and limiting its industrial and culinary usage (Topnikova et al., 2022).

To mitigate oxidative degradation and maintain the nutritional quality and shelf life of linseed oil, appropriate storage conditions are essential. This includes temperature control, protection from light, and limited oxygen exposure (Rudnik et al., 2001). These processing and storage practices collectively influence the stability, functionality, and health benefits of linseed oil, ensuring it remains a valuable component in various applications (Bayrak et al., 2010).

3.2 Health Benefits

Linseeds are a valuable dietary source of both omega-3 and omega-6 fatty acids. In the realm of vegetable oils, linseed oil is particularly noteworthy as it provides a substantial amount of these essential fatty acids, meeting the daily requirements for maintaining optimal health (Katoch & Bhatia, 2021). For a balanced diet, the minimum daily requirement for omega-6 PUFAs is approximately 3% of total energy intake, which equates to about 60 kcal or 6.6 grams for a 2000 kcal diet. Similarly, the minimum requirement for omega-3 PUFAs ranges from 0.6% to 1.2% of total energy intake, translating to approximately 20 kcal or 2.2 grams per day for the same diet (Zuk et al., 2015). Essential PUFAs play crucial roles in the body. Omega-6 PUFAs are predominant in most cells, contributing significantly to the structure of cell membranes. In contrast, omega-3 PUFAs are highly concentrated in brain cells and nerve tissues, highlighting their importance for neurological health and cognitive function (Gandova et al., 2023). Long-chain PUFAs derived from omega-3 and omega-6 fatty acids are vital for growth and development, supporting a range of physiological functions (Goyal et al., 2014).

3.3 Nutraceutical and Therapeutic Properties

Linseed oil's impressive nutraceutical and therapeutic properties are largely attributed to its rich composition of alpha-linolenic acid (ALA) and a diverse array of minor bioactive compounds. ALA, a crucial omega-3 fatty acid, works synergistically with bioactive compounds such as cyclolinopeptides and phytosterols to exert significant anti-inflammatory effects (Campos et al., 2019). This combination makes linseed oil highly beneficial for managing inflammatory conditions, including arthritis and cardiovascular diseases. The high ALA content, in conjunction with phytosterols, supports heart health by reducing blood cholesterol levels, improving lipid profiles, and lowering blood pressure (Prasad, 2009).

Phytosterols in linseed oil play a pivotal role in delaying digestion by preventing bile salts from adhering to oil droplets and inhibiting bile salt-induced lipase interfacial adsorption (Piironen et al., 2000). These compounds also contribute to the prevention and treatment of hypercholesterolemia by lowering total and LDL cholesterol levels. Notably, cycloartenol and 2,4-methylene cycloartenol have shown potential in traditional diabetes treatments, with studies indicating that these compounds can ameliorate symptoms in type II diabetic, suggesting that linseed oil could be valuable for diabetes prevention due to its high bioactive phytochemical content (Shadyro et al., 2020).

Polyphenolic compounds in linseed oil act as metal ion chelators, free radical scavengers, and inhibitors of lipid peroxidation, thereby preventing oxidative damage. (Vereshchagin & Novitskaya, 1965). This action contributes to the prevention of chronic illnesses such as cancer, cardiovascular disease, and neurodegenerative disorders. The presence of flavonoids and phenolic compounds underscores the importance of linseed oil as a nutritional and functional food component with significant therapeutic potential (Cheng et al., 2022).

The health benefits of lignans in linseed oil are notable, mainly due to the antioxidant activities of their metabolites, enterolactone and enterodiol (Xu et al., 2022). These metabolites are believed to prevent the production of oxygen radicals, reducing the risk of atherosclerosis and exhibiting potential anticancer properties (Wu et al., 2022).

Additionally, linseed oil's rich composition of squalene and tocopherols supports skin health by protecting against oxidative damage and promoting hydration (Ali et al., 2019). Cyclolinopeptides, another minor constituent, offer significant functional characteristics, including potential anticancer and immunosuppressive properties. Carotenoids, particularly β-carotene, not only impart color but also act as precursors to vitamin A with antioxidant and immune boosting properties (Parikh et al., 2018).

4 Conclusion

This chapter has explored the detailed composition of linseed oil, focusing on its major and minor constituents and their roles in stability, functionality, and health benefits. The primary fatty acids—linolenic, oleic, and linoleic acids—offer significant health advantages, such as anti-inflammatory properties and cardiovascular protection.

Minor constituents, including phytosterols, phospholipids, tocopherols, polyphenols, and carotenoids, enhance the oil's quality. Phytosterols act as antioxidants and improve emulsification properties, phospholipids stabilize oil droplets and enhance bioavailability, and tocopherols prevent oxidative degradation. Polyphenols and flavonoids provide additional antioxidant protection, and carotenoids protect against photo-oxidation and enhance the oil's visual appeal. Environmental and genetic factors, along with processing and storage conditions, significantly influence linseed oil's composition. Cooler climates and optimal water availability improve oil yield and omega-3 content, while appropriate processing techniques, such as extraction, roasting, and enzyme treatments, refine the oil's bioactive compound levels. Adequate storage conditions are essential to maintain stability and nutritional quality.

Future research and innovation can focus on optimizing cultivation and processing methods to enhance the beneficial properties of linseed oil. Additionally, exploring the synergistic effects of its various constituents can lead to the development of specialized linseed oil products tailored for specific health benefits and industrial applications. The valorization of linseed oil, leveraging its comprehensive nutrient profile, promises to advance its role in nutrition, health, and industry, marking it as a valuable resource in the quest for sustainable and functional food ingredients.

References

Ali, A. H., Zou, X., Abed, S. M., Korma, S. A., Jin, Q., & Wang, X. (2019). Natural phospholipids: Occurrence, biosynthesis, separation, identification, and beneficial health aspects. *Critical Reviews in Food Science and Nutrition, 59*(2), 253–275. https://doi.org/10.1080/10408398.2017.1363714

Alireza, S. M., Trey, S. M., Henriksson, G., & Johansson, M. (2010). Effect of model lignin structures on the oxidation of unsaturated fatty acids. *Polymers from Renewable Resources, 1*(2), 69–90. https://doi.org/10.1177/204124791000100201

Al-Madhagy, S., Ashmawy, N. S., Mamdouh, A., Eldahshan, O. A., & Farag, M. A. (2023). A comprehensive review of the health benefits of flaxseed oil in relation to its chemical composition and comparison with other omega-3-rich oils. *European Journal of Medical Research, 28*(1), 240. https://doi.org/10.1186/s40001-023-01203-6

Bai, G., Ma, C., & Chen, X. (2021). Phytosterols in edible oil: Distribution, analysis and variation during processing. *Grain & Oil Science and Technology, 4*(1), 33–44. https://doi.org/10.1016/j.gaost.2020.12.003

Bayrak, A., Kiralan, M., Ipek, A., Arslan, N., Cosge, B., & Khawar, K. M. (2010). Fatty acid compositions of linseed (*Linum Usitatissimum* L.) genotypes of different origin cultivated in Turkey. *Biotechnology & Biotechnological Equipment, 24*(2), 1836–1842. https://doi.org/10.2478/V10133-010-0034-2

Beema, N., Mukkamula, N., Srinivas, M., Ravinder, T., Azmeera, T., & Kiran Kumar, B. (2022). Comparative analysis of physico-chemical properties and fatty acid composition of linseed (Linum usitatissimum L.) oils of Indian accessions. *Journal of Applied Biology & Biotechnology.* https://doi.org/10.7324/JABB.2023.110112

Bekhit, A. E.-D. A., Shavandi, A., Jodjaja, T., Birch, J., Teh, S., Mohamed Ahmed, I. A., Al-Juhaimi, F. Y., Saeedi, P., & Bekhit, A. A. (2018). Flaxseed: Composition, detoxification, utilization, and opportunities. *Biocatalysis and Agricultural Biotechnology, 13*, 129–152. https://doi.org/10.1016/j.bcab.2017.11.017

Bozan, B., & Temelli, F. (2008). Chemical composition and oxidative stability of flax, safflower and poppy seed and seed oils. *Bioresource Technology, 99*(14), 6354–6359. https://doi.org/10.1016/j.biortech.2007.12.009

Campos, J. R., Severino, P., Ferreira, C. S., Zielinska, A., Santini, A., Souto, S. B., & Souto, E. B. (2019). Linseed essential oil – Source of lipids as active ingredients for pharmaceuticals and nutraceuticals. *Current Medicinal Chemistry, 26*(24), 4537–4558. https://doi.org/10.2174/0929867325666181031105603

Čeh, B., Štraus, S., Hladnik, A., & Kušar, A. (2020). Impact of linseed variety, location and production year on seed yield, oil content and its composition. *Agronomy, 10*(11), 1770. https://doi.org/10.3390/agronomy10111770

Cheng, C., Yu, K., Yu, X., Geng, F., Huang, F., Wang, L., Huang, Q., Quan, S., & Deng, Q. (2022). Optimized endogenous lipid concomitants in flaxseed oil by different oil extraction technologies: Their positive roles in emulsions. *LWT, 155*, 113000. https://doi.org/10.1016/j.lwt.2021.113000

Ciftci, O. N., Przybylski, R., & Rudzińska, M. (2012). Lipid components of flax, perilla, and chia seeds. *European Journal of Lipid Science and Technology, 114*(7), 794–800. https://doi.org/10.1002/ejlt.201100207

Dąbrowski, G., Czaplicki, S., & Konopka, I. (2019). Fractionation of sterols, tocols and squalene in flaxseed oils under the impact of variable conditions of supercritical CO2 extraction. *Journal of Food Composition and Analysis, 83*, 103261. https://doi.org/10.1016/j.jfca.2019.103261

Dixit, S., Kanakraj, S., & Rehman, A. (2012). Linseed oil as a potential resource for bio-diesel: A review. *Renewable and Sustainable Energy Reviews, 16*(7), 4415–4421. https://doi.org/10.1016/j.rser.2012.04.042

Dumarey, C., Sket, D., Joseph, D., & Boquet, P. (1975). [Basic phospholipase of Naja nigricollis venom]. *Comptes Rendus Hebdomadaires Des Seances De l'Academie Des Sciences. Serie D: Sciences Naturelles, 280*(13), 1633–1635.

Farag, M. A., Elimam, D. M., & Afifi, S. M. (2021). Outgoing and potential trends of the omega-3 rich linseed oil quality characteristics and rancidity management: A comprehensive review for maximizing its food and nutraceutical applications. *Trends in Food Science & Technology, 114*, 292–309. https://doi.org/10.1016/j.tifs.2021.05.041

Feng, S., Wang, L., Shao, P., Sun, P., & Yang, C. S. (2022). A review on chemical and physical modifications of phytosterols and their influence on bioavailability and safety. *Critical Reviews in Food Science and Nutrition, 62*(20), 5638–5657. https://doi.org/10.1080/10408398.2021.1888692

Fila, G., Bagatta, M., Maestrini, C., Potenza, E., & Matteo, R. (2018). Linseed as a dual-purpose crop: Evaluation of cultivar suitability and analysis of yield determinants. *The Journal of Agricultural Science, 156*(2), 162–176. https://doi.org/10.1017/S0021859618000114

Franke, S., Fröhlich, K., Werner, S., Böhm, V., & Schöne, F. (2010). Analysis of carotenoids and vitamin E in selected oilseeds, press cakes and oils. *European Journal of Lipid Science and Technology, 112*(10), 1122–1129. https://doi.org/10.1002/ejlt.200900251

Gandova, V., Teneva, O., Petkova, Z., Iliev, I., & Stoyanova, A. (2023). Lipid composition and physicochemical parameters of flaxseed oil (Linum usitatissimum L.) from Bulgaria. *Applied Sciences, 13*(18), 10141. https://doi.org/10.3390/app131810141

Goldstein, N., & Reifen, R. (2022). The potential of legume-derived proteins in the food industry. *Grain & Oil Science and Technology, 5*(4), 167–178. https://doi.org/10.1016/j.gaost.2022.06.002

Goyal, A., Sharma, V., Upadhyay, N., Gill, S., & Sihag, M. (2014). Flax and flaxseed oil: An ancient medicine & modern functional food. *Journal of Food Science and Technology, 51*(9), 1633–1653. https://doi.org/10.1007/s13197-013-1247-9

Gutte, K. B., Sahoo, A. K., & Ranveer, R. C. (2015). Bioactive components of flaxseed and its health benefits. *Reproduct Ion, 09*.

Herchi, W., Arráez-Román, D., Trabelsi, H., Bouali, I., Boukhchina, S., Kallel, H., Segura-Carretero, A., & Fernández-Gutierrez, A. (2014). Phenolic compounds in flaxseed: A review of their properties and analytical methods. An overview of the last decade. *Journal of Oleo Science, 63*(1), 7–14. https://doi.org/10.5650/jos.ess13135

Katoch, M., & Bhatia, N. (2021). Linseed and its basic composition. *International Journal of Advances in Agricultural Science and Technology, 8*, 10–26. https://doi.org/10.47856/ijaast.2021.v08i6.002

Kaur, V., Gomashe, S. S., Aravind, J., Yadav, S. K., Sheela, Singh, D., Chauhan, S. S., Kumar, V., Jat, B., Tayade, N. R., Saroha, A., Kaushik, N., Langyan, S., Singh, M., Wankhede, D. P., Singh, K., Kumar, A., & Singh, G. P. (2023). Multi-environment phenotyping of linseed (Linum usitatissimum L.) germplasm for morphological and seed quality traits to assemble a core collection. *Industrial Crops and Products, 206*, 117657. https://doi.org/10.1016/j.indcrop.2023.117657

Kostik, V., Memeti, S., & Bauer, B. (2013). Fatty acid composition of edible oils and fats. *Journal of Hygienic Engineering and Design, 4*, 112–116.

Langyan, S., Yadava, P., Khan, F. N., Sharma, S., Singh, R., Bana, R. S., Singh, N., Kaur, V., Kalia, S., & Kumar, A. (2023). Trends and advances in pre- and post-harvest processing of linseed oil for quality food and health products. *Critical Reviews in Food Science and Nutrition, 1–24*, 746. https://doi.org/10.1080/10408398.2023.2280768

Lewinska, A., Zebrowski, J., Duda, M., Gorka, A., & Wnuk, M. (2015). Fatty acid profile and biological activities of linseed and rapeseed oils. *Molecules, 20*(12), 12. https://doi.org/10.3390/molecules201219887

Long, J., Fu, Y., Zu, Y., Li, J., Wang, W., Gu, C., & Luo, M. (2011). Ultrasound-assisted extraction of flaxseed oil using immobilized enzymes. *Bioresource Technology, 102*(21), 9991–9996. https://doi.org/10.1016/j.biortech.2011.07.104

Ma, G., Wang, Y., Li, Y., Zhang, L., Gao, Y., Li, Q., & Yu, X. (2023). Antioxidant properties of lipid concomitants in edible oils: A review. *Food Chemistry, 422*, 136219. https://doi.org/10.1016/j.foodchem.2023.136219

Morya, S., Menaa, F., Jiménez-López, C., Lourenço-Lopes, C., BinMowyna, M. N., & Alqahtani, A. (2022). Nutraceutical and pharmaceutical behavior of bioactive compounds of miracle oilseeds: An overview. *Foods, 11*(13), 1824. https://doi.org/10.3390/foods11131824

Mueed, A., Shibli, S., Korma, S. A., Madjirebaye, P., Esatbeyoglu, T., & Deng, Z. (2022). Flaxseed bioactive compounds: Chemical composition, functional properties, food applications and health benefits-related gut microbes. *Foods, 11*(20), 3307. https://doi.org/10.3390/foods11203307

Pali, V., & Mehta, N. (2014). Evaluation of oil content and fatty acid compositions of flax (Linum usitatissimum L.) varieties of India. *Journal of Agricultural Science, 6*. https://doi.org/10.5539/jas.v6n9p198

Parikh, M., Netticadan, T., & Pierce, G. N. (2018). Flaxseed: Its bioactive components and their cardiovascular benefits. *American Journal of Physiology-Heart and Circulatory Physiology, 314*(2), H146–H159. https://doi.org/10.1152/ajpheart.00400.2017

Piironen, V., Toivo, J., & Lampi, A.-M. (2000). Natural sources of dietary plant sterols. *Journal of Food Composition and Analysis, 13*(4), 619–624. https://doi.org/10.1006/jfca.2000.0898

Piłat, B., & Zadernowski, R. (2010). Physicochemical characteristics of linseed oil and flour. *Polish Journal of Natural Science, 25*(1), 106–113. https://doi.org/10.2478/v10020-010-0008-8

Prasad, K. (2009). Flaxseed and cardiovascular health. *Journal of Cardiovascular Pharmacology, 54*(5), 369–377. https://doi.org/10.1097/FJC.0b013e3181af04e5

Rudnik, E., Szczucinska, A., Gwardiak, H., Szulc, A., & Winiarska, A. (2001). Comparative studies of oxidative stability of linseed oil. *Thermochimica Acta, 370*(1), 135–140. https://doi.org/10.1016/S0040-6031(00)00781-4

Saleem, M. H., Ali, S., Hussain, S., Kamran, M., Chattha, M. S., Ahmad, S., Aqeel, M., Rizwan, M., Aljarba, N. H., Alkahtani, S., & Abdel-Daim, M. M. (2020). Flax (Linum usitatissimum L.): A potential candidate for phytoremediation? *Biological and Economical Points of View. Plants, 9*(4), 496. https://doi.org/10.3390/plants9040496

Shadyro, O., Sosnovskaya, A., & Edimecheva, I. (2020). Effect of biologically active substances on oxidative stability of flaxseed oil. *Journal of Food Science and Technology, 57*(1), 243–252. https://doi.org/10.1007/s13197-019-04054-4

Shakya, L., Singh, A., Agnihotri, A., Muyal, J. P., Umar, S., Barwa, S., & Dhiman, S. K. (2023). Various approaches used to increase the growth and yield of linseed linseed crop. *International Journal of Plant and Environment, 9*(04), 291–300.

Sharif, H. R., Williams, P. A., Sharif, M. K., Khan, M. A., Majeed, H., Safdar, W., Shamoon, M., Shoaib, M., Haider, J., & Zhong, F. (2017). Influence of OSA-starch on the physico chemical characteristics of flax seed oil-eugenol nanoemulsions. *Food Hydrocolloids, 66*, 365–377. https://doi.org/10.1016/j.foodhyd.2016.12.002

Sharma, M., Dadhwal, K., Gat, Y., Kumar, V., Panghal, A., Prasad, R., Kaur, S., & Gat, P. (2019). A review on newer techniques in extraction of oleaginous flaxseed constituents. *OCL, 26*, 14. https://doi.org/10.1051/ocl/2019006

Shim, Y. Y., Gui, B., Arnison, P. G., Wang, Y., & Reaney, M. J. T. (2014). Flaxseed (*Linum usitatissimum* L.) bioactive compounds and peptide nomenclature: A review. *Trends in Food Science & Technology, 38*(1), 5–20. https://doi.org/10.1016/j.tifs.2014.03.011

Singh, R., Singh, T. P., & Dutta, M. (2015). Linseed: An oilseed crop with multiple uses. *Indian Farming, 63*(1). https://epubs.icar.org.in/index.php/IndFarm/article/download/53842/22782/133134

Teneva, O. T., Zlatanov, M. D., Antova, G. A., Angelova-Romova, M. Y., & Marcheva, M. P. (2014). Lipid composition of flaxseeds. *Bulgarian Chemical Communications, 46*(3), 465–472.

Tolkachev, O. N., & Zhuchenko, A. A. (2000). No title found. *Pharmaceutical Chemistry Journal, 34*(7), 360–367. https://doi.org/10.1023/A:1005217407453

Tomaszewska-Gras, J., Islam, M., Grzeca, L., Kaczmarek, A., & Fornal, E. (2021). Comprehensive thermal characteristics of different cultivars of flaxseed oil (Linum usittatissimum L.). *Molecules, 26*(7), 7. https://doi.org/10.3390/molecules26071958

Topnikova, E. V., Pirogova, E. N., & Danilova, E. S. (2022). Quality assessment of linseed oil. *IOP Conference Series: Earth and Environmental Science, 1052*(1), 012096. https://doi.org/10.1088/1755-1315/1052/1/012096

Tripathi, V., Abidi, A. B., Marker, S., & Bilal, S. (2013). Linseed and linseed oil: Health benefits – A review. *International Journal of Pharmacy and Biological Sciences, 3*(3), 434.

Vereshchagin, A. G., & Novitskaya, G. V. (1965). The triglyceride composition of linseed oil. *Journal of the American Oil Chemists' Society, 42*(11), 970–974. https://doi.org/10.1007/BF02632457

Wakjira, A., Labuschagne, M. T., & Hugo, A. (2004). Variability in oil content and fatty acid composition of Ethiopian and introduced cultivars of linseed. *Journal of the Science of Food and Agriculture, 84*(6), 601–607. https://doi.org/10.1002/jsfa.1698

Wang, X., Yu, K., Cheng, C., Peng, D., Yu, X., Chen, H., Chen, Y., Julian McClements, D., & Deng, Q. (2021). Effect of sesamol on the physical and chemical stability of plant-based flaxseed oil-in-water emulsions stabilized by proteins or phospholipids. *Food & Function, 12*(5), 2090–2101. https://doi.org/10.1039/D0FO02420A

Wu, L., Zhao, J., Wu, L., Zhang, Y., & Li, J. (2022). Simultaneous determination of squalene, tocopherols and phytosterols in edible vegetable oil by SPE combined with saponification and GC-MS. *LWT, 169*, 114026. https://doi.org/10.1016/j.lwt.2022.114026

Xu, Z., Liu, S., Shen, M., Xie, J., & Yang, J. (2022). Evaluation of *trans* fatty acids, carbonyl compounds and bioactive minor components in commercial linseed oils. *Food Chemistry, 369*, 130930. https://doi.org/10.1016/j.foodchem.2021.130930

Yadav, R. K., Singh, M., Roy, S., Ansari, M., & N., Saeedan, A. S., & Kaithwas, G. (2018). Modulation of oxidative stress response by flaxseed oil: Role of lipid peroxidation and underlying mechanisms. *Prostaglandins & Other Lipid Mediators, 135*, 21–26. https://doi.org/10.1016/j.prostaglandins.2018.02.003

Yang, J., Wen, C., Duan, Y., Deng, Q., Peng, D., Zhang, H., & Ma, H. (2021). The composition, extraction, analysis, bioactivities, bioavailability and applications in food system of flaxseed (*Linum usitatissimum* L.) oil: A review. *Trends in Food Science & Technology, 118*, 252–260. https://doi.org/10.1016/j.tifs.2021.09.025

Yasmeen, M., Nisar, S., Tavallali, V., & Khalid, T. (2018). A review of phytochemicals and uses of flaxseed.

Younas, R., Sahar, A., Sameen, A., Khan, M. I., Ali, M. A., Tahir, M. A., Mohsin, M., Usman, M., & Aadil, R. M. (2023). A narrative review on extraction techniques of phytosterols and their applications in food industry. *Biomass Conversion and Biorefinery, 14*, 30897. https://doi.org/10.1007/s13399-023-05007-w

Zeb, A. (2021). A comprehensive review on different classes of polyphenolic compounds present in edible oils. *Food Research International, 143*, 110312. https://doi.org/10.1016/j.foodres.2021.110312

Zeng, J., Xiao, T., Ni, X., Wei, T., Liu, X., Deng, Z.-Y., & Li, J. (2022). The comparative analysis of different oil extraction methods based on the quality of flaxseed oil. *Journal of Food Composition and Analysis, 107*, 104373. https://doi.org/10.1016/j.jfca.2021.104373

Zhang, D., Li, X., Duan, X., Sun, H., & Cao, Y. (2021). Lipidomics reveals the changes in lipid profile of flaxseed oil affected by roasting. *Food Chemistry, 364*, 130431. https://doi.org/10.1016/j.foodchem.2021.130431

Zhang, Y., Li, T., Xu, Z., Liu, R., Zhang, H., Wang, X., Huang, J., & Jin, Q. (2020). Comparison of the characteristics and oxidation kinetic parameters of flaxseed (*Linum usitatissimum L.*) oil products with different refining degree. *Journal of Food Processing and Preservation, 44*(10). https://doi.org/10.1111/jfpp.14753

Zuk, M., Richter, D., Matuła, J., & Szopa, J. (2015). Linseed, the multipurpose plant. *Industrial Crops and Products, 75*, 165–177. https://doi.org/10.1016/j.indcrop.2015.05.005

Shelf Life of Linseed Oil: Challenges and Mitigation Strategies

Priyanka Kumari Singh and Meenakshi Garg

Abstract

Linseed (*Linum usitatissimum L.*) oil, recognized for its high alpha-linolenic acid content, offers significant health benefits, but high polyunsaturated fatty acid (PUFA) content results in oxidation. This oxidation leads to the accumulation of undesirable compounds, which results in taste deterioration and nutrient loss and is harmful to health. Addressing these challenges is crucial for enhancing the stability of linseed oil in food applications. This chapter explores strategies to mitigate lipid oxidation in flaxseed oil, focusing on recent advancements such as novel oil extraction technology, oil modification technology (blending and inter-esterification), encapsulation, and antioxidant enrichment. Research efforts aimed at improving oxidative stability through innovative approaches are reviewed, highlighting the potential of these strategies to sustain the nutritional integrity and quality of linseed oil products in various food formulations.

Keywords

Lipid oxidation · Oxidative stability · Oil modification · Encapsulation · Antioxidant enrichment

P. Kumari Singh
Department of Food and Nutrition and Food Technology, Institute of Home Economics, University of Delhi, New Delhi, India

M. Garg (✉)
Department of Food Technology, Bhaskaracharya College of Applied Sciences, University of Delhi, New Delhi, India
e-mail: meenakshi.garg@bcas.du.ac.in

© The Author(s), under exclusive license to Springer Nature Singapore Pte Ltd. 2025

R. Chopra et al. (eds.), *Dynamics of Linseed and its Valorization*,
https://doi.org/10.1007/978-981-96-8927-9_7

1 Introduction

Linseed (*Linum usitatissimum L.*), also referred as flaxseed, stands out as a primitive plant species renowned for its diverse applications and nutritional advantages, notably its rich in omega-3 fatty acids content (Douny et al., 2016). Omega-3 is an essential fatty acid crucial for regulating cholesterol levels, blood pressure, and cognitive function in the human body (Simopoulos & DiNicolantonio, 2016). Despite its nutritional richness, ensuring the shelf life of linseed oil, a beneficial omega-3-rich food along with polyphenols and various bioactive compounds, presents significant challenges due to its susceptibility to oxidation. Lipid oxidation degrades the nutritional and sensory quality of linseed oil and limits its use in the food industry.

Recent research has increasingly focused on mitigation strategies aimed at extending the shelf-life of linseed oil. Innovative approaches such as active packaging, oil modification methods, novel extraction technology and antioxidant incorporation have garnered attention for their potential to retard oxidation processes. These strategies function by either creating protective barriers or directly scavenging free radicals that initiate lipid oxidation. Implementing effective mitigation strategies is crucial not only to extend the shelf life of linseed oil but also for preserving its health-promoting properties and meeting consumer expectations for high-quality, stable products.

This chapter explores recent advancements in reducing oxidation in linseed oil to preserve its nutritional and sensory characteristics. Given its high susceptibility to lipid oxidation, various strategies have been developed to enhance its shelf life and stability. Various key strategies involving oil modification techniques like blending and interesterification, active packaging to minimize oxygen exposure, and antioxidant incorporation to counteract free radicals contribute to preserving the oil's quality. These methods enhance its stability, ensuring its effectiveness as a health-promoting ingredient. By reviewing these innovative techniques, this chapter highlights their significance in sustaining the linseed functionality of oil in food applications while achieving consumer demand for high-quality and stable products.

2 Linseed Oil and Oxidation

There is a rising demand for nutritious, healthier, more natural foods in modern lifestyles. However, the dietary imbalance between excessive intake of omega-6 fatty acids and insufficient omega-3 PUFAs has raised concerns about health risks like atherosclerosis and obesity (Zhang et al., 2019). Consequently, there's growing interest in food commodities enriched in omega-3 fatty acids. Linseed oil, known for ALA-rich, serves as a significant omega-3 PUFA source. Yet, its susceptibility to oxidation due to its PUFA content compromises its nutritional value. Additionally, its lipophilic nature and limited oral bioavailability have restricted its application in hydrophilic food matrices (Ayelign & Alemu, 2016).

There is a rising demand for healthier, more natural foods in contemporary lifestyles. However, concerns have emerged about health risks such as atherosclerosis and obesity due to the dietary imbalance between excessive consumption of omega-6 PUFA and inadequate omega-3 PUFAs (Zhang et al., 2019). Consequently, there is growing interest in food products enriched with ω-3 PUFAs. Linseed oil, renowned for its high levels of α-linolenic acid (ALA), represents a significant source of ω-3 PUFAs. Nevertheless, its susceptibility to oxidation, stemming from its PUFA content, compromises its nutritional value. Moreover, its lipophilic nature and limited oral bioavailability have constrained its utilization in hydrophilic food matrices (Ayelign & Alemu, 2016).

Linseed oil is rich in USFAs, comprising between 87.8% and 89.8%, and contains only a small proportion of saturated fatty acids (SFAs), which range from 7% to 8%. It also has a moderate amount of monounsaturated fatty acids, ranging from 16% to 18% (Goyal et al., 2014). The primary fatty acids in linseed oil include ALA (C18:3, n-3), which constitutes 49% to 53%, linoleic acid (C18:2, n-6) at 15% to 17%, and oleic acid (C18:1, n-9) at around 16% to 21%. These levels can vary due to different environmental factors and growth conditions (Rubilar et al., 2010). Linseed oil is also abundant in various phytosterols and phenolic compounds, contributing to its antioxidant properties. It contains a significant amount of sterols, ranging from 4720 to 7550 mg/kg of oil, including β-sitosterols (240 mg/100 g), campesterol (110 mg/100 g), and stigmasterol (50 mg/100 g) (Dąbrowski et al., 2019; Han et al., 2015). Additionally, linseed oil is rich in γ-tocopherols (460–610 mg/kg) and tocochromanols (154–934 mg/kg) along with the lower level of plastochromanol-8, a and α-tocopherol (Mène-Saffrané & DellaPenna, 2010; Obranović et al., 2015). Linseed oil has been reported to contain specific phenolics, such as p-hydroxybenzoic, p-coumaric, and vanillic acids, and ferulic, either in free or conjugated forms (Hasiewicz-Derkacz et al., 2015; Herchi et al., 2011).

2.1 Mechanism of Oxidation

The oxidation of linseed oil presents a significant challenge, impacting its quality and suitability for consumption. Similar to other fats and oils, linseed oil is susceptible to oxidation, resulting in the development of off-flavors, degradation of essential nutrients and bioactive compounds, and the potential formation of harmful substances, thereby compromising its safety (Barden & Decker, 2016). This process leads to the development of unpleasant flavors, degradation of essential nutrients and bioactive compounds, and can even generate harmful substances, rendering lipid-containing foods unsuitable for consumption.

The mechanisms of fat and oil oxidation primarily fall into three categories: autoxidation, photosensitized oxidation, and enzymatic oxidation, depending on the oxygen species involved (Shahidi & Zhong, 2010). Atmospheric triplet oxygen ($^3O_2$) initiates autoxidation, characterized by a chain reaction involving free radicals. In contrast, singlet oxygen ($^1O_2$), an energized state of oxygen, can be formed from triplet oxygen through various processes, including chemical, photochemical,

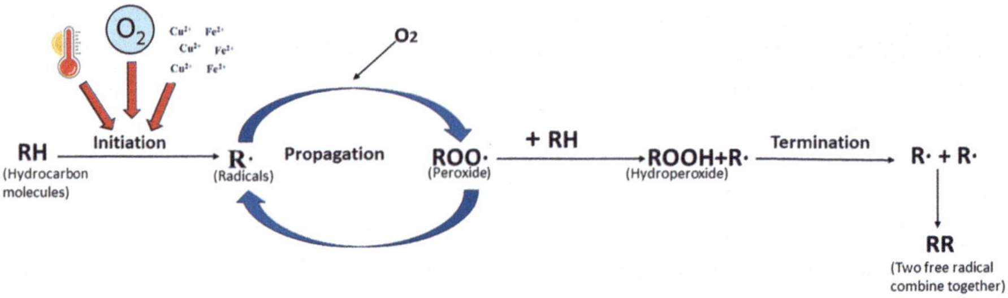

Fig. 1 A scheme showing steps of oxidation in linseed oil

and enzymatic pathways. Additionally, singlet oxygen can arise from the decomposition of hydroperoxides during photosensitized oxidation. These mechanisms highlight the diverse pathways through which oxidation can occur in fats and oils, emphasizing the need for comprehensive strategies to mitigate its detrimental effects (Diaz-Uribe et al., 2022; Van Dyck, 2010). Initially, hydroperoxides (ROOH) decompose bimolecularly to produce alkyl and peroxyl radicals (R•, ROO•). In the propagation step, these radicals react with oxygen (O_2) and the substrate (RH) (Fig. 1). The final termination reaction involves the combination of radical species to form inert products. The following equation illustrates these reactions, shedding light on the detailed mechanisms of linseed oil oxidation.

2.2 Factors Affecting Lipid Oxidation

During the processing and storage of fats and oils, a variety of chemical reactions take place, resulting in the formation of potentially detrimental compounds. The primary pathways of degradation involve oxidation, hydrolysis, and thermal degradation. Elevated temperatures can induce oxidation, decomposition, polymerization, and condensation of lipids, generating free fatty acids (FFA), hydroperoxides, aldehydes, as well as dimers and trimers, contributing to a deterioration in food quality. The oxidation of fats and oils involves complex reactions, with common methods being autoxidation, photooxidation, and enzymatic oxidation (Choe & Min, 2006; Shahidi & Zhong, 2010). These oxidation processes, facilitated by oxygen, significantly impact the quality of food during both storage and processing.

Research on the oxidation of linseed oil has been extensive, employing various analytical methods. Empirical models highlight the influence of environmental factors like oxygen levels, humidity, temperature, and exposure time on the oxidative behavior of the oil (Afik et al., 2020). Linseed oil oxidation typically progresses through initiation, propagation, and termination stages, involving radical generation, oxygen absorption, and decomposition product formation, respectively (Juita et al., 2012). Higher temperatures have been observed to markedly accelerate the oxidation of linseed oil, whereas humidity exerts minimal influence. However, research on linseed oil oxidation at ambient or low temperatures in the absence of catalysts remains limited. Current kinetic models primarily focus on elucidating the oil curing process, involving multiple reactions that can complicate their practical use across various conditions. Simplifying these models is essential to enhance their applicability and effectiveness in capturing the autoxidation behavior of linseed oil (Farhoosh, 2020).

3 Mitigation Strategies

The rising demand for premium, long-lasting products has propelled progress in packaging and preservation technologies. Consumers are more frequently seeking minimally processed, additive-free items with a stable shelf life. This increasing demand for top-quality, durable products has driven innovation in packaging and preservation methods. Awareness among consumers results in the consumption of minimally processed, preservative products that offer improved shelf life. Residual oxygen in package headspace is a key factor influencing food shelf life, as it promotes lipid oxidation, enzymatic reactions, and microbial growth, leading to quality deterioration and shortened shelf life (Sun et al., 2021; Kaur & Srinivasa Rao, 2018).

Preventing complete oil oxidation poses a challenge, but effective strategies can slow down the oxidation process. Various approaches have been explored to minimize hydrolytic reactions or delay autoxidation. These methods involve the incorporation of antioxidants, such as plant extracts or approved synthetic preservatives. Physical lipid modifications through processes like hydrogenation, blending, and interesterification are also utilized. Additionally, optimizing storage conditions using techniques like vacuum or modified atmosphere packaging and cold storage proves to be effective. An alternative strategy involves employing novel technologies such as encapsulation. This approach aims to prevent direct contact between PUFAs and environmental factors like oxygen, light, moisture, and heat. Encapsulation serves as a protective barrier, mitigating the impact of these stressors and thereby contributing to the preservation and stability of PUFAs in various applications (Choe & Min, 2006; Jurić et al., 2022; Zhang et al., 2023). Figure 2 summarizes the effective strategies to inhibit the oxidation of linseed oil.

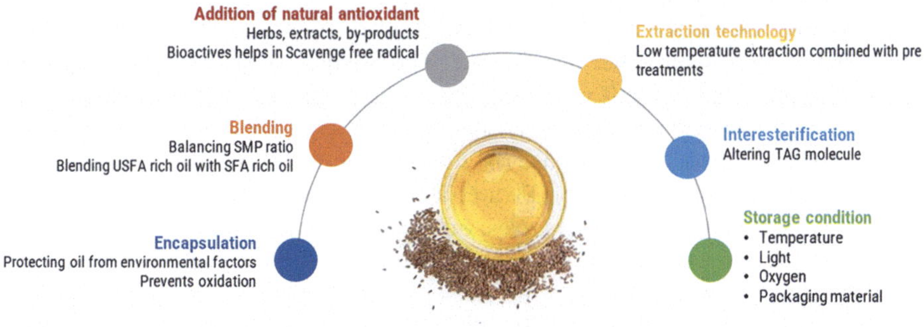

Fig. 2 Mitigation strategies to inhibit oxidation in linseed oil

PUFA-rich oils pose significant challenges in food processing and storage due to their inherent instability. The presence of multiple double bonds in PUFAs renders these molecules highly susceptible to oxidation reactions, which can lead to the deterioration of product quality. Unlike SFAs, PUFAs are more susceptible to chemical transformations, including metal-catalyzed autoxidation and hydrogenation, due to their vulnerable C=C bonds. This susceptibility to oxidation not only results in the production of undesirable flavors but also compromises the nutritional value of the oils. Additionally, efforts to incorporate omega-3 fatty acids into food products may face challenges due to their low solubility in many food systems and their high susceptibility to oxidation, which can reduce their effectiveness. Therefore, addressing the challenges associated with PUFA-rich oils in food processing and storage requires careful consideration of oxidation prevention strategies and formulation techniques to maintain product quality and nutritional integrity.

Numerous factors influence lipid oxidation, including energy input (light and heat), the fatty acids profile, degree of unsaturation, the oxygen type ($^3O_2$ & $^1O_2$), and the presence of pro-oxidants or antioxidant or minor compounds such as metals, chlorophyll, carotenoids, tocopherol, phospholipids, FFA, monoacylglycerol (MAG), diacylglycerol (DAG), and thermally oxidized compounds present in the oil or added to it. A substantial body of research has been dedicated to understanding and improving the thermo-oxidative stability of oils by exploring the influence of these factors.

3.1 Extraction Method and Processing of Linseed Oil

Various extraction methods are used to extract oil from linseed, typically yielding between 35% and 45%. Conventional methods, such as pressing at high or low temperatures, are popular due to their cost efficiency and convenience. Hot pressing of linseed results in a better yield compared to cold pressing; however, it can result in deterioration of thermolabile compounds, including bioactive and phenolic compounds, which reduces the oil's nutritive value and oxidative stability (Zhang et al., 2018). Conversely, cold pressing results in a lower yield but offers better stability, as it produces oil with lower peroxide and free fatty acid values compared to hot pressing (Kulkarni et al., 2017; Zeng et al., 2022).

Alternative methods for extracting linseed oil involve the use of nonpolar solvents such as petroleum ether or n-hexane. The Soxhlet extraction technique with these solvents ensures a uniform composition, helps preserve PUFA content, and retains a high antioxidant capacity (Adam Omer Ishag et al., 2020; Zhang et al., 2018). However, these solvents pose risks due to flammability, health hazards, and environmental pollution (Sabadin Piva et al., 2018; Tan et al., 2016). Ethanol or acetone extraction are safer alternatives, offer similar yield and quality (Johnson & Lusas, 1983; Liang et al., 2020). Ethanol extraction results in high purity and acceptable bioactive compound levels, while acetone provides the highest yield and efficiently extracts polar lipids. Additionally, to accelerate the extraction process, accelerated solvent extraction (ASE) is used, which employs high pressure and temperature to speed up the extraction rate and reduce the time required (Khattab & Zeitoun, 2013).

The transition to green chemistry involves embracing eco-friendly methods, with an emphasis on minimizing solvent usage, employing less harmful alternatives, and cutting down on energy consumption. It's crucial to emphasize that in modern extraction techniques, careful consideration of specific extraction parameters is essential. In extraction methods, cautious adjustment of several factors is vital for optimal results. These include temperature and pressure in supercritical-fluid extraction (SFE), microwave power in microwave-assisted extraction (MAE), ultrasound power and frequency in ultrasound-assisted extraction (UAE), and the toxicity of the solvent in pressurized liquid extraction (PLE). SFE is the most suitable extraction process for quality and eco-friendliness, as it eliminates solvent traces from the final product. Despite higher costs, it maintains high levels of valuable ingredients and allows complete oil recovery without solvent residues (Bozan & Temelli, 2002; Özkal & Yener, 2016).

Pretreatment of seed material before oil extraction is crucial for maintaining oil stability, quality, and yield. Various pretreatments, such as drying, dehulling, crushing, thermal treatments, and enzymatic methods, aid in cellular degradation, facilitating the extraction process (Zhang et al., 2020). Techniques like steam explosion and ultrasonic-assisted extraction enhance yield and stability by increasing the bioactive compound content and reducing extraction time. Enzymatic pretreatment improves oil yield and preserves physicochemical properties, while methods like microwave roasting and infrared-assisted drying enhance yield but may affect stability by increasing peroxide values (Domínguez et al., 1994). However, excessive preheating can degrade thermolabile components, and improper optimization of pretreatment methods can reduce antioxidant activity and overall oil quality. Combining multiple pretreatments can dramatically improve yield and quality, but the specific conditions must be carefully managed to avoid negative effects (Ren et al., 2015).

3.1.1 Oil Modification Methods

Blending

Blending various vegetable oils with varying fatty acid profiles and phytochemicals is a strategic method to produce oils with specific functionalities and better resistance to oxidation (Hashempour-Baltork et al., 2016; Pattnaik & Mishra, 2022). This blending technique seeks to boost antioxidant capacity by combining oils abundant in PUFA with more stable oils, such as those rich in SFA like palm olein, groundnut oil, and rice bran oil (Dhyani et al., 2023; Pattnaik & Mishra, 2021). Research indicates that mixing linseed oil with corn, sesame, canola, and bitter almond oils can significantly enhance its oxidative stability. Blends containing 66% of these oils show notable improvements, with the highest stability achieved in the blend containing 66% corn oil (Golmakani et al., 2020b). Additionally, combining linseed oil with avocado oil results in a well-balanced ratio of n-6 to n-3 fatty acids. This blend positively influences atherogenic and thrombogenic index values while also improving oxidative stability (Moura et al., 2023). In another study, co-pressing low omega-3 rich peanut oil with high omega-3 black cumin and linseed oil improved both the nutritional content and oxidative stability of the blended oil, as evidenced by enhanced induction periods (Suri et al., 2023). Numerous other studies reported increased oxidative stability of linseed oil when blended with other types of oil in different proportions (Bhardwaj et al., 2015; Hashempour-baltork et al., 2018; Sharma et al., 2009; Srivastava et al., 2024). Table 1 summarizes the recent studies on blending linseed oil with other oils to improve oxidative stability and nutritional composition. This blending approach offers a cost-effective means to enhance the nutritional, physical, and sensory attributes of linseed oil, achieving a balanced composition of SFA and USFA. At the same time, intrinsic antioxidant compounds further contribute to inhibiting oxidation.

Interesterification

The interesterification process results in the disruption of ester bonds in TAGs, liberating fatty acids (FAs) that are then rearranged and re-esterified onto either the same glycerol molecule or another glycerol molecule (Singh et al., 2022; Sivakanthan & Madhujith, 2020). Interesterification has proven valuable in producing customized lipids with higher essential PUFA and modifying TAG to possess specific structures and FAs. Its applications extend to the production of commercial margarine or butter equivalents, substitutes for milk fat, and low-calorie fats (Albuquerque da Silva et al., 2023; Alfieri et al., 2017). These are not limited to food products; they are also used in medicine to create specialized foods for infants or patients with fat malabsorption, enhancing the bioavailability of poorly absorbed oils (Alfieri et al., 2017). Some studies reported that structurally modified lipids prepared from interesterification may exhibit lower stability due to prolonged high heat exposure and enzymatic/chemical processing (Singh et al., 2023; Sivakanthan et al., 2019; Zhang et al., 2022). A study by Giet et al. (2009) and Aguedo et al. (2008) reported improved oxidative stability when linseed oil interesterified with anhydrous milk and rapeseed oil. A study blend of linseed oil, cotton seed oil, and palm stearin subjected to enzymatic interesterification resulted in an improved omega-6 to omega-3 ratio, along with better solid fat content and wide melting range. Various other researchers also used the interesterification process to improve the oxidative stability of linseed oil (Baoyindugurong et al., 2024; Farfán et al., 2013; Sharma & Lokesh, 2012).

Encapsulation

Novel technologies such as encapsulation are a straightforward method to prolong the shelf life of oil preventing detrimental factors from interacting with bioactive components. Recent technological advancements have led to the development of oil encapsulation, wherein lipids are enclosed within a coating, referred to as a wall or shell, or embedded into a heterogeneous or homogeneous matrix (Rashid et al., 2022; Sagiri et al., 2016). Encapsulation transforms liquid oil into minute-sized capsules, facilitating easier handling and expanding the potential applications of the oil for nutraceuticals and food fortification and is also a promising strategy for

Table 1 Summary of recent study (2019–2024) on the impact of blending on thermo-oxidative stability of linseed oil

Oil blend	Ratio and blending type	Methodology	Findings	References
Linseed oil with peanut and black cumin seeds oil	10, 20, 30, 40%, and binary blends	Physicochemical properties, chlorophylls, carotenoids, total phenolic content, antioxidant activity	↑ OSI, level of pigment, TPC Balanced n-6/n-3 ratio ↑ Antioxidant activity	Khormizi et al. (2019)
Linseed oil with corn, canola, sesame, and bitter almond oil	33% or 66% and binary blending	Oxidative kinetics, PV OSI, FAC, CD, CT	↑ Oxidation stability when blended with 66% of other oil Improved shelf life	Golmakani et al. (2020a)
Linseed Oil with cold pressed Nigella sativa (NO)	80:20 (w/w) and binary blend	FAC, PV, FFA, CD, and CT	↑ Oxidation stability Inhibited formation of PV, CD, CT and p-AV	Khormizi et al. (2019)
Sunflower seed oil: Linseed oil	100:0–80:20 (v/v) & binary blend	Frying cycle, FFA, PV, TPM	Improved SMP ratio Better thermal stability	Khanna and Chopra (2020)
Linseed oil: canola oil, LO: soybean oil	25: 75, 35: 65 to 45: 55 (v/v) and binary blend	FAC	Improved SMP and n-6 to n-3 ratio	Hasanov et al. (2022)
Linseed oil (LO): soybean (SBO) LO: mustard (MO), LO: coconut (CO), LO: olive (OO), LO: sunflower oil (SFO)	20:80, 30:70, 40:60, 50:50, 60:40, 70:30, and 80:20 (v/v) and binary	AV, PV, IV, FAC, and storage study for 4 months	Balanced FA 1.5:1:3.1 for LO and CO (80:20), 1:1.4:4.6 for LO and SBO (20:80), and 1:1.9:3.4 for LO and OO (80:20) Poor oxidative stability in blend with ↑ PUFA	Grover et al. (2020)
Flaxseed: avocado oil	0:100100:0 (v/v) & binary	FAC, tocopherol, PV, CD, CT, antioxidant properties	Unbalanced ratio of ω6-ω3 fatty acids of 18.40:1 ↑Oxidative Stability	Moura et al. (2023)
Rice Bran Oil (RBO): Palmolein (PO): Linseed Oil (LO)	50:40:10, 55:40:5, 60:30:10, 65:30:5, 70:20:10, 75:20:5	FA composition, PV, AV, tocopherols,	↑Oxidative Stability Oil blend with 75% RBO, 20% PO and 5% LO showed highest oxidative stability	Pattnaik and Mishra (2021)

(continued)

Table 1 (continued)

Oil blend	Ratio and blending type	Methodology	Findings	References
Sunflower: Linseed Oil	0:90, 20:80, 30:70, 40:60, 50:50, 60:40, 70:30, 80:20, 90:10 (v/v) & binary	FAC, tocopherol	↑ Carotenoids and ALA Balance fatty acid composition.	Romanić et al. (2021)
Linseed Oil: Palm olein	20:80, 10:90 and 5:95 (v/v) & binary	9-month storage stability of blends (FAC, PV, FFA, p-AV, Smoke point)	Blending improved n-6:n-3 ratio ↑ Thermal and oxidative stability nine-month storage	Joshi et al. (2022)

PV peroxide value, *p-AV* p anisidine value, *CD* conjugated diene, *CT* conjugated trienes, *FFA* free fatty acid, *OSI* oxidative stability index, *FAC* fatty acid composition, ↑ increase, ↓ decrease

long-term oil protection (Delshadi et al., 2020). Nano-based encapsulation systems, such as liposomes, offer advantages such as masking unpleasant tastes, odors, and colors (Wang et al., 2022). Studies demonstrate that encapsulation significantly increases the oxidative stability of PUFA-rich oils while preserving phenolic and antioxidant compounds, maintaining nutritional quality, and ensuring economic feasibility. Choosing the right encapsulation process can substantially enhance the functionality, acceptability, and shelf life of omega-3 oils. Encapsulation addresses issues related to low bioaccessibility of PUFA in bulk oil forms, improving therapeutic potential through controlled release in the gastrointestinal tract, enhanced bioavailability, and increased uptake during intestinal digestion (Jurić et al., 2022; Timilsena et al., 2017).

Carneiro et al. (2013) investigated how different combinations of encapsulation materials affect the microencapsulation of flaxseed oil using the spray drying method. They found that combining maltodextrin with whey protein concentrate yielded superior oxidative stability over extended storage periods. Similarly, other researchers have identified whey protein concentrate as a promising method for stabilizing linseed oil, making it an effective delivery system for omega-3 fatty acids and for fortifying food products (Goyal et al., 2015; Abaee et al., 2017). In a recent study, microencapsulation using flax mucilage nanofibers effectively reduced the accumulation of oxidation products (primary and secondary) compared to free oil (Hadad & Goli, 2019). Avramenko et al. (2016) assessed the stability of microencapsulated flaxseed oil and found that using lentil protein and maltodextrin as encapsulating agents extended the oil's stability by 30 days. Additional research has focused on enhancing the oxidative stability of microencapsulated linseed oil, supporting microencapsulation as a viable strategy for improving its stability and facilitating its use in various food applications (Barroso et al., 2014; Fioramonti et al., 2019; Shiga et al., 2017).

3.1.2 Addition of Synthetic and Natural Antioxidant

To combat oxidation in edible oils, various mitigation strategies have been implemented, with the addition of antioxidants emerging as the most effective, economical and convenient method to prevent oxidation of fats and oil. Antioxidants play a crucial role in controlling oxidation, even at low concentrations, by capturing and neutralizing FFAs and hydroperoxides generated in the initial stages of oil degradation (Viana da Silva et al., 2022). Oils rich in PUFAs benefit significantly from antioxidants that either scavenge free radicals or chelate metal ions, thereby extending their shelf life. Antioxidants are classified into primary and secondary types based on their mechanisms of action. Primary antioxidants work by neutralizing radical intermediates, thereby interrupting the oxidation chain reaction. Secondary antioxidants, on the other hand, prevent the regeneration of oxidation initiators or promoters (Ribeiro et al., 2019). Commonly used synthetic antioxidant, including tocopherol, butylated hydroxyanisole (BHA), butylated hydroxytoluene (BHT), and tertiary butylhydroquinone (TBHQ), are widely employed in edible oil to protect against oxidative and thermal degradation (Mishra et al., 2021). While TBHQ is currently permitted as a safe preservative at 200 ppm (EFSA, 2011; Prasad et al., 2015), the use of BHA and BHT has been discontinued due to their recognized cardiotoxic and carcinogenic properties (Xu et al., 2021). Therefore, its potential to cause DNA damage and health concerns has led to a preference for natural antioxidants (Eskandani et al., 2014; Oikawa et al., 1998).

Thus, the exploration of alternative antioxidants, particularly those sourced from natural origins, remains a primary objective in the quest for both effective and safe oil preservation methods. Natural antioxidants, derived from various sources, including isolates, extracts, or bioactive compounds, such as vitamins A, C, and E, as well as polyphenols, have demonstrated efficacy in safeguarding oils (Erickson et al., 2022; Viana da Silva et al., 2022). The oxidative stability of linseed oil is greatly affected by both the chemical properties and the amount of added antioxidants, as well as the oil's intrinsic composition (Choe & Min, 2009). For instance, a comparative analysis of natural antioxidants with varying polarities—from hydrophilic to hydrophobic to intermediate—demonstrated their effectiveness in reducing linseed oil oxidation during extended storage under different conditions (Mohanan et al., 2018).

In a separate study, researchers studied the effect of combining natural and herbal extracts rich in polyphenols to reduce and stabilize linseed oil. The addition of phytic acid, tocopherol, ascorbyl palmitate, and tea polyphenol palmitate extended the oil's shelf life by 3.2 times, highlighting the synergistic effects of these antioxidants (Lu et al., 2020). Numerous researchers have studied the impact of bioactive substances on the oxidative stability of linseed oil. Table 2 discusses recent studies on linseed oil enhancement using various extracts and herbs. Shadyro et al. (2020) investigated the effects of compounds such as carotenoids and lutein on linseed oil during accelerated lipid oxidation, finding that β-carotene significantly inhibited oxidation at very low concentration, indicating that the antioxidant or pro-oxidant

Table 2 Recent studies (2019–2024) on the effect of natural antioxidants on the oxidative stability of linseed oil

Natural antioxidant	Level of antioxidant and addition method	Type of study	Parameters	Key findings	References
Rosemary extract	5%w/w, Maceration (48 h, 25 °C)	Storage study (T- RT t-6 month)	FFA, PV, TPC, DPPH, microbiological, and sensory analysis	*↑FFA & TPC *↓PV *↑ Stronger bitterness *Microbiological content varied	Odeh et al. (2021)
Commercial Rosemary extract	200 mg/kg and direct addition	Accelerated storage (30, 40, and 50 °C, intervals of 2 days until 14 days)	PV, TBARS, free radicals, and shelf life prediction	*↑ IP value *Better antioxidant activity	Lu et al. (2021)
Tomato lycopene-rich extract (TLE)	80 mg lycopene/kg	Rancimat study (110 °C) and stability kinetics study	Moisture, color, refractive index, fatty acid composition, and antioxidants	*↑ Shelf-life by 31% (Rancimat) and by 42% (stability kinetics during storage)	Varas Condori et al. (2020)
Combination of tocopherol, ascorbyl palmitate (AP), phytic acid (PA), and a source of polyphenol (antioxidant of bamboo leaves (AOB), rosemary extract (RE), tea polyphenols extract (TP), and tea polyphenol palmitate (TPP))	Tocopherol-100-80 mg/kg AP- 40-80 mg/kg PA-40-80 mg/kg AOB-125 mg/kg RE-75 mg/kg TP-100 mg/kg TPP-120-240 mg/kg	Accelerated storage (60 °C) study and shelf life prediction	PV, TBARS, free radicals, and Rancimat (IP)	*80 mg/kg tocopherol, 40 mg/kg AP, 40 mg/kg PA, and 240 mg/kg TPP showed ↑ stability * 3.22-fold ↑ in shelf life compared to control oil	Lu et al. (2020)
Basil, fennel, oregano, rosemary, and chili	5 g/100 g and maceration (140 rpm for 48 h at 25 °C)	Storage study for 6 months at RT	FFA, PV, DPPH, Phenolic compound using HPLC and microbiological assay	*↑Improved phenolic and antioxidant activity *↓PV	Odeh et al. (2021)

Black elderberry and spirulina extracts	0.10, 0.25, 0.50, 0.75%	Accelerated study,40 °C for 35 days	PV, p-AV, TPC, antioxidant activity	*Better oxidative stability of flaxseed oil than BHT and gallic acid	Kahraman and Özdemir (2021)
Hydrophilic mixture (HM), sinapic, ascorbic, and citric acid; and a lipophilic mixture (LM) composed of α-tocopherol, ascorbyl palmitate, and citric acid	Varying concentration	Direct analysis of oxidative indices	PV, MDA, Fatty acid composition, tocopherol content and volatile content	*HM is more effective than LM *↑ Oxidative stability than synthetic antioxidant	Roschel et al. (2019)
Biologically active compounds (coenzyme Q_{10}, β-carotene, lutein, zeaxanthin, α-tocopherol, α-tocopherol acetate, cholecalciferol, selenomethionine)	0.2% and 1%	Accelerated kinetic model and rancimat	FFA, PV, p-AV, IV, IP value	β-Carotene at 5 mg/100 g inhibits oxidation in flaxseed oil, whereas coenzyme Q10 (100 mg/100 g), carotenoids (10 mg/100 g), and selenomethionine (0.5 mg/100 g) accelerate it	Shadyro et al. (2020)

FFA free fatty acid, *PV* peroxide value, *p-AV* -p anisidine value, *IV* iodine value, *CD* conjugated diene, *CT* -conjugated trienes, *IP* induction period, *OSI* oxidative stability index, *FAC* fatty acid composition, ↑ increase, ↓ decrease

effects of a compound depend on its concentration. Additionally, research has shown that apple pomace (Śpitalniak-Bajerska et al., 2018), lycopene from tomato extract (Varas Condori et al., 2020), and rosemary extract (Wang et al., 2018) can also stabilize linseed oil. The combination of tea polyphenols (200 mg/kg) and TBHQ (100 mg/kg) achieved the lowest PV and p-AV during storage (Omar et al., 2010). A combination of tea polyphenols, TBHQ, and monoglyceride citrate (200, 100, and 100 mg/kg, respectively) demonstrated the highest oxidative stability in rancimat tests, possibly due to accelerated aeration, which requires further optimization. Additionally, an optimized mixture of oleoresin rosemary (0.06–0.08%), oleoresin sage (0.05–0.08%), and citric acid (0.03–0.05%) effectively reduced linseed oil deterioration during frying, highlighting the synergistic benefits of these natural antioxidants (Jaswir et al., 2005).

3.1.3 Packaging Technologies

Packaging plays a crucial role in food manufacturing by facilitating transportation throughout the supply chain, safeguarding against physical damage, preventing tampering, and ensuring food quality and safety. It serves as a protective barrier, protecting food from environmental factors like oxygen, moisture, light, odors, and both chemical and microbial contaminants (Robertson, 2012). Current advancements in packaging technologies, particularly active packaging, have significantly enhanced these protective functions. This innovation responds to growing consumer preferences for minimally processed, high-quality foods with extended shelf life (Vilela et al., 2018).

Active packaging seeks to prolong the shelf life of food products by utilizing various mechanisms. These include systems that either remove unwanted compounds from the food or its surroundings or systems that release beneficial compounds into the packaged food or its environment (Carpena et al., 2021). This technology provides numerous advantages, such as slowing down ripening, inhibiting microbial growth, and enhancing oxidative stability (Yildirim et al., 2018). Active packaging offers an alternative to encapsulating oil within a polymer matrix to mitigate oxidation. By integrating antioxidants into the packaging materials, these antioxidants can migrate to the food and neutralize free radicals generated during lipid oxidation, thereby preventing oxidation on the food's surface (Rangaraj et al., 2021). Recent research has highlighted the efficacy of gelatin-based films in delaying oil oxidation. For instance, research by Kchaou et al. (2020) demonstrated that gelatin-based pouches significantly reduced oxidation in linseed oil, maintaining stable peroxide levels and lower TBARs content compared to unpackaged oil. Notably, non-heated glucose-supplemented pouches provided the best preservation results, suggesting their potential as biodegradable and sustainable packaging options. Additionally, PuOC-based films were shown to ensure improved stability and better sensory attributes of oil without significant changes in oil nutritional composition (Hromiš et al., 2022).

3.2 Future Challenges and Perspectives

Enhancing the oxidative stability of microencapsulated linseed oil presents several challenges and promising perspectives. One key challenge is optimizing encapsulation techniques to achieve consistent and reproducible results across different encapsulating materials and processing conditions. Improving the scalability and cost-effectiveness of microencapsulation methods is essential to facilitate widespread adoption in the food industry. Furthermore, understanding the interactions between encapsulating materials and linseed oil components under various environmental and storage conditions remains critical. Future research should focus on developing novel extraction technology that offer enhanced oxidative stability while preserving the nutritional integrity of linseed oil, which are also low cost and feasible for industry. Additionally, exploring sustainable and eco-friendly approaches such as addition of natural extract aligns with current trends toward environmentally responsible food processing technologies. The level of natural antioxidant, method of addition, toxicity level and effect on human health on long-term consumption can be explored. Addressing these challenges unlock new opportunities for utilizing linseed oil as a functional ingredient in a broader range of food and nutraceutical products.

4 Conclusion

Enhancing the shelf life of linseed oil is vital to preserve its nutritional and sensory qualities, making it more viable for various food applications. There are several advanced strategies, including oil modification technologies and encapsulation, which effectively mitigate lipid oxidation. Incorporating natural antioxidants and innovative encapsulation techniques has shown significant promise in maintaining the stability and integrity of linseed oil during processing and storage. Industries can use low-cost and feasible methods to meet consumer demand for PUFA-rich food products. Continued research and development in these areas are essential to create effective solutions that meet consumer demand for high-quality, stable, functional foods. By implementing these strategies, the food industry can better leverage the health benefits of linseed oil, offering products that are both nutritious and long-lasting.

References

Abaee, A., Mohammadian, M., & Jafari, S. M. (2017). Whey and soy protein-based hydrogels and nano-hydrogels as bioactive delivery systems. *Trends in Food Science & Technology, 70*, 69–81. https://doi.org/10.1016/j.tifs.2017.10.011

Adam Omer Ishag, O., Khalid, A. A., Abdi, A., Yaagoub Erwa, I., Babiker Omer, A., & Nour, A. H. (2020). Proximate composition, physicochemical properties and antioxidant activity of flaxseed. *Annual Research & Review in Biology*, 1–10. https://doi.org/10.9734/arrb/2019/v34i230148

Afik, N., Yadgar, O., Volison-Klimentiev, A., Peretz-Damari, S., Ohayon-Lavi, A., Alatawna, A., Yosefi, G., Bitton, R., Fuchs, N., & Regev, O. (2020). Sensing exposure time to oxygen by applying a percolation-induced principle. *Sensors, 20*(16), 4465. https://doi.org/10.3390/s20164465

Aguedo, M., Hanon, E., Danthine, S., Paquot, M., Lognay, G., Thomas, A., Vandenbol, M., Thonart, P., Wathelet, J.-P., & Blecker, C. (2008). Enrichment of anhydrous milk fat in polyunsaturated fatty acid residues from linseed and rapeseed oils through enzymatic interesterification. *Journal of Agricultural and Food Chemistry, 56*(5), 1757–1765. https://doi.org/10.1021/jf0722203

Albuquerque da Silva, D., Manoel da Cruz Rodrigues, A., Oliveira dos Santos, A., Salvador-Reyes, R., & Meller da Silva, L. H. (2023). Physicochemical and technological properties of pracaxi oil, cupuassu fat and palm stearin blends enzymatically interesterified for food applications. *LWT, 184*, 114961. https://doi.org/10.1016/j.lwt.2023.114961

Alfieri, A., Imperlini, E., Nigro, E., Vitucci, D., Orrù, S., Daniele, A., Buono, P., & Mancini, A. (2017). Effects of plant oil interesterified triacylglycerols on lipemia and human health. *International Journal of Molecular Sciences, 19*(1), 104. https://doi.org/10.3390/ijms19010104

Avramenko, N. A., Chang, C., Low, N. H., & Nickerson, M. T. (2016). Encapsulation of flaxseed oil within native and modified lentil protein-based microcapsules. *Food Research International, 81*, 17–24. https://doi.org/10.1016/j.foodres.2015.12.028

Ayelign, A., & Alemu, T. (2016). The functional nutrients of flaxseed and their effect on human health: A review. *European Journal of Nutrition & Food Safety, 6*(2), 83–92. https://doi.org/10.9734/EJNFS/2016/16318

Baoyindugurong, J., Hou, J., Ren, Y., Li, Y., Heshuote, M., Hugejiletu, Ohara, N., Naito, Y., & Tatematsu, K. (2024). Lipase-catalyzed interesterification of Sunite sheep tail fat and flaxseed oil provides a fat having a unique fatty acid content and favorable physicochemical and nutritional properties. *Food Science & Nutrition, 12*(6), 4443–4458. https://doi.org/10.1002/fsn3.4111

Barden, L., & Decker, E. A. (2016). Lipid oxidation in low-moisture food: A review. *Critical Reviews in Food Science and Nutrition, 56*(15), 2467–2482. https://doi.org/10.1080/10408398.2013.848833

Barroso, A. K. M., Pierucci, A. P. T. R., Freitas, S. P., Torres, A. G., & da Rocha-Leão, M. H. M. (2014). Oxidative stability and sensory evaluation of microencapsulated flaxseed oil. *Journal of Microencapsulation, 31*(2), 193–201. https://doi.org/10.3109/02652048.2013.824514

Bhardwaj, K., Verma, N., & Bhardwaj, S. (2015). A novel approach for improvement of oxidative stability of flaxseed oil by blending with palm oil. *International Journal of Advanced Research, 3*(11), 1399–1407.

Bozan, B., & Temelli, F. (2002). Supercritical CO 2 extraction of flaxseed. *Journal of the American Oil Chemists' Society, 79*(3), 231–235. https://doi.org/10.1007/s11746-002-0466-x

Carneiro, H. C. F., Tonon, R. V., Grosso, C. R. F., & Hubinger, M. D. (2013). Encapsulation efficiency and oxidative stability of flaxseed oil microencapsulated by spray drying using different combinations of wall materials. *Journal of Food Engineering, 115*(4), 443–451. https://doi.org/10.1016/j.jfoodeng.2012.03.033

Carpena, M., Nuñez-Estevez, B., Soria-Lopez, A., Garcia-Oliveira, P., & Prieto, M. A. (2021). Essential oils and their application on active packaging systems: A review. *Resources, 10*(1), 7. https://doi.org/10.3390/resources10010007

Choe, E., & Min, D. B. (2006). Mechanisms and factors for edible oil oxidation. *Comprehensive Reviews in Food Science and Food Safety, 5*(4), 169–186. https://doi.org/10.1111/j.1541-4337.2006.00009.x

Choe, E., & Min, D. B. (2009). Mechanisms of antioxidants in the oxidation of foods. *Comprehensive Reviews in Food Science and Food Safety, 8*(4), 345–358. https://doi.org/10.1111/j.1541-4337.2009.00085.x

Dąbrowski, G., Czaplicki, S., & Konopka, I. (2019). Fractionation of sterols, tocols and squalene in flaxseed oils under the impact of variable conditions of supercritical CO2 extraction. *Journal of Food Composition and Analysis, 83*, 103261. https://doi.org/10.1016/j.jfca.2019.103261

Delshadi, R., Bahrami, A., Tafti, A. G., Barba, F. J., & Williams, L. L. (2020). Micro and nano-encapsulation of vegetable and essential oils to develop functional food products with improved nutritional profiles. *Trends in Food Science & Technology, 104*, 72–83. https://doi.org/10.1016/j.tifs.2020.07.004

Dhyani, A., Chopra, R., Singh, P. K., & Garg, M. (2023). Palm olein and perilla seed oil blends for the improvement of nutritional and thermal stability. *Grasas y Aceites, 74*(3), e511. https://doi.org/10.3989/gya.0220221

Diaz-Uribe, C., Vallejo, W., De la Hoz, T., Florez, J., Muñoz-Acevedo, A., Zarate, X., & Schott, E. (2022). Theoretical and kinetic study of the singlet oxygen quenching reaction by hesperidin isolated from mandarin (Citrus reticulata) fruit peels. *Chemical Papers, 76*(1), 169–178. https://doi.org/10.1007/s11696-021-01825-2

Domínguez, H., Núñez, M. J., & Lema, J. M. (1994). Enzymatic pretreatment to enhance oil extraction from fruits and oilseeds: A review. *Food Chemistry, 49*(3), 271–286. https://doi.org/10.1016/0308-8146(94)90172-4

Douny, C., Razanakolona, R., Ribonnet, L., Milet, J., Baeten, V., Rogez, H., Scippo, M.-L., & Larondelle, Y. (2016). Linseed oil presents different patterns of oxidation in real-time and accelerated aging assays. *Food Chemistry, 208*, 111–115. https://doi.org/10.1016/j.foodchem.2016.04.010

EFSA. (2011). Scientific opinion on the re-evaluation of butylated hydroxyanisole – BHA (E 320) as a food additive. *EFSA Journal, 9*(10), 2392. https://doi.org/10.2903/j.efsa.2011.2392

Erickson, M. D., Yevtushenko, D. P., & Lu, Z. X. (2022). Oxidation and thermal degradation of oil during frying: A review of natural antioxidant use. *Food Reviews International*, 1–32. https://doi.org/10.1080/87559129.2022.2039689

Eskandani, M., Hamishehkar, H., & Ezzati Nazhad Dolatabadi, J. (2014). Cytotoxicity and DNA damage properties of tert-butylhydroquinone (TBHQ) food additive. *Food Chemistry, 153*, 315–320. https://doi.org/10.1016/j.foodchem.2013.12.087

Farfán, M., Villalón, M. J., Ortíz, M. E., Nieto, S., & Bouchon, P. (2013). The effect of interesterification on the bioavailability of fatty acids in structured lipids. *Food Chemistry, 139*(1–4), 571–577. https://doi.org/10.1016/j.foodchem.2013.01.024

Farhoosh, R. (2020). A reconsidered approach providing kinetic parameters and rate constants to analyze the oxidative stability of bulk lipid systems. *Food Chemistry, 327*, 127088. https://doi.org/10.1016/j.foodchem.2020.127088

Fioramonti, S. A., Stepanic, E. M., Tibaldo, A. M., Pavón, Y. L., & Santiago, L. G. (2019). Spray dried flaxseed oil powdered microcapsules obtained using milk whey proteins-alginate double layer emulsions. *Food Research International, 119*, 931–940. https://doi.org/10.1016/j.foodres.2018.10.079

Giet, J.-M., Aguedo, M., Danthine, S., Paquot, M., Thomas, A., Vandenbol, M., Thonart, P., Wathelet, J.-P., Blecker, C., & Lognay, G. (2009). Enzymatic interesterification of anhydrous milk fat with rapeseed and/or linseed oil: Oxidative stability. *Journal of Agricultural and Food Chemistry, 57*(15), 6787–6794. https://doi.org/10.1021/jf9007955

Golmakani, M. T., Keramat, M., & Zare Darniyani, L. (2020a). A kinetic approach to the oxidation of linseed oil as influenced by fruit peel and seeds of pomegranate. *European Journal of Lipid Science and Technology, 122*(2), 1–7. https://doi.org/10.1002/ejlt.201900084

Golmakani, M. T., Soltani, A., Hosseini, S. M. H., & Keramat, M. (2020b). Improving the oxidation kinetics of linseed oil using the blending approach. *Journal of Food Processing and Preservation, 44*(12), e14964. https://doi.org/10.1111/jfpp.14964

Goyal, A., Sharma, V., Upadhyay, N., Gill, S., & Sihag, M. (2014). Flax and flaxseed oil: An ancient medicine & modern functional food. *Journal of Food Science and Technology, 51*(9), 1633–1653. https://doi.org/10.1007/s13197-013-1247-9

Goyal, A., Sharma, V., Upadhyay, N., Singh, A. K., Arora, S., Lal, D., & Sabikhi, L. (2015). Development of stable flaxseed oil emulsions as a potential delivery system of ω-3 fatty acids. *Journal of Food Science and Technology, 52*(7), 4256–4265. https://doi.org/10.1007/s13197-014-1370-2

Grover, S., Kumari, P., Kumar, A., Soni, A., Shegal, S., & Sharma, V. (2020). Preparation and quality evaluation of different oil blends. *Letters in Applied NanoBioScience, 10*(2), 2126–2137. https://doi.org/10.33263/LIANBS102.21262137

Hadad, S., & Goli, S. A. H. (2019). Improving oxidative stability of flaxseed oil by encapsulation in electrospun flaxseed mucilage nanofiber. *Food and Bioprocess Technology, 12*(5), 829–838. https://doi.org/10.1007/s11947-019-02259-1

Han, H., Ma, H., Rong, S., Chen, L., Shan, Z., Xu, J., Zhang, Y., & Liu, L. (2015). Flaxseed oil containing flaxseed oil ester of plant sterol attenuates high-fat diet-induced hepatic steatosis in apolipoprotein-E knockout mice. *Journal of Functional Foods, 13*, 169–182. https://doi.org/10.1016/j.jff.2014.12.046

Hasanov, J. H., Mirzahmedov, S. D., Berdiev, N., & Salikhov, S. I. (2022). Formation of preliminary oil blends based on fatty acid compositions of oil-bearing sources. *Journal of Chemistry and Technologies, 30*(4), 513–519. https://doi.org/10.15421/jchemtech.v30i4.263838

Hashempour-Baltork, F., Torbati, M., Azadmard-Damirchi, S., & Savage, G. P. (2016). Vegetable oil blending: A review of physicochemical, nutritional and health effects. *Trends in Food Science & Technology, 57*, 52–58. https://doi.org/10.1016/j.tifs.2016.09.007

Hashempour-baltork, F., Torbati, M., Azadmard-damirchi, S., & Savage, G. P. (2018). Olive oils blended with linseed oil. *Tabriz University of Medical Sciences, 8*(1), 107–113. https://doi.org/10.15171/apb.2018.013

Hasiewicz-Derkacz, K., Kulma, A., Czuj, T., Prescha, A., Żuk, M., Grajzer, M., Łukaszewicz, M., & Szopa, J. (2015). Natural phenolics greatly increase flax (Linum usitatissimum) oil stability. *BMC Biotechnology, 15*(1), 62. https://doi.org/10.1186/s12896-015-0178-0

Herchi, W., Sawalha, S., Arráez-Román, D., Boukhchina, S., Segura-Carretero, A., Kallel, H., & Fernández-Gutierrez, A. (2011). Determination of phenolic and other polar compounds in flaxseed oil using liquid chromatography coupled with time-of-flight mass spectrometry. *Food Chemistry, 126*(1), 332–338. https://doi.org/10.1016/j.foodchem.2010.10.070

Hromiš, N., Lazić, V., Popović, S., Šuput, D., Bulut, S., Kravić, S., & Romanić, R. (2022). The possible application of edible pumpkin oil cake film as pouches for flaxseed oil protection. *Food Chemistry, 371*, 131197. https://doi.org/10.1016/j.foodchem.2021.131197

Jaswir, I., Kitts, D. D., Man, Y. B. C., & Hassan, T. H. (2005). Physico-chemical stability of flaxseed oil with natural antioxidant mixtures during heating. *Journal of Oleo Science, 54*(2), 71–79. https://doi.org/10.5650/jos.54.71

Johnson, L. A., & Lusas, E. W. (1983). Comparison of alternative solvents for oils extraction. *Journal of the American Oil Chemists' Society, 60*(2Part1), 229–242. https://doi.org/10.1007/BF02543490

Joshi, A., Hegde, M., & Zanwar, A. (2022). Flaxseed oil and palm olein blend to improve omega-6: Omega-3 ratio. *Journal of Food Science and Technology, 59*(2), 498–509. https://doi.org/10.1007/s13197-021-05033-4

Juita, Dlugogorski, B. Z., Kennedy, E. M., & Mackie, J. C. (2012). Low temperature oxidation of linseed oil: A review. *Fire Science Reviews, 1*(1), 3. https://doi.org/10.1186/2193-0414-1-3

Jurić, S., Jurić, M., Siddique, M. A. B., & Fathi, M. (2022). Vegetable oils rich in polyunsaturated fatty acids: Nanoencapsulation methods and stability enhancement. *Food Reviews International, 38*(1), 32–69. https://doi.org/10.1080/87559129.2020.1717524

Kahraman, G., & Özdemir, K. S. (2021). Effects of black elderberry and spirulina extracts on the chemical stability of cold pressed flaxseed oil during accelerated storage. *Journal of Food Measurement and Characterization, 15*(5), 4838–4847. https://doi.org/10.1007/s11694-021-01004-7

Kaur, B. P., & Srinivasa Rao, P. (2018). Effect of storage temperature and packaging on quality and shelf-life of high pressure processed black tiger shrimp (Penaeus monodon). *Journal of Food Processing and Preservation, 42*(1), e13366. https://doi.org/10.1111/jfpp.13366

Kchaou, H., Jridi, M., Nasri, M., & Debeaufort, F. (2020). Design of gelatin pouches for the preservation of flaxseed oil during storage. *Coatings, 10*(2), 150. https://doi.org/10.3390/coatings10020150

Khanna, P., & Chopra, R. (2020). Oxidative and thermal stability of linseed oil blend and its. *Annals: Food Science & Technology, 21*(4).

Khattab, R. Y., & Zeitoun, M. A. (2013). Quality evaluation of flaxseed oil obtained by different extraction techniques. *LWT – Food Science and Technology, 53*(1), 338–345. https://doi.org/10.1016/j.lwt.2013.01.004

Khormizi, A. B., Asadollahi, S., Khorshidpoor, B., & Hosseini, E. (2019). Effect of added black cumin seed (Nigella sativa L) oil on oxidative stability of flaxseed oil. *Asian Food Science Journal*, 1–9. https://doi.org/10.9734/afsj/2019/v7i429975

Kulkarni, N. G., Kar, J. R., & Singhal, R. S. (2017). Extraction of flaxseed oil: A comparative study of three-phase partitioning and supercritical carbon dioxide using response surface methodology. *Food and Bioprocess Technology, 10*(5), 940–948. https://doi.org/10.1007/s11947-017-1877-4

Liang, S., Li, X., Cai, Z., Zhang, N., Reaney, M. J. T., & Wang, Y. (2020). A wet-screening strategy for flaxseed dehulling and compositional quantification of the separated fractions. *LWT, 127*, 109386. https://doi.org/10.1016/j.lwt.2020.109386

Lu, T., Shen, Y., Wang, J., Xie, H., Wang, Y., Zhao, Q., Zhou, D., & Shahidi, F. (2020). Improving oxidative stability of flaxseed oil with a mixture of antioxidants. *Journal of Food Processing and Preservation, 44*(3). https://doi.org/10.1111/jfpp.14355

Lu, T., Shen, Y., Wu, Z.-X., Xie, H.-K., Li, A., Wang, Y.-F., Song, L., Zhou, D.-Y., & Wang, T. (2021). Improving the oxidative stability of flaxseed oil with composite antioxidants comprising gallic acid alkyl ester with appropriate chain length. *LWT, 138*, 110763. https://doi.org/10.1016/j.lwt.2020.110763

Mène-Saffrané, L., & DellaPenna, D. (2010). Biosynthesis, regulation and functions of tocochromanols in plants. *Plant Physiology and Biochemistry, 48*(5), 301–309. https://doi.org/10.1016/j.plaphy.2009.11.004

Mishra, S. K., Belur, P. D., & Iyyaswami, R. (2021). Use of antioxidants for enhancing oxidative stability of bulk edible oils: A review. *International Journal of Food Science & Technology, 56*(1), 1–12. https://doi.org/10.1111/ijfs.14716

Mohanan, A., Nickerson, M. T., & Ghosh, S. (2018). Oxidative stability of flaxseed oil: Effect of hydrophilic, hydrophobic and intermediate polarity antioxidants. *Food Chemistry, 266*, 524–533. https://doi.org/10.1016/j.foodchem.2018.05.117

Moura, M. D. S., da Silva, C. A. M., & Braga, M. B. (2023). Flaxseed and avocado oil blends: Physical and physicochemical characterization, nutritional quality and oxidative stability. *Applied Food Research, 3*(2), 100370. https://doi.org/10.1016/j.afres.2023.100370

Obranović, M., Škevin, D., Kraljić, K., Pospišil, M., Neđeral, S., Blekić, M., & Putnik, P. (2015). Influence of climate, varieties and production process on tocopherols, plastochromanol-8 and pigments in flaxseed oil. *Food Technology and Biotechnology, 53*, 496. https://doi.org/10.17113/ftb.53.04.15.4252

Odeh, D., Kraljić, K., Benussi Skukan, A., & Škevin, D. (2021). Oxidative stability, microbial safety, and sensory properties of flaxseed (Linum usitatissimum L.) oil infused with spices and herbs. *Antioxidants, 10*(5), 785. https://doi.org/10.3390/antiox10050785

Oikawa, S., Nishino, K., Oikawa, S., Inoue, S., Mizutani, T., & Kawanishi, S. (1998). Oxidative DNA damage and apoptosis induced by metabolites of butylated hydroxytoluene. *Biochemical Pharmacology, 56*(3), 361–370. https://doi.org/10.1016/S0006-2952(98)00037-9

Omar, K. A., Shan, L., Wang, Y. L., & Wang, X. (2010). Stabilizing flaxseed oil with individual antioxidants and their mixtures. *European Journal of Lipid Science and Technology, 112*(9), 1003–1011. https://doi.org/10.1002/ejlt.200900264

Özkal, S. G., & Yener, M. E. (2016). Supercritical carbon dioxide extraction of flaxseed oil: Effect of extraction parameters and mass transfer modeling. *The Journal of Supercritical Fluids, 112*, 76–80. https://doi.org/10.1016/j.supflu.2016.02.013

Pattnaik, M., & Mishra, H. N. (2021). Oxidative stability of ternary blends of vegetable oils: A chemometric approach. *LWT, 142*(January), 111018. https://doi.org/10.1016/j.lwt.2021.111018

Pattnaik, M., & Mishra, H. N. (2022). Amelioration of the stability of polyunsaturated fatty acids and bioactive enriched vegetable oil: Blending, encapsulation, and its application. *Critical Reviews in Food Science and Nutrition, 62*(23), 6253–6276. https://doi.org/10.1080/10408398.2021.1899127

Prasad, N., Siddaramaiah, B., & Banu, M. (2015). Effect of antioxidant tertiary butyl hydroquinone on the thermal and oxidative stability of sesame oil (sesamum indicum) by ultrasonic studies. *Journal of Food Science and Technology, 52*(4), 2238–2246. https://doi.org/10.1007/s13197-014-1276-z

Rangaraj, V. M., Rambabu, K., Banat, F., & Mittal, V. (2021). Natural antioxidants-based edible active food packaging: An overview of current advancements. *Food Bioscience, 43*, 101251. https://doi.org/10.1016/j.fbio.2021.101251

Rashid, R., Masoodi, F. A., Wani, S. M., Manzoor, S., & Gull, A. (2022). Ultrasound assisted extraction of bioactive compounds from pomegranate peel, their nanoencapsulation and application for improvement in shelf life extension of edible oils. *Food Chemistry, 385*, 132608. https://doi.org/10.1016/j.foodchem.2022.132608

Ren, G., Zhang, W., Sun, S., Duan, X., & Zhang, Z. (2015). Enhanced extraction of oil from flaxseed (Linum usitatissimum L.) using microwave pre-treatment. *Journal of Oleo Science, 64*(10), 1043–1047. https://doi.org/10.5650/jos.ess15099

Ribeiro, J. S., Santos, M. J. M. C., Silva, L. K. R., Pereira, L. C. L., Santos, I. A., da Silva Lannes, S. C., & da Silva, M. V. (2019). Natural antioxidants used in meat products: A brief review. *Meat Science, 148*, 181–188. https://doi.org/10.1016/j.meatsci.2018.10.016

Robertson, G. L. (2012). Overall status of shelf life studies. *Italian. Journal of Food Science, 24*(SUPPL), 3–8.

Romanić, R. S., Lužaić, T. Z., & Radić, B. Đ. (2021). Enriched sunflower oil with omega 3 fatty acids from flaxseed oil: Prediction of the nutritive characteristics. *LWT, 150*, 112064. https://doi.org/10.1016/j.lwt.2021.112064

Roschel, G. G., da Silveira, T. F. F., Cajaiba, L. M., & Castro, I. A. (2019). Combination of hydrophilic or lipophilic natural compounds to improve the oxidative stability of flaxseed oil. *European Journal of Lipid Science and Technology, 121*(5). https://doi.org/10.1002/ejlt.201800459

Rubilar, M., Gutiérrez, C., Verdugo, M., Shene, C., & Sineiro, J. (2010). Flaxseed as a source of functional ingredients. *Journal of Soil Science and Plant Nutrition, 10*(3). https://doi.org/10.4067/S0718-95162010000100010

Sabadin Piva, G., Weschenfelder, T. A., Franceschi, E., Cansian, R. L., Paroul, N., & Steffens, C. (2018). Flaxseed (Linum usitatissimum) oil extraction using different solvents. *Food Technology and Biotechnology, 56*(3), 366. https://doi.org/10.17113/ftb.56.03.18.5318

Sagiri, S. S., Anis, A., & Pal, K. (2016). Review on encapsulation of vegetable oils: Strategies, preparation methods, and applications. *Polymer-Plastics Technology and Engineering, 55*(3), 291–311. https://doi.org/10.1080/03602559.2015.1050521

Shadyro, O., Sosnovskaya, A., & Edimecheva, I. (2020). Effect of biologically active substances on oxidative stability of flaxseed oil. *Journal of Food Science and Technology, 57*(1), 243–252. https://doi.org/10.1007/s13197-019-04054-4

Shahidi, F., & Zhong, Y. (2010). Lipid oxidation and improving the oxidative stability. *Chemical Society Reviews, 39*(11), 4067. https://doi.org/10.1039/b922183m

Sharma, M., & Lokesh, B. R. (2012). Effect of enzymatic trans- and interesterification on the thermal properties of groundnut and linseed oils and their blends. *Journal of the American Oil Chemists' Society, 89*(5), 805–813. https://doi.org/10.1007/s11746-011-1985-7

Sharma, M., Rastogi, N. K., & Lokesh, B. R. (2009). Synthesis of structured lipid with balanced omega-3: Omega-6 ratio by lipase-catalyzed acidolysis reaction: Optimization of reaction using response surface methodology. *Process Biochemistry, 44*(11), 1284–1288. https://doi.org/10.1016/j.procbio.2009.07.005

Shiga, H., Loon Neoh, T., Ninomiya, A., Adachi, S., Pasten, I. L., Adachi, S., & Yoshii, H. (2017). Effect of oil droplet size on the oxidative stability of spray-dried flaxseed oil powders. *Bioscience, Biotechnology, and Biochemistry, 81*(4), 698–704. https://doi.org/10.1080/09168451.2017.1281720

Simopoulos, A. P., & DiNicolantonio, J. J. (2016). The importance of a balanced ω-6 to ω-3 ratio in the prevention and management of obesity. *Open Heart, 3*(2), e000385. https://doi.org/10.1136/openhrt-2015-000385

Singh, P. K., Chopra, R., Garg, M., Dhiman, A., & Dhyani, A. (2022). Enzymatic interesterification of vegetable oil:A review on physicochemical and functional properties, and its health effects. *Journal of Oleo Science, 71*(12), ess22118. https://doi.org/10.5650/jos.ess22118

Singh, P. K., Chopra, R., Dhiman, A., Chuahan, K., & Garg, M. (2023). Development of omega-3-rich structured lipids using perilla seed oil and palm olein: Optimization and characterization. *Biomass Conversion and Biorefinery, 14*, 23857. https://doi.org/10.1007/s13399-023-04422-3

Sivakanthan, S., & Madhujith, T. (2020). Current trends in applications of enzymatic interesterification of fats and oils: A review. *LWT, 132*, 109880. https://doi.org/10.1016/j.lwt.2020.109880

Sivakanthan, S., Jayasooriya, A. P., & Madhujith, T. (2019). Optimization of the production of structured lipid by enzymatic interesterification from coconut (Cocos nucifera) oil and sesame (Sesamum indicum) oil using response surface methodology. *LWT, 101*(4), 723–730. https://doi.org/10.1016/j.lwt.2018.11.085

Śpitalniak-Bajerska, K., Szumny, A., Kucharska, A. Z., & Kupczyński, R. (2018). Effect of natural antioxidants on the stability of linseed oil and fish stored under anaerobic conditions. *Journal of Chemistry, 2018*, 1–8. https://doi.org/10.1155/2018/9375085

Srivastava, Y., Singh, B., Kaur, B., Ubaid, M., & Semwal, A. D. (2024). Kinetic study of thermal degradation of flaxseed oil and moringa oil blends with physico-chemical, oxidative stability index (OSI) and shelf-life prediction. *Journal of Food Science and Technology, 61*(4), 675–687. https://doi.org/10.1007/s13197-023-05868-z

Sun, C., Shan, Y., Tang, X., Han, D., Wu, X., Wu, H., & Hosseininezhad, M. (2021). Effects of enzymatic hydrolysis on physicochemical property and antioxidant activity of mulberry (Morus atropurpurea Roxb.) leaf protein. *Food Science & Nutrition, 9*(10), 5379–5390. https://doi.org/10.1002/fsn3.2474

Suri, K., Singh, B., Kaur, A., & Yadav, M. P. (2023). Physicochemical characteristics, oxidative stability, pigments, fatty acid profile and antioxidant properties of co-pressed oil from blends of peanuts, flaxseed and black cumin seeds. *Food Chemistry Advances, 2*, 100231. https://doi.org/10.1016/j.focha.2023.100231

Tan, Z., Yang, Z., Yi, Y., Wang, H., Zhou, W., Li, F., & Wang, C. (2016). Extraction of oil from flaxseed (Linum usitatissimum L.) using enzyme-assisted three-phase partitioning. *Applied Biochemistry and Biotechnology, 179*(8), 1325–1335. https://doi.org/10.1007/s12010-016-2068-x

Timilsena, Y. P., Wang, B., Adhikari, R., & Adhikari, B. (2017). Advances in microencapsulation of polyunsaturated fatty acids (PUFAs)-rich plant oils using complex coacervation: A review. *Food Hydrocolloids, 69*, 369–381. https://doi.org/10.1016/j.foodhyd.2017.03.007

Van Dyck, S. (2010). The impact of singlet oxygen on lipid oxidation in foods. In *Oxidation in foods and beverages and antioxidant applications* (pp. 57–75). Elsevier. https://doi.org/10.1533/9780857090447.1.57

Varas Condori, M. A., Pascual Chagman, G. J., Barriga-Sanchez, M., Villegas Vilchez, L. F., Ursetta, S., Guevara Pérez, A., & Hidalgo, A. (2020). Effect of tomato (Solanum lycopersicum L.) lycopene-rich extract on the kinetics of rancidity and shelf-life of linseed (Linum usitatissimum L.) oil. *Food Chemistry, 302*, 125327. https://doi.org/10.1016/j.foodchem.2019.125327

Viana da Silva, M., Santos, M. R. C., Alves Silva, I. R., Macedo Viana, E. B., Dos Anjos, D. A., Santos, I. A., Barbosa de Lima, N. G., Wobeto, C., Jorge, N., & Lannes, S. C. D. S. (2022). Synthetic and natural antioxidants used in the oxidative stability of edible oils: An overview. *Food Reviews International, 38*(sup1), 349–372. https://doi.org/10.1080/87559129.2020.1869775

Vilela, C., Kurek, M., Hayouka, Z., Röcker, B., Yildirim, S., Antunes, M. D. C., Nilsen-Nygaard, J., Pettersen, M. K., & Freire, C. S. R. (2018). A concise guide to active agents for active food packaging. *Trends in Food Science & Technology, 80*, 212–222. https://doi.org/10.1016/j.tifs.2018.08.006

Wang, Y.-Z., Fu, S.-G., Wang, S.-Y., Yang, D.-J., Wu, Y.-H. S., & Chen, Y.-C. (2018). Effects of a natural antioxidant, polyphenol-rich rosemary (Rosmarinus officinalis L.) extract, on lipid stability of plant-derived omega-3 fatty-acid rich oil. *LWT, 89*, 210–216. https://doi.org/10.1016/j.lwt.2017.10.055

Wang, H., Hu, L., Peng, L., Du, J., Lan, M., Cheng, Y., Ma, L., & Zhang, Y. (2022). Dual encapsulation of β-carotene by β-cyclodextrin and chitosan for 3D printing application. *Food Chemistry, 378*, 132088. https://doi.org/10.1016/j.foodchem.2022.132088

Xu, X., Liu, A., Hu, S., Ares, I., Martínez-Larrañaga, M.-R., Wang, X., Martínez, M., Anadón, A., & Martínez, M.-A. (2021). Synthetic phenolic antioxidants: Metabolism, hazards and mechanism of action. *Food Chemistry, 353*, 129488. https://doi.org/10.1016/j.foodchem.2021.129488

Yildirim, S., Röcker, B., Pettersen, M. K., Nilsen-Nygaard, J., Ayhan, Z., Rutkaite, R., Radusin, T., Suminska, P., Marcos, B., & Coma, V. (2018). Active packaging applications for food. *Comprehensive Reviews in Food Science and Food Safety, 17*(1), 165–199. https://doi.org/10.1111/1541-4337.12322

Zeng, J., Xiao, T., Ni, X., Wei, T., Liu, X., Deng, Z.-Y., & Li, J. (2022). The comparative analysis of different oil extraction methods based on the quality of flaxseed oil. *Journal of Food Composition and Analysis, 107*, 104373. https://doi.org/10.1016/j.jfca.2021.104373

Zhang, Z., Liu, Y., & Che, L. (2018). Effects of different drying methods on the extraction rate and qualities of oils from demucilaged flaxseed. *Drying Technology, 36*(13), 1642–1652. https://doi.org/10.1080/07373937.2017.1421220

Zhang, T.-T., Xu, J., Wang, Y.-M., & Xue, C.-H. (2019). Health benefits of dietary marine DHA/EPA-enriched glycerophospholipids. *Progress in Lipid Research, 75*, 100997. https://doi.org/10.1016/j.plipres.2019.100997

Zhang, W., Peng, H., Sun, H., Hua, X., Zhao, W., & Yang, R. (2020). Effect of acidic moisture-conditioning as pretreatment for aqueous extraction of flaxseed oil with lower water consumption. *Food and Bioproducts Processing, 121*, 20–28. https://doi.org/10.1016/j.fbp.2020.01.017

Zhang, Z., Lee, W. J., Sun, X., & Wang, Y. (2022). Enzymatic interesterification of palm olein in a continuous packed bed reactor: Effect of process parameters on the properties of fats and immobilized Thermomyces lanuginosus lipase. *LWT, 162*, 113459. https://doi.org/10.1016/j.lwt.2022.113459

Zhang, Y., Wang, M., Zhang, X., Qu, Z., Gao, Y., Li, Q., & Yu, X. (2023). Mechanism, indexes, methods, challenges, and perspectives of edible oil oxidation analysis. *Critical Reviews in Food Science and Nutrition, 63*(21), 4901–4915. https://doi.org/10.1080/10408398.2021.2009437

Nutritional Benefits of Linseed Oil-Based Omega-3 Fatty Acids

Snigdha Homroy, Reena Malongil Bapputty, Rajni Chopra, Richa Soni, Deepa Sanglekar, and Vidhi Shah

Abstract

This chapter explores the critical role of omega-3 polyunsaturated fatty acids (PUFA), focusing on α-linolenic acid from linseed oil. It begins by explaining the types of omega-3 fatty acids (FA), including α-linolenic acid (ALA), stearidonic acid (SDA), eicosapentaenoic acid (EPA), and docosahexaenoic acid (DHA), detailing their distinct health benefits. The following sections provide an in-depth analysis of the digestion, absorption, and metabolism of omega-3 FA, elucidating how they are processed within the body. Special emphasis is placed on the extensive health benefits of linseed oil across various body systems. In terms of cardiovascular health, omega-3 FAs improve serum lipid profiles and regulate signal transduction pathways. For brain health, their potential in reducing the risk of stroke and Alzheimer's disease is highlighted. The chapter also discusses omega-3 FA's anti-inflammatory properties and their role in immune system modulation, as well as oxidative stress reduction. Furthermore, there are discussions about hepatoprotective effects against nonalcoholic fatty liver disease with antidiabetic benefits through serum triglyceride regulation. This chapter also addresses metabolic syndrome improvement along with contributions to skin, hair, and digestive health. This holistic review highlights the significant benefits of including linseed oil in dietary regimens to improve overall health.

S. Homroy · R. Chopra
Department of Food Science and Technology, National Institute of Food Technology Entrepreneurship and Management, Kundli, Haryana, India

R. M. Bapputty (✉)
Department of Pediatrics, Case Western Reserve University, Cleveland, OH, USA

R. Soni · D. Sanglekar · V. Shah
Department of Life Science and Food Science and Nutrition, University School of Science, Gujarat University, Ahmedabad, Gujarat, India

© The Author(s), under exclusive license to Springer Nature Singapore Pte Ltd. 2025

R. Chopra et al. (eds.), *Dynamics of Linseed and its Valorization*,
https://doi.org/10.1007/978-981-96-8927-9_8

Keywords

Health benefits · Linseed oil · Linolenic acid · EPA · DHA · PUFA

1 Introduction

Cardiovascular diseases are now better understood, and improving cardiovascular health has become a priority in recent years. Despite concerted efforts to raise awareness and encourage healthier lifestyles, South Asia continues to have the highest global prevalence of cardiovascular disease, affecting people at younger ages. Key contributing factors for developing chronic heart disease include poor dietary habits such as higher intake of saturated and trans fats, sugar, and salt; excessive animal-sourced foods; snacking; and low consumption of "healthier fats," whole grains, legumes, fruits, and vegetables (Homroy et al., 2024). Epidemiological and clinical studies demonstrate that consuming long-chain omega-3 fatty acids (FA) provide health benefits, including reduced CVD related morbidity and mortality, improved eye and brain development and function, and reduced inflammation (Casula et al., 2020; Saini et al., 2021). α-linolenic acid (ALA, 18:3 omega−3) is the predominant omega-3 FA for people following plant-based diet and do not take concentrated eicosapentaenoic acid (EPA, 20:5 omega−3) or docosahexaenoic acid (DHA, 22:6 omega−3) supplements. Dietary sources of ALA include nuts and seeds (walnut, almond, chia, echium, linseeds, perilla, soybean, and rapeseed/canola). Although the dietary intake of ALA is higher, the proportion of ALA in plasma, tissue, and cells is lower compared to EPA and DHA on average. EPA and DHA are the main long-chain omega-3 fatty acids that the body uses. ALA is the precursor that is then converted into EPA and DHA (Chaudhary et al., 2021; Homroy et al., 2024; Shang et al., 2017). Apart from metabolic conversion, the source of EPA and DHA is through diet, mostly from oily fish and other seafood.

They are present in smaller quantities in other animal-based foods. The World Health Organization (WHO) and various other authorities advocate consuming oily fish once or twice weekly to ensure adequate dietary intake of EPA and DHA, given their health benefits. However, concerns exist about the sustainability of fish consumption due to mercury and other heavy metal contamination (Venugopalan et al., 2021). Moreover, growing concerns about sustainability have led to increased research into alternative sources of PUFA, such as plant-based and microalgae. Plant-based PUFA also effectively caters to the needs of the vegetarian/vegan population. Linseed oil is one such plant-based oil containing nearly 50–55% ALA. Numerous studies support the consumption of linseed and its oil for its health-promoting effects (Kouamé et al., 2021). This chapter focuses on linseed oil and its health benefits owing to its rich ALA content. It discusses the role of ALA as a precursor to EPA and DHA and its impact on cardiovascular health, neurological development, and inflammation.

2 Health Benefits of Omega-3 PUFA

Omega-3 FAs are those fatty acids where the first encountered methylene-separated double bond is at the third position from the methyl terminus (Wang et al., 2021a). Major omega-3 fatty acids of dietary origin are ALA, stearidonic acid (SDA), EPA, and DHA. These are fatty acids with 18 or more carbons with 3 or more double bonds. EPA and DHA along with omega-6, ARA, are long chain PUFAs known for their significant biological functions. ALA and SDA are natural precursors for EPA, docosapentaenoic acid (DPA; 22:5), and DHA. From the research conducted to date, ALA and SDA need to be converted to EPA, DPA, or DHA to be biologically effective. These FAs are involved in many biological processes, and their inadequacy in the body strains the self-regulating actions and disrupts homeostasis. There is promising evidence linking regular consumption of omega-3 lipids to preventing and treating some widely recognized and chronic diseases, including age-related macular degeneration and cardiometabolic diseases. Myocardial infarction, severe adverse cardiovascular events, and cardiac death are considerably decreased by omega-3 PUFA intake. These FAs also lower the elevated blood pressure and plasma triglycerides and reduce the risk of CVD and type-2 diabetes. They are a proven solution to prevent inflammatory and autoimmune diseases and cancer. They have also shown potential to treat depression, anxiety, dementia, schizophrenia, and Alzheimer's disease. Unlike omega-3 PUFA, the accompanying omega-6 FA (omega-6 PUFA) has debatable health benefits. Higher levels of omega-6 PUFA have been associated with negative health effects. However, maintaining a balanced ratio of omega-6 to omega-3 FAs, typically between 2:1 and 5:1, has been shown to have protective antioxidant, anti-inflammatory, and anti-arrhythmic properties and can help prevent metabolic disorders (Blanco-Llamero et al., 2022; Casula et al., 2020; Chamorro et al., 2022; Saini et al., 2021; Wang et al., 2022b).

EPA and DHA are the two most studied bioactive forms of omega-3 PUFA. ALA is mostly converted to EPA and DHA, which play their roles. DHA is typically recognized for its favorable effects on the heart, nervous system, and brain, owing to its ability to regulate cell and membrane activities, thereby bringing various advantages. It is a structural component of the cortical gray matter and retinal photoreceptors and play a critical role in visual function. Its significance is further highlighted during gestation as its DHA content dramatically increases in the retinal membrane synapses and neural cortex during the third trimester of pregnancy and is essential for eye development. DHA improves neurological activity by promoting neurogenesis and synaptic plasticity, as well as decreasing neuroinflammation, linking high DHA levels in the body with a reduced risk of myocardial infarction and cardiovascular disease. The anti-inflammatory action of DHA is carried out mainly through its derivatives, such as oxidized FA metabolites called oxylipins such as resolvins, maresins, and protectins (Homroy et al., 2024; Wang et al., 2022b). The cardioprotective effect of EPA is mediated mainly through its antithrombotic activities. Increased EPA in cell membranes alters the availability of omega-6 FA, arachidonic acid (C20:4 ω-6, ARA) and inhibits the production of eicosanoids with pro-inflammatory (leukotrienes, thromboxanes, and prostaglandins) activities and thereby regulate blood flow, ion transport, inflammation, and immunological response. Furthermore, EPA-derived E-series resolvins confers protection against inflammatory attacks (Wang et al., 2021a, b). Docospentanoic acid (DPA) is an intermediary omega-3 FA formed from EPA prior its conversion to DHA. Studies have demonstrated that DPA and EPA can also be formed from DHA by its retro-conversion after dietary supplementation (Arterburn et al., 2006). The rapid conversion between EPA and DPA indicates the possibility that DPA can be a potential storage form for EPA. Studies have been reported that omega-3 DPA effectively inhibits platelet aggregation and has cardioprotective effect. Moreover, it is the most abundant omega-3 long chain PUFA in the brain after DHA and has shown to provide neuroprotection.

The average daily intake of total fat and omega-6 PUFA linoleic acid (LA, 18:2 omega-6) is generally in line with the recommended values for most populations. However, many people have inadequate intake of long chain omega-3 PUFA, as well as ALA, leading to an imbalanced omega-6/omega-3 ratio. Adequate omega-3 PUFA intake is crucial, especially during critical growth stages like infancy and adolescence. The maternal diet and body stores during pregnancy and breastfeeding play a vital role in supplying FAs to the fetus and infant, influencing breast milk's omega-6 and omega-3 composition. These FA are essential for human metabolism and physiology, with ARA and DHA particularly important for infant development. They play a crucial role in the flexibility and fluidity of neuronal membranes, supporting processes like signal transduction, neuronal growth, and synaptic plasticity during the infant developmental stage. Furthermore, these PUFAs can impact muscle and adipose tissue energy metabolism by influencing insulin action and inflammatory response (Barrera et al., 2018; Chamorro et al., 2022).

Governments have provided dietary recommendations for omega-3 intake based on research. For instance, the US National Academy of Medicine suggests 1.1–1.6 gram/day omega-3 for adults, while the WHO recommends 250–500 mg/day of EPA and DHA for European adults. The National Institute of Nutrition-Indian Council of Medical Research (NIN-ICMR) has set the Recommended Dietary Allowance (RDA) for ALA at 1.6 gram per day for men and 1.1 gram per day for women. Intake recommendations vary depending on age, gender, and health conditions. Individuals with certain conditions, such as cardiovascular disease, may require higher doses of omega-3 supplementation for therapeutic benefits. The Food and Agriculture Organization (FAO) advises adults to consume 300 mg of EPA + DHA daily, which can be obtained from 250 grams of marine fish per week. Meeting these recommendations can be challenging, especially for vegetarians/vegans. Additionally, fish oils have a strong fishy flavor, making them less popular, and fish consumption presents risks of toxic metal exposure. Fortunately, various vegetable and plant-based oils, such as linseed, walnut, canola, and soybean, are rich sources of omega-3 PUFA, which can boost ALA intake (precursor of EPA and DHA) (ICMR, 2024; NIH, 2005; Venugopalan et al., 2021).

3 Digestion, Absorption, and Metabolism of Omega-3 PUFA in Body

Humans cannot synthesize omega-3 FA within their bodies and must obtain these from dietary sources, hence called essential FAs. Omega-3 FAs, such as ALA, are further desaturated and elongated into long-chain FA, namely, EPA and DHA. The conversions of PUFAs are primarily observed in the liver, with relatively lower levels detected in the brain, testicles, and kidneys. However, no detectable biosynthetic activity of these essential FAs was found in the heart and lungs (Valenzuela et al., 2023). EPA and DHA are formed through the conversion of ALA, while ARA is produced from LA with assistance from desaturases and elongase enzymes. The human body can convert merely 0.5% to 8% of the ingested ALA into long-chain omega-3 FA, which is a relatively low rate of conversion. Evidence indicates that the conversion rate of ALA to EPA is approximately 4–8%, while the conversion to DHA is much lower, at around 1% (Burdge et al., 2003; Burdge & Wootton, 2002; Gerster, 1998; Plourde & Cunnane, 2007; Saini et al., 2021). Therefore, it is strongly advised to include long-chain omega-3-rich oils, such as those from marine sources, in recommended amounts within diets or from supplements. This is because consuming these long-chain omega-3 FAs directly has the added advantage of bypassing the conversion processes in the body, allowing them to be absorbed directly into the bloodstream. This helps to ensure adequate intake of these essential FA (Blanco-Llamero et al., 2022; Panda et al., 2022; Saini et al., 2021; Venugopalan et al., 2021; Videla et al., 2022; Wang et al., 2022b).

The conversion rate of omega-3 FAs also varies depending on a multitude of factors such as age, sex, and genetic or epigenetic variations. An individual's physiological or nutritional status plays a vital role in the metabolism of PUFA and the conversion rate. The rising prevalence of obesity and nonalcoholic fatty liver disease (NAFLD) has been associated with a decline in the production of long-chain omega-3 PUFA. Furthermore, the activity of desaturase enzymes, which are crucial for converting shorter-chain PUFAs into their long-chain counterparts, is significantly reduced when individuals consume a high-fat diet. This reduction is accompanied by a decreased accumulation of long-chain omega-3 PUFAs in various tissues, including the liver. The underlying cause is the oxidative stress induced by NAFLD, which disrupts both the expression and activity of these essential enzymes, thereby impairing the body's ability to produce and store long-chain omega-3 PUFAs effectively. This disruption further reduces omega-3 PUFA levels through free-radical-dependent peroxidation processes (Valenzuela et al., 2017; Videla et al., 2022; Yang et al., 2022).

Following ingestion, the food matrix containing PUFAs enters the stomach, where it is subjected to the low pH and digestive enzymes of the gastric fluids, which facilitate breakdown. The gastric lipase enzyme degrades the oil globules and triglycerides (TAG), releasing free FA. The primary absorption of oils and fats occurs in the small intestine, where the peristaltic motion of the gastrointestinal tract breaks down the lipid globules into smaller units. These smaller lipid particles are then acted upon by bile salts and juices, forming an emulsion. This increased solubility and surface area provides a favorable environment for the lipase enzymes to act on the lipids resulting in release of FA, which are then absorbed by the intestinal epithelium, where they bind to transport proteins, forming chylomicrons that enter the circulatory system via the lymph through the lacteal. ALA is absorbed from the gut and enter the circulatory system after being esterified into TAG molecules, which are picked and transported within chylomicrons (Homroy et al., 2024). The chylomicron-TAG are then hydrolyzed by lipoprotein lipase present on endothelial cells. Additionally, adipose tissue is stimulated to increase lipoprotein lipase during the postprandial period to facilitate the uptake and storage of meal FA. The hydrolysis of TAGs results in the formation of diacylglycerol and chylomicron remnants. These remnants are primarily taken up from the circulation through hepatic receptor-mediated pathways. The FAs from these chylomicron remnants are then processed within the liver, where they can be made available for incorporation into cellular membranes, storage (within adipose tissue), energy production (β-oxidation), or conversion to long-chain omega-3 PUFAs (Baker et al., 2016). Figure 1 summarizes the metabolic fates of dietary ALA in human body.

ALA is the most abundant omega-3 PUFA in human adipose tissue, accounting for approximately 1% of total FA, while there are only trace amounts of DHA and EPA (Baker et al., 2016). During fasting, hormone-triggered lipase breaks down TAG stores in adipose tissue, releasing free FA into the plasma. Interestingly, studies have detected ALA within the nonesterified FA pool in the plasma shortly after digestion, suggesting a rapid release of nonesterified ALA, potentially from chylomicron-TAG. The relatively low entrapment of ALA in adipose tissue may enhance its availability for conversion into EPA and DHA. Similar trend has been observed for EPA and DHA with very small amounts in adipose tissue. Furthermore, lower uptake of DHA into adipose tissue compared to EPA has also been studied, where DHA levels were twice than EPA in the plasma after a meal. There are

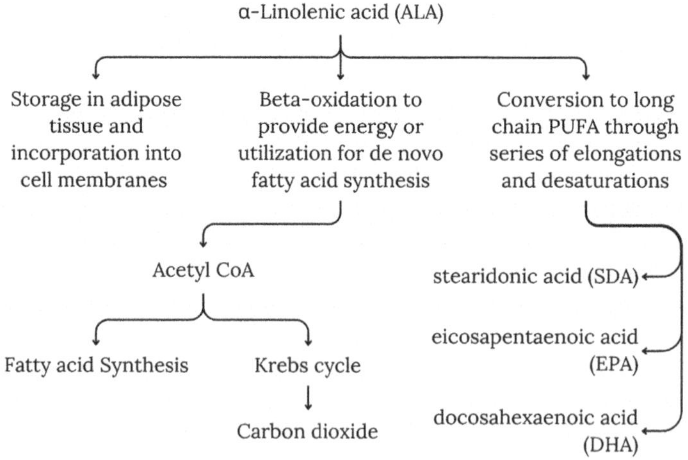

Fig. 1 Metabolic pathways of alpha-linolenic acid in humans

notable differences in ALA metabolism and storage between men and women. Due to a higher percentage of adipose tissue, women may store more ALA than men (Baker et al., 2016; Walker et al., 2014). Studies have shown that ALA, among the unsaturated FAs examined, undergoes β-oxidation at the highest rate. Tracer studies indicate that the conversion of consumed ALA to carbon dioxide via β-oxidation within the first hour accounts for 15–35% of the ALA intake. In contrast, the oxidation of the omega-6 PUFA LA after consumption represents 12% of the consumed linoleic acid (McCloy et al., 2004).

ALA undergoes conversion into long-chain omega-3 FA, namely, EPA and DHA, through a sequence of biochemical reactions. This process involves elongation and desaturation, which predominantly occurs within the endoplasmic reticulum. However, the final step of β-oxidation, which is crucial for the formation of DHA, takes place in the peroxisomes. (as shown in Fig. 2). Primarily, this metabolic pathway occurs in the liver. However, some evidence suggests that the brain, retina, and testes also exhibit significant expression of the genes responsible for producing the required enzymes (Baker et al., 2016; Homroy et al., 2024; Nakamura & Nara, 2004). The initial step of ALA's conversion to SDA is catalyzed by the enzyme Δ-6-desaturase (Δ6D, encoded by the fatty acid desaturase 2 gene; Fads2). This enzyme introduces a double bond at the Δ6 position of ALA, resulting in the formation of SDA (18:4 ω-3). Following this, enzyme elongase-5 (encoded by the fatty acid elongase 5 gene; Elovl5) adds two additional carbon atoms to SDA to produce eicosatetraenoic acid (ETA, 20:4 ω-3). The conversion of ETA to eicosapentaenoic acid (EPA) occurs through the action of Δ-5-desaturase, which inserts an additional double bond at the Δ5 position of the carbon chain. The efficiency of SDA to EPA conversion is higher compared to conversion of ALA to EPA because the conversion

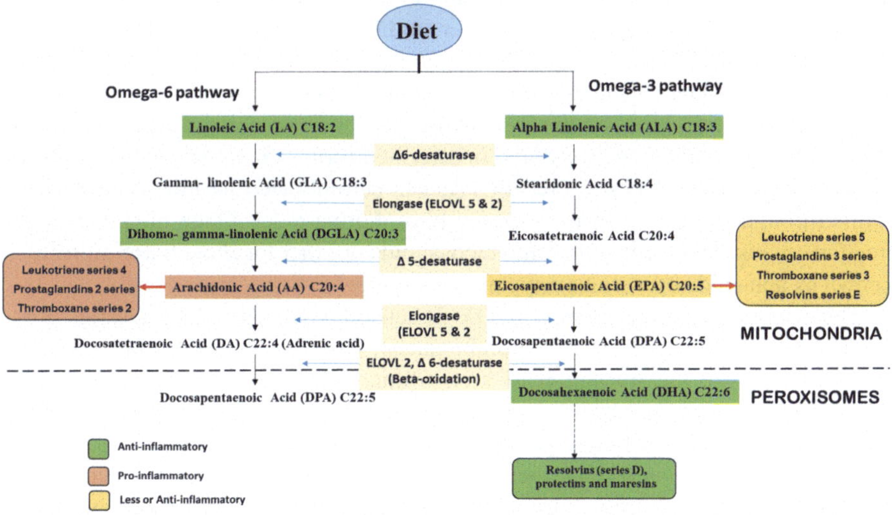

Fig. 2 The pathway of metabolic conversion of omega-6 and omega-3 PUFA to long chain omega-3 PUFAs body. (Source: Chisaguano et al. (2013), Mathias et al. (2010))

from SDA does not require the initial Δ-6-desaturation step. As a result, SDA is often referred to as "pro-EPA" due to its enhanced role in facilitating this conversion. (Gregory et al., 2011). EPA undergoes further elongation through the action of enzymes elongases 2 or elongases 5, leading to the formation of docosapentaenoic acid (DPA; 22:5 ω-3). DPA, in turn, is elongated by elongase 2 to produce a longer-chain fatty acid, specifically 24:5 ω-3. Following this, the enzyme Δ-6-desaturase (Δ6D), which was initially involved in the conversion of ALA to SDA, also catalyzes the desaturation of 24:5 ω-3 to form 24:6 ω-3. This desaturation step is crucial for the further metabolism and functional roles of these long-chain omega-3 fatty acids. This 24:6ω-3 is then transported to peroxisomes, where the final β-oxidation reaction takes place to produce the end-product DHA.

Delta-6-desaturase (encoded by Fads2) is considered a rate-limiting enzyme in the conversion of dietary ALA to DHA. This is evidenced by the observations where patients with Δ6D deficiency were unable to desaturate either ALA or 24:5ω-3. The enzyme, Δ6D preferentially acts on ALA over LA. However, competition occurs between the conversion of omega-6 and omega-3 FAs, as both utilize this shared metabolic pathway. When LA is much more readily available than ALA, the metabolism of LA exceeds that of ALA (Baker et al., 2016; Williard et al., 2001). Increasing dietary ALA or the direct Fads2 product, SDA, enhances tissue levels of EPA and DPA, but not DHA. These observations indicate the existence of regulatory control points apart from the ALA metabolism through Fads2. One potential control point could be the second reaction involving Fads2, as Δ6D catalyzes the desaturation of both ALA to SDA and 24:5ω-3 to 24:6ω-3. Furthermore, the metabolism of EPA and DPA also requires elongation reactions. Recent research indicates that the conversion of EPA to DHA could be limited by the availability of the fatty acid 24:5 ω-3. Additionally, it appears that other stages of this metabolic pathway may be regulated, especially the process involving the translocation of 24:6 ω-3 into the peroxisome. This suggests that further studies focusing on the role and regulatory mechanisms of elongase 2 (Elovl2) could be essential for a comprehensive understanding of DHA synthesis (Gregory et al., 2011).

PUFAs that are either synthesized within the body or derived from metabolic conversions are predominantly stored in esterified forms, either as phospholipids or as neutral glycerides. These stored PUFAs can be mobilized into their unesterified forms through the action of the enzyme phospholipase A2. Once liberated, these free fatty acids can be converted into eicosanoids or other local mediator molecules known as autacoids by various oxygenase enzymes.

The enzyme cyclooxygenase-2 (COX-2) acts on ARA to produce 2-series prostaglandins (PG) and 2-series thromboxanes, whereas lipoxygenase (5-LOX) enzymes catalyze the formation of series four leukotrienes (or LTs), including LTB4, LTC4, LTD4, and LTE4. Conversely, EPA is metabolized to produce series three prostaglandins (or PGs), specifically PGD3, PGE3, PGF3, and PGI3, as well as series five leukotrienes (LT), including LTB5, LTC5, and LTD5. These products of EPA metabolism are known for their potent anti-inflammatory, vasodilatory, and anti-aggregative properties. Furthermore, DHA metabolism yields autacoids such as protectins, D-series resolvins, and maresins, which also contribute to the body's regulatory and protective functions.

4 Health Benefits of Linseed Oil on Various Body Systems

Evidence suggests that dietary omega 3 FA beneficially affect health by modulating numerous biological processes including maintaining cardiovascular function by regulating blood lipid levels and thrombosis, brain and visual system development, inflammation, membrane fluidity, and signal transduction. The health benefits of linseed oil are mainly attributed to the omega-3 FA it contains and the presence of lignans in it. The following sections elucidate the various health benefits imparted by ALA-rich linseed oil while Table 1 summarizes a few notable randomized control trials validating the beneficial effects of linseed oil.

4.1 Cardiovascular Health

According to Global Burden of Disease Study, CVD are the leading cause of mortality all over the world, accounting for 32% of total global deaths in 2019 (Roth et al., 2020). Evidence from prospective and case control studies indicate that increased intake of omega-3 FA alone can have tremendous beneficial effect on the CVD risk as its intake helps reduce the impact of many other modifiable risk factors such as atherosclerosis, hyperlipidemia, thrombosis, inflammation, hypertension, and arrhythmia of the heart. The most effective way to enrich omega-3 is by incorporating oily fish in the diet. However, the consumption of fish is low among the majority of the populations and is not a choice for populations looking for a plant-based diet. Here comes the importance of an omega-3-rich fat source that would provide cardio protection (Fig. 3).

Linseed oil is one of the richest sources of omega-3, alpha-linolenic acid. It contains phytoestrogen, lignans, along with other minor constituents. ALA's beneficial effect is mediated via its long chain conversion products: EPA, DPA, and DHA. The efficacy of ALA conversion to EPA and DHA are analyzed by measuring the omega-3 index of erythrocyte membrane and serum phospholipids. Several clinical trials have demonstrated that ALA intake results in accumulation of EPA and DPA in erythrocytes and serum with minor quantities of DHA. Healthy human subjects supplemented with 3.5 g linseed oil for 8 weeks have shown to increase erythrocyte membrane EPA to 133% and DPA to 120% of the baseline (Cao et al., 2006).

The cardioprotective effect of linseed oil is mainly due to the hypolipidemic, antithrombotic, anti-atherosclerotic, and anti-inflammatory effects and these effects are contributed by both lignans and omega-3 ALA it contains. Studies have demonstrated that lignan complex (40 mg/kg body weight) isolated from linseed was effective in modulating cholesterol levels in experimental hypercholesterolemic rabbits. It inhibited both serum total and LDL-cholesterol and upregulated the antioxidant lipoprotein, HDL-cholesterol, which might provide additional antioxidant effects. Moreover, lignan complex have shown to be effective in reducing oxidative stress markers such as malondialdehyde formation in serum and isolated aorta and inhibited aortic atherosclerotic plaque formation and prevented atherosclerosis (Prasad, 2005). However, the lignan complex did not affect the triglyceride levels in these rabbits.

Table 1 Randomized controlled trials (RCT) proving health benefits associated with regular linseed consumption

Health benefits observed	Details of clinical trial	Major findings to support the observation	References
Alleviation of CVD risk	The 12-week study evaluated the metabolic syndrome-related parameters in 64 subjects with mild-to-moderate ulcerative colitis. Participants were randomly assigned to an intervention group (30 g ground linseed powder each day) or a control group. Biochemical variables were measured at the start and final stage of the intervention	Linseed supplementation over 12 weeks resulted in significant decreases in insulin, HOMA-IR, triglycerides, total cholesterol, and a significant increase in HDL. After linseed supplementation, significant improvements were observed in serum TNF-α and CRP. Overall, linseed supplementation led to greater improvements in certain metabolic syndrome-related parameters	Morshedzadeh et al. (2021a)
	A total of 1107 participants were evaluated through a meta-analysis of 14 RCTs	Incorporation of linseed was associated with improved lipid parameters, including reductions in total cholesterol, low-density lipoprotein cholesterol, and triglycerides, among dyslipidemic patients compared to the control group. However, no significant changes were observed in high-density lipoprotein levels. Conversely, in healthy individuals, linseed consumption significantly increased HDL-C, LDL-C, and triglycerides. Subgroup analysis of healthy subjects revealed that linseed improved LDL-C specifically in overweight individuals with a BMI greater than 25	Sadat Masjedi et al. (2022)
	A 12-week triple-blind clinical trial in hypertension subjects with two intervention groups receiving 10 or 30 grams of linseed per day compared to control group	The group that consumed 30 g of linseed exhibited the most favorable outcomes, demonstrating a 13.38-unit decline in systolic blood pressure compared to a 1.72-unit increase in the placebo group, and a 5.6-unit decrease in diastolic blood pressure compared to a 2.39-unit increase in the placebo group. Additionally, the linseed group experienced a 0.86-unit reduction in BMI, contrasted with a 0.06-unit decrease in the placebo group. Total cholesterol levels also decreased by 20.4 units in the linseed group, in contrast to an 11.86-unit decrease in the placebo group	Toulabi et al. (2022)
Anti-inflammatory properties	Thirty-four hemodialysis patients were given 6 grams of linseed oil per day for 8 weeks. Their serum levels of high-sensitivity C-reactive protein (hs-CRP) and soluble vascular cell adhesion molecule-1 (sVCAM-1) were measured after fasting for 12–14 h	Serum levels of hs-CRP, a marker of systemic inflammation, and sVCAM-1, a marker of vascular inflammation, decreased significantly in the linseed oil group by the end of week 8 compared to baseline. Furthermore, these reductions were statistically significant when compared to the control group. This study indicates that daily consumption of linseed oil reduces two risk factors for CVD	Mirfatahi et al. (2016)
	The study examined the impact of ground linseed (30 grams/day) and linseed oil (10 grams/day) on clinical markers, quality of life, and disease severity in patients with ulcerative colitis, a chronic inflammatory bowel condition. Seventy-five ulcerative colitis patients over 12 weeks participated in an open-label RCT design and were randomly assigned to two intervention groups receiving ground linseed or linseed oil, as well as a control group. Data were collected from participants before and 12 weeks after the intervention	Following the intervention, hs-CRP (a marker of inflammation) and Mayo scores (measure the severity of ulcerative colitis) decreased significantly in the groups that consumed linseed products compared to the control group. A notable increase in IL-10 concentration was observed in the linseed oil-fed group, but no significant change was found in serum IL-10 levels in the control group. Additionally, the decrease in Mayo score was more pronounced in patients with more severe disease	Morshedzadeh et al. (2021b)

Improvement and maintenance of brain health	Sixty healthy older adults (65–80 years without cognitive impairment or depression) were randomly divided into two groups; either they received 3.7 gram/day of linseed oil or an isocaloric placebo for 12 weeks. The primary parameters were six cognitive functions closely related to everyday life	After 12 weeks, the intervention group showed significantly greater improvements in verbal fluency scores on the frontal assessment compared to the control group. Daily intake of linseed oil, rich in antioxidants and ALA, improved cognitive function, specifically verbal fluency, in healthy individuals despite age-related cognitive decline and without any cognitive abnormalities	Ogawa et al. (2023)
	The impact of two short-term oral administrations of linseed oil (0.26 and 0.52 mL/kg) was assessed through tests on Wistar rats with hyperammonemia, evaluating its effects on short-term and long-term visuospatial memory as well as motor coordination, and the neuronal morphology of the prefrontal cortex	Compared to an ammonium-rich diet, linseed oil and normal foods helped sustain cognition or motor function, as demonstrated by short-term and visuospatial memory tests. Additionally, the linseed oil preserved the normal neuronal morphology of the prefrontal cortex, indicating a neuroprotective effect	Ocaña-Sánchez et al. (2023)
Hepatoprotective effects	This study investigated the effects of linseed oil treatment against diazinon-induced liver toxicity. Twenty-five Wistar rats were randomly divided into five groups: control, diazinon-fed, linseed oil-fed, co-treatment group (diazinon 70 mg/kg/day and linseed oil at doses of 100mg/kg/day), and co-treatment group (diazinon 70 mg/kg/day and linseed oil at doses of 200 mg/kg/day). Oxidative stress markers were analyzed, including liver and serum levels of malondialdehyde, catalase, total antioxidant capacity, and total thiol group. Liver function tests, such as serum alanine aminotransferase, alkaline phosphatase, aspartate aminotransferase, and liver histological examination were also evaluated	Diazinon significantly increased markers of oxidative stress in the liver and serum, as well as levels of liver enzymes compared to the control group. Linseed oil consumption significantly improved oxidative stress status and liver function tests in a dose-dependent manner. Furthermore, linseed oil ameliorated the liver histopathological alterations induced by diazinon. Linseed supplementation had a liver-protective effect by decreasing oxidative stress markers and improving antioxidative status, thereby reducing diazinon-induced alterations in the liver	Lotfi et al. (2023)
	The study evaluated the hypolipidemic and hepatoprotective effects of linseed. Thirty-six Albino Wistar rats were divided into six groups (control, medication control, and different doses of Linseed extract; 100 mg/kg, 200 mg/kg and 400 mg/kg). Blood samples were taken at the end of 2 months	The results demonstrate a significant decrease in lipid parameters and liver enzymes after 2 months in all three groups receiving the linseed extract. The highest dose of the extract was comparable to the standard drug. This suggests that adding linseed to the diet may help mitigate the rise in circulating cholesterol levels caused by a high-cholesterol diet, likely due to its ALA and lignin content. The study also provides evidence for the hepatoprotective role of linseed in hypercholesterolemia	Pattanayak et al. (2021)

(continued)

Table 1 (continued)

Health benefits observed	Details of clinical trial	Major findings to support the observation	References
Improvement in mental health status	Sixty depressed women aged 18–45 were randomly assigned to two groups. One group took a 1000 mg linseed oil capsule twice daily for 10 weeks, while the other group took a placebo. Serum brain-derived neurotrophic factor (BDNF), Beck Depression Inventory-II scores, and anthropometric measures were assessed before and after the intervention	The results showed that serum BDNF levels increased significantly in the linseed oil group (1.12 ± 0.6 pg/ml) compared to the placebo group (0.2 ± 0.56 pg/ml). The total BDI-II score was significantly lower after linseed oil supplementation (−16.62) compared to placebo (−8.45)	Poorbaferani et al. (2020)
	Seventy-two overweight and obese children and adolescents were randomly assigned to two groups: one receiving 20 grams per day of linseed and the other receiving 25 grams per day of puffed wheat; for 4 weeks	Consumption of linseed led to a significant decrease in mental fatigue. However, general fatigue, motivation, activity, and mood feelings did not differ significantly between the two groups	Gholami and Akhlaghi (2021)
Improvement in skin condition and wound healing rate	Twenty-six women with sensitive skin were given four capsules of linseed oil (555.32 mg/capsule) per day opposed to control group (four capsules of safflower oil per day) for 12-week intervention	Significant decrease in sensitivity, skin roughness, scaling, and transepidermal water loss, while epidermal hydration and smoothness were increased in the intervention group	Neukam et al. (2011)
	The study included 60 participants diagnosed with grade 3 diabetic foot syndrome. The intervention lasted 12 weeks, with the treatment group receiving 1000 mg of linseed oil twice daily	Significant reduction in the length and depth of ulcers in the intervention group	Soleimani et al. (2017)

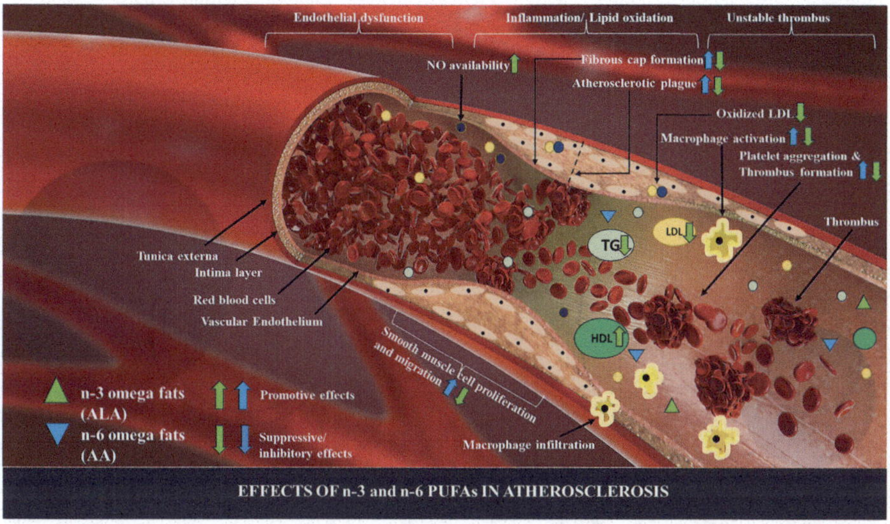

Fig. 3 Effects of omega-3 and omega-6 PUFAs on initiation of atherosclerosis. (*Source*: Budoff et al. (2020), Mathias et al. (2010))LDL Low-density lipoprotein, NO Nitric oxide, TG Triglycerides, HDL High density lipoprotein, ALA Alpha-linolenic acid, AA Arachidonic acid

Several clinical trials and experiments in animal models have shown that omega-3 fatty acids exert hypolipidemic properties. Supplementation of 30 g ground linseed powder for 12 weeks resulted in decrease in serum total cholesterol and triglycerides in subjects with mild-to-moderate ulcerative colitis (Morshedzadeh et al., 2021b). Meta-analysis of 14 randomized clinical trials indicated that linseed was effective in lowering total cholesterol, LDL cholesterol, and triglycerides in dyslipidemic subjects (Sadat Masjedi et al., 2022). Enriching dietary fat with ALA or ALA containing linseed oil improved serum and liver lipid profiles in experimental rats. Decreased serum triglycerides and serum and liver cholesterol were observed in these rats compared to rats fed with omega-6-rich groundnut oil (Chopra & Sambaiah, 2009; Sharma & Lokesh, 2013). Decreased serum and liver cholesterol levels observed in rats were associated with the decreased HMG CoA activity, indicating that the cholesterol lowering effect is mediated through reduction in cholesterol synthesis (Sharma & Lokesh, 2013). Even though many human trials showed positive effects, some of them failed to show the hypolipidemic effect of omega-lipids from linseed oil. One of the reasons for this might be due to the inadequate amount of omega-3 FAs and lignans. It may also be due to the high amount of omega-6 linoleic FA in the diet. Increased amounts of LA in the diet compete with omega-3 for desaturase and elongase enzymes and make them less available for their conversion into long chain bioactive molecules EPA, DPA, and DHA. The ratio of omega-3 to omega-6 should be ideal for achieving the optimum benefits from omega-3 (Simopoulos, 2006).

The anti-inflammatory effect exerted by the dietary linseed oil can provide a significant cardioprotective effect (Fig. 4). Most human trials reported that ALA

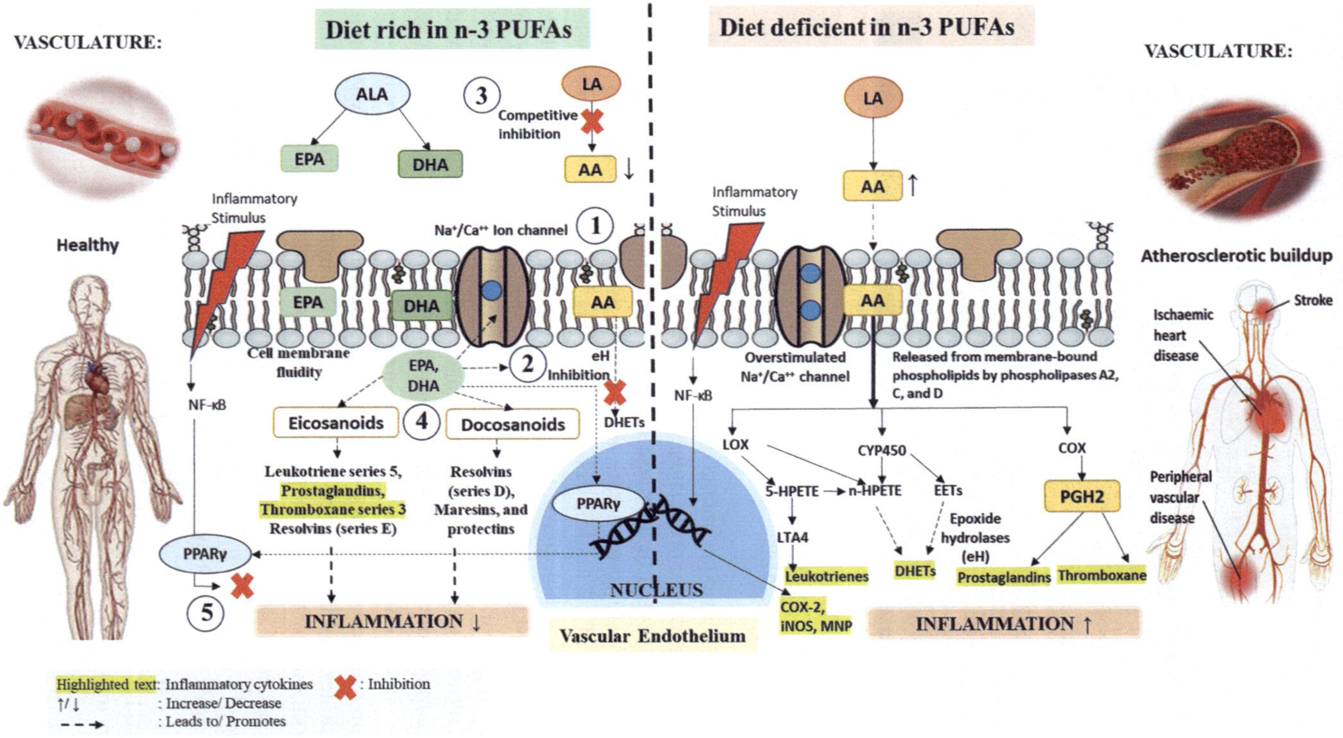

Fig. 4 Anti-inflammatory effects of linseed oil consumption. (*Source*: Endo and Arita (2016), Wang et al. (2021a, b))PUFA Polyunsaturated fatty acid, DHETs Dihydroxy eicosatrienoic acids, ALA Alpha-linolenic acid, LOX Lipoxygenase, LA Linoleic acid, CYP450 Cytochrome P450, AA Arachidonic acid, COX-1/COX-2 Cyclooxygenase 1 & 2, EPA Eicosapentaenoic acid, n-HPETE n-hydroperoxy eicosatetraenoic acid, DHA Docosahexaenoic acid, EETs Epoxy eicosatrienoic acid, eH Epoxide hydrolase, LTA4 Leukotriene A_4, PPARγ Peroxisome proliferator-activated receptor gamma, PGH2 Prostaglandin H_2, NF-κB Nuclear factor kappa-light-chain-enhancer of activated B cells, iNOS Nitric Oxide Synthase, MNP Mononuclear Phagocytes

intake increases tissue EPA and DPA level significantly (Cao et al., 2006). Increased levels of EPA, DPA, and DHA in membrane phospholipids is associated with decreased levels of n-6 ARA. This decreases the availability of ARA for the synthesis of proinflammatory, proatherogenic eicosanoids such as leukotrienes (LT-4 series), prostaglandins (PG-2 series), and thromboxane (TX- 2 series). The eicosanoid counterparts produced from EPA (LT-5 series, PG-3 series, and TX- 3 series) are relatively less inflammatory and less atherogenic. For example, the leukotriene B5 has protective effects compared to the proinflammatory leukotriene B4, which induce ICAM1 and NF-kB, the inflammatory transcription factor that induce expression of proinflammatory genes. ICAM1, the adhesion molecule mediates leukocyte adhesion to the endothelium, an initiation step in atherosclerosis. Similarly, TXA3 produced from EPA is a much weaker platelet aggregator compared to the TXA2 from ARA. The REDUCE-IT (Reduction of Cardiovascular Events with Icosapent Ethyl Intervention Trial) reported the effectiveness of EPA on the cardioprotective effect recently. EPA-only formulation called icosapent ethyl showed a 25% reduction in cardiovascular events in patients with established cardiovascular disease or diabetes mellitus and other cardiovascular risk factors (Manson et al., 2019). EPA is effective in reducing the triglyceride concentration in CVD with marginal to high triglyceride concentration. EPA (2-4 g/d) inhibited the amount of oxidized LDL formed and reduced the high-sensitivity C-reactive protein, the two important makers for atherosclerosis and inflammation in CVD patients with high triglycerides (Bays et al., 2013).

Specialized pro-resolving molecules (SPMs), resolvins (Rv), protectin, and maresins produced from EPA and DHA play critical roles in resolution of inflammation and immune function. Resolvins are produced from DHA, DPA, and EPA. The metabolic products of EPA include 18-hydroxy eicosapentaenoic acid, (18-HEPE), RvE1, RvE2, and RvE3. They counter-regulate proinflammatories and promote resolution via macrophage uptake of debris (18-HEPE), apoptotosis of neutrophils (RvE1), and killing and clearing microbes (Serhan & Levy, 2018). D-series resolvins (RvD1-RvD6) from DHA are involved in organ protection by bacterial killing and clearance and aid protection against PMN-mediated reperfusion injury. Resolvins play a significant role in cardio protection as they regulate lipid-macrophages-PMNs-loaded foam cells of atherosclerosis plaque clearance.

Studies have demonstrated DPA accumulation in cell membranes with ALA containing diet. Increased levels of serum DPA has been observed with linseed oil diet in humans (Cao et al., 2006). DPA provides additional benefits in that it can get retroconverted to EPA. Therefore, the DPA in cells can be a supplier of EPA. Moreover, DPA metabolites are shown to exert cardio protection by inhibiting platelet aggregation (Drouin et al., 2019). Apart from the anti-inflammatory actions through SPMs, DHA have been shown to be involved in many other protective effects. DHA and EPA affect gene expression through regulation of transcription factor activity. Transcription factors that regulate cholesterol/FA metabolism (PPAR, LXR, SREBP) and inflammation (NF-kB) have a LCPUFA-binding domain (Balić et al., 2020). Altogether linseed oil with its lignans and ALA-derived EPA,

DPA, and DHA and their metabolites is a natural source that help prevent the development of cardiovascular diseases.

4.2 Brain and Eye Health

Omega-3 FA, particularly EPA and DHA, are critical for sustaining long-term brain health. DHA is a major structural component of neuronal membranes, particularly in the cerebral cortex, retina, and synaptosomes, where it maintains membrane fluidity and function. This fluidity is essential for the proper functioning of neurotransmitter receptors and transporters, which impact synaptic plasticity and cognitive processes. DHA is particularly important for the development and maintenance of the central nervous system. During fetal development, DHA accumulates rapidly in the brain, highlighting its significance for prenatal brain health. Adequate DHA levels are associated with improved cognitive development and visual acuity in infants (Homroy et al., 2024; Jin et al., 2020).

After absorption into the brain, DHA and arachidonic acid (AA) are activated by a long-chain-fatty-acid-CoA synthetase called ACSL19, after they are incorporated into phospholipid membranes. Meanwhile, LA, ALA, and EPA undergo beta-oxidation; however, the amount of energy or ATP produced from beta-oxidation is less than that produced by glucose oxidation, partly due to the excessive oxidative stress generated during this process (Bazinet & Layé, 2014). PUFA and their metabolic derivatives exert their effects in the brain through a variety of mechanisms. These mechanisms encompass the modulation of membrane dynamics, where PUFAs influence the fluidity and organization of cellular membranes, thereby affecting their functionality. Additionally, PUFAs interact with specific receptors on neuronal cells, leading to the activation of various intracellular signaling pathways. This receptor engagement triggers a cascade of biochemical events that can alter cellular processes and impact brain function (Bazinet & Layé, 2014; Layé et al., 2018). Free PUFAs and their derivatives function as agonists for a range of receptors, such as the oxysterol receptor LXR, peroxisome proliferator-activated receptors (PPAR), and hepatic nuclear factor 4A (HNF4A), among others. These fatty acids can also activate protein kinase C (PKC) and suppress the activity of nuclear factor-κB (NF-κB). Additionally, PUFAs play a role in brain function by affecting the endocannabinoid system, given that endocannabinoids are synthesized from PUFAs. Endocannabinoids act as retrograde transmitters at synapses, thus modulating neuronal activity and various brain functions and behaviors including memory, reward and addiction, motor coordination, pain perception, feeding and appetite, stress, schizophrenia, and epilepsy (Bazinet & Layé, 2014).

Studies have demonstrated DHA's crucial role in maintaining synaptic integrity and its involvement in the assembly of the SNARE (soluble N-ethylmaleimide-sensitive fusion (NSF) protein attachment protein receptor) protein complex. This is supported by the finding that DHA is present in high concentrations within synapses. DHA has been observed to mitigate the altered expression of postsynaptic dendritic proteins (PSD95), NMDA receptors, and Ca2+–calmodulin-dependent protein kinase 2 (CAMK2) in Alzheimer's disease investigations. Furthermore, DHA regulates the SNARE fusion machinery responsible for presynaptic exocytosis and endocytosis. The SNARE complex is the core component of the protein machinery that facilitates the fusion of synaptic vesicles with presynaptic terminals, enabling neurotransmitter release (Bazinet & Layé, 2014; Jin et al., 2020).

Studies have shown that learning and memory are deeply influenced by serum DHA levels, but the exact cellular and molecular mechanisms are not fully understood. The most notable observation of DHA' role in the brain was its ability to promote neuronal survival and neurogenesis. DHA, the major FA in phosphatidylserine, enhances its synthesis. Depletion of DHA from the membrane impairs the translocation and activation of AKT and RAF1, which are important for neurogenesis. The positive effects of DHA and its mediators on cell survival and neurogenesis are proven in preclinical models of neurological diseases (Bazinet & Layé, 2014; Fuentes-Albero et al., 2019).

Compelling evidence over the decades firmly establishes the defining role of PUFAs such as EPA and DHA, in not only the development of the nervous system of infants but also in the growth phase of children and adolescents, and the maintenance of nerve membranes, enzymatic functions, and electrophysiological parameters within the nervous system of adults and the elderly (Melo et al., 2019). PUFAs such as DHA are essential and effective in driving morpho-anatomical changes in the nervous system, by contributing to astrocyte maturation, nerve signal conduction, release of neurotransmitters, and formative changes in the hippocampal region for motor functions, memory development, and growth. ALA bioconversion to form EPA and DHA is pivotal, considering the human brain weighs roughly 55% lipids. To ensure optimum PUFA levels for brain development, rapid accumulation of DHA in the brain (especially in the gray matter) has been observed during the last trimester of pregnancy and in the early stages of infancy (Dighriri et al. 2022). The significance of EPA and DHA lies in their ability to produce specialized pro-resolving lipid mediators (SMPs) that actively resolve inflammation.

Chronic neuroinflammation contributes to the development of various neurodegenerative disorders, such as Alzheimer's disease and Parkinson's disease. Omega-3 PUFAs, particularly DHA reduce the production of pro-inflammatory cytokines such as interleukin-1β (IL-1β), interleukin-6 (IL-6), and tumor necrosis factor-alpha (TNF-α) through the modulation of NF-κB signaling pathways. DHA's anti-inflammatory effects might be due to its direct interaction with invading macrophages or microglia. Evidence from both in vitro and in vivo studies indicates that DHA effectively blocks the activation of NF-κB triggered by macrophages and microglia in the central nervous system (CNS). EPA and DHA influence gene expression related to brain health through the activation of PPARs. PPARα and PPARγ, when activated by omega-3 PUFA, upregulate genes involved in antioxidant defense and anti-inflammatory pathways, further contributing to neuronal protection and overall brain health. Both EPA and DHA-derived resolvins, protectins, and maresins are specialized pro-resolving mediators that facilitate the resolution of inflammation (Layé et al., 2018). In patients with Alzheimer's and age-related dementia, supplementing the diet with linseed oil have proven effective in reducing the symptoms associated with cognitive impairment and demonstrated protective effects against further brain damage (Dighriri et al. 2022; Kalmijn et al. 1997).

Omega-3 FA have been shown to improve behavior and cognitive function affected by neuroinflammation. For example, dietary EPA reduced memory problems and anxiety-like behavior caused by exposure to interleukin-1β, and also improved impairment of long-term potentiation by lipopolysaccharide and amyloid-β. EPA and DHA exhibit anti-inflammatory and neuroprotective effects, which also benefit mental health. Studies show that higher dietary intake of ALA and DHA is linked to a lower risk of depression and anxiety disorders. This is likely due to the FAs' ability to modulate neurotransmitter pathways, particularly serotonin and dopamine, as well as reduce inflammatory markers often elevated in depression. Furthermore, lower levels of ARA and DHA in the blood are associated with higher cortisol levels and have been observed in patients with depression (Bazinet & Layé, 2014; Fuentes-Albero et al., 2019; Joffre, 2019). A recent clinical trial (Gholami and Akhlaghi 2021) in overweight/obese individuals documented relief in mood disturbances and fatigue even though the general feelings of anxiety or depression did not alter at a dose of 20 g flaxseeds/day in the 4-week duration. Another study where 60 women with clinical depression were supplemented with flaxseed oil (1000 mg capsule twice/day) for 10 weeks improved serum brain-derived neurotropic factor to confer beneficial results (Poorbaferani et al. 2020).

Omega-3 FAs play an important role in the development of the eye and for maintenance of visual function. DHA content dramatically increases in the retinal membrane synapses and neural cortex during the third trimester of pregnancy and is essential for eye development (Judge et al., 2007). Many sight-threatening eye diseases are associated with the dysfunction in the omega-3 FA metabolism. Impaired omega-3 metabolism is observed in age-related macular degeneration, which causes impairment in central vision. Highest body concentrations of DHA per unit weight are found in phospholipids of retinal photoreceptor outer segments where the phototransduction takes place (SanGiovanni & Chew, 2005). DHA is also present in retinal vascular cells and glia. Vascular endothelial cells are particularly rich in EPA. Vision-threatening diseases including diabetic retinopathy and retinopathy of prematurity initiate with a vascular vessel loss followed by hypoxia-induced neovascularization. Studies have demonstrated that EPA, DHA (2 g% omega 3), and their bioactive products such as neuroprotectin (NPD1), Resolvin D1, and Resolvin E1 inhibit pathologic neovascularization through enhanced vessel regrowth after vascular loss and injury. In the retina, omega-3 fatty acids inhibited TNF production by activated macrophages (Connor et al., 2007). Intake of omega-3 FAs (180 mg of eicosapentaenoic acid and 120 mg docosahexaenoic acid) improved symptoms such as reduction in tear film osmolarity, and increase in Schirmer, tear film breakup time, and goblet cell density in patients with dry eye disease (Bhargava et al., 2023). These studies indicate that incorporating omega-3 FAs improve eye health and function.

4.3 Inflammation and Immune System

Immune cell membranes contain long-chain PUFA (LCPUFAs), including arachidonic acid (AA, C20:4 ω-6), EPA, and DHA. Typically, AA is the most abundant LCPUFA, whereas DHA is the dominant omega-3 LCPUFA. In adults, AA makes up 15–20% of total FAs in blood mononuclear cells, whereas EPA and DHA account for 0.5–1% and 2–3%, respectively. Due to their unsaturations, LCPUFAs affect the physical properties of cell membranes and the function of membrane proteins, including their mobility and signaling systems. This influences the activation of transcription factors and gene expression, regulating the function of various immune cells including neutrophils, monocytes, macrophages, dendritic cells, T cells, and B cells. Upon cell stimulation, often due to phospholipase A_2 activity, PUFAs can be released and enter the COX, LOX, or cytochrome P450 pathways. As mentioned before, the COX pathway produces 2-series PGs such as PGE2 and PGF2α, and several of AA-derived mediators influence immunity. PGE2 has various pro-inflammatory effects, including inducing fever. LTB4 is a chemoattractant involved in leukocyte recruitment to the site of inflammation (Calder, 2018; Miles et al., 2021; Stulnig, 2003). Cysteinyl leukotrienes are known to cause vascular permeability and airway inflammation in asthma patients. AA metabolism also leads to the production of anti-inflammatory lipoxins via the combined actions of 5-LOX and either 15-LOX or 12-LOX. Hence, eicosanoids exhibit both pro- and anti-inflammatory actions to switch on and switch off complex inflammatory events (Folco & Murphy, 2006).

The conversion of EPA to 5-series leukotrienes 3-series PGs and thromboxanes and E-series resolvins, and DHA to D-series resolvins, protectins, and maresins, promotes an inflammatory resolution. Eicosanoids derived from EPA are less potent than those derived from AA. A balanced supply of omega-6 and omega-3 PUFA precursors is important for optimal immune cell membrane composition, to provide protection against pathogens while avoiding excessive inflammation. EPA and DHA reduce the production of AA-derived eicosanoids, partly by replacing AA in cell membranes and reducing substrate availability (Calder, 2018; Miles et al., 2021; Stulnig, 2003). An increased intake of ALA has been demonstrated to elevate the levels of EPA and DPA in the membranes of inflammatory cells, such as neutrophils, monocytes, and lymphocytes. This suggests that omega-3 PUFAs derived from linseed have the potential to mitigate inflammation and offer protection against chronic inflammatory conditions. Derivatives from LC omega-3 PUFAs EPA, DPA, and DHA, including resolvins and protectins, resolve inflammatory processes. In a study on patients undergoing hemodialysis, an increase in ALA intake led to significant reductions in plasma inflammatory markers, including C-reactive protein (CRP) concentrations, after just 8 weeks of consuming 40 g/day of ground linseed (Khalatbari Soltani et al., 2013).

4.4 Myogenesis and Anabolic Resistance

Myogenesis or muscle regeneration is an important process for maintaining muscle mass, skeletal movement, and combating age-related muscle wasting. Myogenesis occurs in response to muscle injury (e.g., exercise-related contraction) by the muscle stem cells or satellite cells, which respond to the anabolic stimuli (e.g., resistance exercise, protein feeding) and start to proliferate and differentiate into myocytes that further fuse with the damaged myofibers (measured via "fusion index") for muscle fiber regeneration. With age, the satellite cells that are key to this regenerative process become unresponsive (lose sensitivity) to anabolic stimulus (termed as "anabolic resistance"), and loss of skeletal muscle mass or "sarcopenia" predominates (Dao et al., 2020; Tezze et al., 2023). Other contributory factors for anabolic resistance include lack of physical activity, low circulating sex hormones, and persistent low-grade inflammation in the body.

Omega-3 PUFAs play an active role in mitigating this low-grade systemic inflammation by counteracting the pro-inflammatory cytokine "flood," thus actively resolving inflammation (Taheri et al., 2023). Since higher inflammation levels are characteristic in old age, flaxseed supplementation has revealed significant improvements in the musculoskeletal features of the elderly than in younger adults. Flaxseed supplementation also helps improve the fusion index, modulate muscle protein synthesis and increase muscle strength, via its role in nerve signal conduction (Batool et al., 2024).

4.5 Liver Health

Dietary ALA has a crucial metabolic and physiological function through the metabolism and synthesis of EPA and DHA. By reducing inflammation, balancing lipid oxidation, and regulating blood lipid levels, PUFA appears to mitigate hepatocyte oxidative damage. The effects of these omega-3 PUFA on lipid metabolism may be linked to gene expression and metabolic changes, thereby partially alleviating the severity of lipid metabolism disorders and liver injury (Bae et al., 2020; Lv & Xu, 2022; Scorletti & Byrne, 2013; Shang et al., 2017). The liver plays a central role in lipid metabolism, encompassing cholesterol synthesis, de novo lipogenesis, and the production of apolipoprotein B100. However, it is not intended for lipid storage, and the accumulation of lipids in hepatocytes can lead to toxicity. Nonalcoholic fatty liver disease (NAFLD) includes various fat-related conditions. The initial phase is characterized by the accumulation of triglyceride droplets in the cytoplasm of over 5% of hepatocytes. This condition, known as steatosis, can advance to nonalcoholic steatohepatitis (NASH), where hepatocyte injury is exacerbated by inflammation and collagen deposition. As collagen tissue replaces hepatocytes, the disease progresses to cirrhosis, which can eventually develop into hepatocellular carcinoma (Scorletti & Byrne, 2013).

Plasma hypertriglyceridemia has been shown to be associated with increased risk for NAFLD. Omega 3 fatty acids, EPA + DHA or EPA, alone has been recommended for effective in reducing triglyceride levels (Bays et al., 2013). Intake of 4 g EPA + DHA can inhibit TAG synthesis by 35% and increase mitochondrial FA oxidation (Chan et al., 2003). Elevated sphingolipids levels in plasma are linked to the development of obesity, NAFLD, and insulin resistance (Scorletti & Byrne, 2013). Ceramide plays a role in the development and progression of NASH. Regular high intake of long chain saturated fatty acids and omega-6 PUFA supplies substrate for de novo ceramide synthesis (Frangioudakis et al., 2010). Ceramide contributes to liver inflammation through NF-κB, TNF-α, and various proinflammatory cytokines-mediated cascades. Its accumulation in the liver also leads to increased production of reactive oxygen species, which, along with cytokines, further aggravates liver steatosis. Additionally, ceramide disrupts insulin function by inhibiting the phosphorylation and activation of Akt, a protein kinase essential for regulating glucose and lipid metabolism, thereby promoting insulin resistance. In contrast, omega-3 FA can enhance metabolism of lipids and reduce insulin resistance by stimulating the phosphorylation of adenosine monophosphate-activated protein kinase (AMPK) in both the liver and adipose tissue. Specifically, AMPK is activated by DHA, which leads to lipid oxidation in hepatocytes, skeletal muscle, and adipocytes, thereby influencing the body's lipid as well as glucose metabolism. Similarly, EPA's activation of AMPK boosts glucose uptake in muscles, thereby enhancing insulin sensitivity. Peroxisome proliferator-activated receptors (PPARs) are a group of transcription factors that regulate gene expression related to lipid and carbohydrate metabolism. PPARα, which is predominantly expressed in the liver, governs FA uptake, transport, and oxidation. Omega-3 FA act as potent PPAR ligands, with activation of PPARα-promoting mitochondrial and peroxisomal FA oxidation, thus reducing intracellular FA accumulation. In liver cells, omega-3 FAs lower the expression of genes involved in fat synthesis by inhibiting SREBP-1c and enhance fat burning by activating PPARα, which facilitates fatty acid transport into mitochondria. Notably, DHA specifically reduces the expression of SREBP-1c (Bae et al., 2020; Lv & Xu, 2022; Scorletti & Byrne, 2013; Shang et al., 2017).

4.6 Blood Glucose Regulation and Insulin Sensitivity

Type 2 Diabetes Mellitus (T2DM) is characterized by insulin resistance in skeletal muscle and adipose tissue, along with the dysregulation of hepatic gluconeogenesis and excessive insulin secretion as compensation for impaired insulin sensitivity. Chronic inflammation significantly contributes to the development of insulin resistance. Increased interaction between macrophages and adipocytes also plays a critical role in decreasing insulin sensitivity. Resident macrophages in adipose tissue produces inflammatory substances such as TNF-α and interleukin-6 (IL-6) (Weisberg et al., 2003), which play a role in activating intracellular pathways and triggering insulin resistance. Therefore, the anti-inflammatory potential of omega-3 PUFA may enhance insulin sensitivity (Homroy et al., 2024; Scorletti & Byrne, 2013).

Omega-3 FA can function as signaling molecules, influencing crucial cellular and immunological processes. These molecules activate G-protein-coupled receptors (GPCR), triggering various cellular responses through secondary messenger systems. Long-chain FAs, including EPA and DHA, bind to the GPR40 and GPR120 receptors. The binding of omega-3 PUFAs to these receptors can directly and indirectly stimulate insulin secretion. Insulin is secreted in response to increased blood glucose levels. The G-protein-coupled receptor GPR40 is highly expressed in pancreatic β-cells and directly stimulates insulin release. In diabetic individuals, high glucose concentrations further increase insulin secretion, a process stimulated by linoleic acid. The GPR120 receptor is found in pro-inflammatory macrophages, adipose tissue, and gastrointestinal tract (particularly in enteroendocrine L cells). When PUFA binds to GPR120, it indirectly promotes secretion of insulin by stimulating glucagon-like peptide-1 (GLP-1) release. Individuals with T2DM have lower levels of the glucose transporter type 4 (GLUT4). Furthermore, PUFA binding to GPR120 increases GLUT4 translocation, enhancing glucose uptake by fat cells. Insulin also promotes the translocation of GLUT4-containing vesicles and increases GLUT4 expression on the muscle cell membrane. Thus, ALA consumption indirectly increases insulin secretion while stimulating glucose uptake via GLUT4 in fat cells (Bhat et al., 2023; Coelho et al., 2017; Jiang et al., 2022).

PPARγ agonists promote FA removal in adipose tissue, reduction of free FAs in circulation and lowering their transport to the muscle and liver, thereby enhancing insulin sensitivity. Additionally, PPARγ ligands downregulate pro-inflammatory markers, further promoting insulin sensitization. Moreover, PPARγ agonists induce the production of the insulin-sensitizing hormone adiponectin (Coelho et al., 2017; Scorletti & Byrne, 2013).

4.7 Reproductive Health

Linseed consumption exerts a critical influence on male and female reproductive physiology. Due to its PUFA and phytoestrogen content, and its effect on energy production and lipid metabolism, flaxseed has modulatory effects on the production of the steroidal sex hormones (Sirotkin, 2023). In female physiology, body fats assist pregnancy and fetal development. Optimum levels of PUFAs such as EPA and DHA are also essential in the maternal body to nourish and support the rapidly developing fetus and its emerging nervous system (Lauritzen et al. 2016). Several in vitro studies have documented both promoter and inhibitory effects of flaxseeds on ovarian follicle development, oocyte maturation, and length and consistency of the reproductive cycles (Sirotkin, 2023). For example Tou et al. (1999), validated the promotor or inhibitory effects and found them dose dependent. Higher doses (10%) correlated with higher relative ovarian weight, higher serum estradiol levels, early onset of puberty, and increased length of estrous cycles in female rats. On the contrary, when the rats were supplemented with 5% flaxseed extract, the effects were starkly contradictory, such as delayed puberty onset and reduced folliculogenesis. Similarly, in male rats, a 10% dose correlated with higher relative testicular weight increased prostate cell proliferation and raised serum testosterone levels. However, on a lifetime exposure (at 5%), the effects were inhibitory, such as reduced adult relative prostate weight and proliferation. No decrease in sex hormone levels was observed. Authors validated the efficacy of linseed supplementation in altering reproductive developments and changes in higher animals, based on the time and dose and duration of exposure to linseed in diet (Tou et al., 1999).

Studies in bovine models also validate these findings, suggesting the modulatory action of linseed on reproductive cycles and a positive effect in reducing instances of pregnancy losses (Ambrose et al., 2006). In humans, the findings have been mixed, with some suggesting a therapeutic impact in the treatment of subjects with polycystic ovarian syndrome, while others reporting no clinically significant outcomes. A recent clinical trial with PCOS patients registered indirect improvements in their endocrine health by reducing serum triglycerides, CRP, insulin concentration, and increasing HDL and adiponectin levels compared to the control group (Haidari et al., 2020). Perhaps, the variable dose, the duration of treatment, and the indirect mechanism of action may explain some of the contradictory findings. Furthermore, the lignan content and molecular derivatives such as 2-methoxy estradiol in flaxseeds have been shown to suppress tumor development through their pro-apoptotic and cytotoxic effects against abnormal cell growth, thereby protecting against breast tumors and ovarian cancer (Carreau et al., 2008; Pal et al., 2019).

Due to the immense significance of ALA and DHA in the development of the nervous system, significant DHA accumulates in the brain and retinal membranes. PUFAs are also crucial for cell proliferation and immune activation, thus mandating optimum omega FA intake during pregnancy and early childhood (Coletta et al., 2010). Flaxseeds, a rich source of omega-3 PUFA, may be preferred over fatty fish intakes due to the risk of heavy metal toxicity, such as methylmercury, which can be especially detrimental with teratogenic effects on the developing fetus (Oken et al., 2008).

Emerging studies implicate the beneficial effects of linseed supplementation on male fertility and improved breeding outcomes in livestock. For example, in a recent 10-week trial with Simmental Bulls, combination therapy of flaxseed and vitamin E resulted in improved sperm motility parameters, along with increased levels of testosterone, estradiol, and glutathione peroxidase and catalase enzymes. The dual supplementation also reduced oxidative stress in the seminal plasma and the sperms demonstrated higher in vitro fertilization rates with improved success in embryogenesis.

4.8 Skin and Hair Health

Omega-3 PUFA such as ALA, AA, EPA, and DHA are metabolized to eicosanoids, docosanoids, endocannabinoids, and related bioactive lipid species, known to mediate inflammatory and immune reactions in many tissues, including skin (Kendall et al., 2017). The epidermis, apart from cells, is made of extracellular lipid matrix with linoleic acid being a prominent fatty acid. Linoleic acid serves as a precursor to ceramides, which are essential in forming the permeability barrier of the stratum corneum. The barrier of the stratum corneum has three main components: the lipid-rich extracellular matrix, the cornified coating or envelop, and keratin-based fibrils aggregated by the filaggrin protein. Ceramides make up half of the extracellular matrix and the rest comprises cholesterol (25%) and free fatty acids (15%). Additionally, between lamellar bodies in the upper epidermis are lipids, enzymes, and antimicrobial peptides. This extracellular lipid matrix, which overlays the cornified envelope proteins, establishes a robust and water-tight barrier. Defects in the stratum corneum barrier can result from mutations in genes encoding the relevant proteins and enzymes, or from lipid deficiencies. During long-chain PUFA deficiency, the abnormal appearance of the extracellular lipid membrane corresponds with impaired barrier function, which reflects failure to synthesize these ceramide families (Balić et al., 2020; Kendall et al., 2017).

Omega-3 PUFAs are essential for improving dermatitis symptoms due to their anti-inflammatory effects. These include inhibiting lymphocyte proliferation, cytokine and antibody production, adhesion molecule expression, natural killer cell activity, and triggering apoptosis. DHA and EPA act as anti-inflammatory agents in treating atopic dermatitis, acting as agonists of PPAR-γ, requiring higher concentrations to activate the receptor. DHA and EPA may also reduce inflammation by regulating TLR-2 and TLR-4 and their downstream signaling pathways. Additionally, docosahexaenoyl ethanolamide, a naturally produced metabolite of DHA, can inhibit mast cell degranulation and mitigate IgE-mediated allergic reactions, suggesting its potential as an anti-allergic agent. Psoriasis is characterized by the abnormal proliferation of skin cells, known as keratinocyte hyperproliferation, which results from T cell activation. This T cell activation triggers the production of arachidonic acid, leading to the generation of various inflammatory substances such as prostaglandins and leukotrienes. Omega-3 PUFAs mitigate skin inflammation by competing with arachidonic acid, thereby inhibiting the production of pro-inflammatory eicosanoids. The therapeutic effects of omega-3 PUFA supplementation in psoriasis are attributed to changes in the lipid composition of serum, epidermal, and blood cell membranes. Increased dietary intake of omega-3 PUFAs, for example, through regular linseed consumption, enhances their incorporation into cell membranes. The metabolites of omega-3 PUFAs suppress the production of pro-inflammatory cytokines, such as IL-6 and TNF-α, which are elevated in psoriasis patients (Balić et al., 2020; Boelsma et al., 2001; Li et al., 2019).

EPA and DHA play a significant role in promoting hair health. These essential fatty acids help to maintain the integrity and hydration of the scalp by supporting the lipid barrier, which can prevent dryness and flakiness. Omega-3 LC-PUFAs also possess anti-inflammatory properties, which can reduce scalp inflammation and alleviate conditions like dandruff and psoriasis. Additionally, EPA and DHA promote blood circulation to the scalp, ensuring that hair follicles receive adequate nutrients and oxygen, fostering stronger and healthier hair growth. Their role in modulating sebum production further helps in maintaining a balanced and healthy scalp environment, ultimately contributing to overall hair health (Le Floc'h et al., 2015; Li et al., 2019). Figure 5 illustrates the multiple benefits of regular linseed oil consumption and their underlying mechanism.

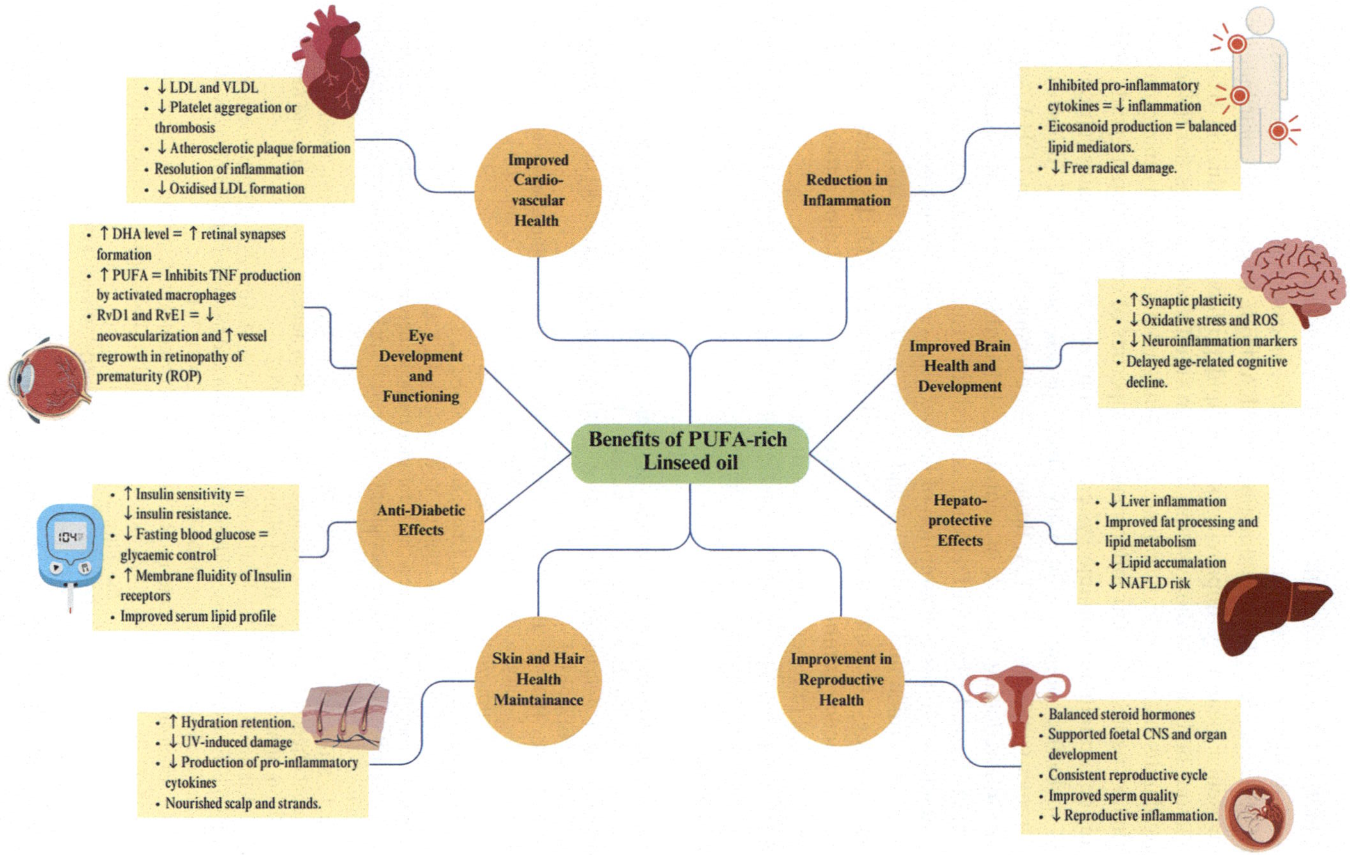

Fig. 5 Benefits of PUFA-rich linseed oil consumption

5 Conclusion

Incorporating linseed oil into the daily diet offers extensive health benefits, primarily due to its high α-linolenic acid (ALA) content, an essential omega-3 polyunsaturated fatty acid. Regular consumption of ALA from linseed oil contributes to cardiovascular health by improving serum lipid profiles and reducing oxidative stress in our body across the systems. This can significantly reduce the risk of cardiovascular diseases (CVD), which are prevalent globally, especially in regions with poor dietary habits. The anti-inflammatory properties of omega-3 fatty acids in linseed oil help modulate immune system functions and protect against chronic diseases, including nonalcoholic fatty liver disease and type-2 diabetes. The neuroprotective benefits of ALA, through its conversion to EPA and DHA, support brain health, reducing the risk of neurological disorders such as Alzheimer's disease. ALA-derived EPA and DHA is essential for visual system development and visual function. Higher consumption of linseed oil, as part of a balanced diet rich in whole grains, fruits, and vegetables and low in saturated and trans fats, can be a powerful strategy to combat the rising incidence of CVD. By addressing the omega-3 deficiency common in many diets, linseed oil can help restore a healthier dietary fatty acid ratio, enhancing its cardioprotective effects.

References

Ambrose, D. J., Kastelic, J. P., Corbett, R., Pitney, P. A., Petit, H. V., Small, J. A., & Zalkovic, P. (2006). Lower pregnancy losses in lactating dairy cows fed a diet enriched in α-linolenic acid. *Journal of Dairy Science, 89*(8), 3066–3074. https://doi.org/10.3168/JDS.S0022-0302(06)72581-4

Arterburn, L. M., Hall, E. B., & Oken, H. (2006). Distribution, interconversion, and dose response of n−3 fatty acids in humans. *The American Journal of Clinical Nutrition, 83*(6), 1467S–1476S. https://doi.org/10.1093/ajcn/83.6.1467S

Bae, S. J., Kim, J. E., Choi, H. J., Choi, Y. J., Lee, S. J., Gong, J. E., Seo, S., Yang, S. Y., An, B.-S., Lee, H. S., Kim, D. S., Lee, C. Y., & Hwang, D. Y. (2020). A-Linolenic acid-enriched cold-pressed perilla oil suppress high-fat diet-induced hepatic steatosis through amelioration of the ER stress-mediated autophagy. *Molecules, 25*(11), 2662. https://doi.org/10.3390/molecules25112662

Baker, E. J., Miles, E. A., Burdge, G. C., Yaqoob, P., & Calder, P. C. (2016). Metabolism and functional effects of plant-derived omega-3 fatty acids in humans. *Progress in Lipid Research, 64*, 30–56. https://doi.org/10.1016/j.plipres.2016.07.002

Balić, A., Vlašić, D., Žužul, K., Marinović, B., & Bukvić Mokos, Z. (2020). Omega-3 versus omega-6 polyunsaturated fatty acids in the prevention and treatment of inflammatory skin diseases. *International Journal of Molecular Sciences, 21*(3), 741.

Barrera, C., Valenzuela, R., Chamorro, R., Bascuñán, K., Sandoval, J., Sabag, N., Valenzuela, F., Valencia, M.-P., Puigrredon, C., & Valenzuela, A. (2018). The impact of maternal diet during pregnancy and lactation on the fatty acid composition of erythrocytes and breast milk of Chilean women. *Nutrients, 10*(7), 839. https://doi.org/10.3390/nu10070839

Batool, I., Altemimi, A. B., Munir, S., Imran, S., Khalid, N., Khan, M. A., Abdi, G., et al. (2024). Exploring flaxseed's potential in enhancing bone health: Unveiling osteo-protective properties. *Journal of Agriculture and Food Research, 15*, 101018.

Bays, H. E., Ballantyne, C. M., Braeckman, R. A., Stirtan, W. G., & Soni, P. N. (2013). Icosapent ethyl, a pure ethyl ester of eicosapentaenoic acid: Effects on circulating markers of inflammation from the MARINE and ANCHOR studies. *American Journal of Cardiovascular Drugs: Drugs, Devices, and Other Interventions, 13*(1), 37–46. https://doi.org/10.1007/s40256-012-0002-3

Bazinet, R. P., & Layé, S. (2014). Polyunsaturated fatty acids and their metabolites in brain function and disease. *Nature Reviews Neuroscience, 15*(12), 771–785. https://doi.org/10.1038/nrn3820

Bhargava, R., Pandey, K., Ranjan, S., Mehta, B., & Malik, A. (2023). Omega-3 fatty acids supplements for dry eye—Are they effective or ineffective? *Indian Journal of Ophthalmology, 71*(4), 1619–1625. https://doi.org/10.4103/IJO.IJO_2789_22

Bhat, S., Sarkar, S., Zaffar, D., Dandona, P., & Kalyani, R. R. (2023). Omega-3 fatty acids in cardiovascular disease and diabetes: A review of recent evidence. *Current Cardiology Reports, 25*(2), 51–65. https://doi.org/10.1007/s11886-022-01831-0

Blanco-Llamero, C., Fonseca, J., Durazzo, A., Lucarini, M., Santini, A., Señoráns, F. J., & Souto, E. B. (2022). Nutraceuticals and food-grade lipid nanoparticles: From natural sources to a circular bioeconomy approach. *Foods, 11*(15), 2318. https://doi.org/10.3390/foods11152318

Boelsma, E., Hendriks, H. F., & Roza, L. (2001). Nutritional skin care: Health effects of micronutrients and fatty acids. *The American Journal of Clinical Nutrition, 73*(5), 853–864.

Budoff, M. J., Bhatt, D. L., Kinninger, A., Lakshmanan, S., Muhlestein, J. B., Le, V. T., May, H. T., et al. (2020). Effect of icosapent ethyl on progression of coronary atherosclerosis in patients with elevated triglycerides on statin therapy: Final results of the EVAPORATE trial. *European Heart Journal, 41*(40), 3925–3932. https://doi.org/10.1093/EURHEARTJ/EHAA652

Burdge, G. C., & Wootton, S. A. (2002). Conversion of α-linolenic acid to eicosapentaenoic, docosapentaenoic and docosahexaenoic acids in young women. *British Journal of Nutrition, 88*(4), 411–420. https://doi.org/10.1079/BJN2002689

Burdge, G. C., Finnegan, Y. E., Minihane, A. M., Williams, C. M., & Wootton, S. A. (2003). Effect of altered dietary *n* -3 fatty acid intake upon plasma lipid fatty acid composition, conversion of [^{13} C]α-linolenic acid to longer-chain fatty acids and partitioning towards β-oxidation in older men. *British Journal of Nutrition, 90*(2), 311–321. https://doi.org/10.1079/BJN2003901

Calder, P. C. (2018). Metabolism of polyunsaturated fatty acids by cells of the immune system. In *Polyunsaturated fatty acid metabolism* (pp. 135–155). Elsevier. https://doi.org/10.1016/B978-0-12-811230-4.00008-9

Cao, J., Schwichtenberg, K. A., Hanson, N. Q., & Tsai, M. Y. (2006). Incorporation and clearance of omega-3 fatty acids in erythrocyte membranes and plasma phospholipids. *Clinical Chemistry, 52*(12), 2265–2272. https://doi.org/10.1373/clinchem.2006.072322

Carreau, C., Flouriot, G., Bennetau-Pelissero, C., & Potier, M. (2008). Enterodiol and enterolactone, two major diet-derived polyphenol metabolites have different impact on ERα transcriptional activation in human breast cancer cells. *The Journal of Steroid Biochemistry and Molecular Biology, 110*(1–2), 176–185. https://doi.org/10.1016/J.JSBMB.2008.03.032

Casula, M., Olmastroni, E., Gazzotti, M., Galimberti, F., Zambon, A., & Catapano, A. L. (2020). Omega-3 polyunsaturated fatty acids supplementation and cardiovascular outcomes: Do formulation, dosage, and baseline cardiovascular risk matter- An updated meta-analysis of randomized controlled trials. *Pharmacological Research, 160*, 105060. https://doi.org/10.1016/j.phrs.2020.105060

Chamorro, R., Bascuñán, K. A., Barrera, C., Sandoval, J., Puigrredon, C., & Valenzuela, R. (2022). Reduced n-3 and n-6 PUFA (DHA and AA) concentrations in breast milk and erythrocytes phospholipids during pregnancy and lactation in women with obesity. *International Journal of Environmental Research and Public Health, 19*(4), 1930. https://doi.org/10.3390/ijerph19041930

Chan, D. C., Watts, G. F., Mori, T. A., Barrett, P. H. R., Redgrave, T. G., & Beilin, L. J. (2003). Randomized controlled trial of the effect of n–3 fatty acid supplementation on the metabolism of apolipoprotein B-100 and chylomicron remnants in men with visceral obesity. *The American Journal of Clinical Nutrition, 77*(2), 300–307. https://doi.org/10.1093/ajcn/77.2.300

Chaudhary, V., Nigam, A. K., Paliwal, A., Singh, M. K., Gour, J. K., & Sinha, V. B. (2021). Omega 3 PUFA. In *Naturally occurring chemicals against Alzheimer's disease* (pp. 65–82). Elsevier. https://doi.org/10.1016/B978-0-12-819212-2.00005-0

Chisaguano, A. M., Montes, R., Pérez-Berezo, T., Castellote, A. I., Guerendiain, M., Bustamante, M., Morales, E., et al. (2013). Gene expression of desaturase (FADS1 and FADS2) and Elongase (ELOVL5) enzymes in peripheral blood: Association with polyunsaturated fatty acid levels and atopic eczema in 4-year-old children. *PLoS One, 8*(10), e78245. https://doi.org/10.1371/JOURNAL.PONE.0078245

Chopra, R., & Sambaiah, K. (2009). Effects of rice bran oil enriched with n-3 PUFA on liver and serum lipids in rats. *Lipids, 44*(1), 37–46. https://doi.org/10.1007/s11745-008-3240-z

Coelho, O. G. L., Da Silva, B. P., Rocha, D. M. U. P., Lopes, L. L., & Alfenas, R. D. C. G. (2017). Polyunsaturated fatty acids and type 2 diabetes: Impact on the glycemic control mechanism. *Critical Reviews in Food Science and Nutrition, 57*(17), 3614–3619. https://doi.org/10.1080/10408398.2015.1130016

Coletta, J. M., Bell, S. J., & Roman, A. S. (2010). Omega-3 fatty acids and pregnancy. *Reviews in Obstetrics and Gynecology, 3*(4), 163. https://doi.org/10.3909/riog0137

Connor, K. M., SanGiovanni, J. P., Lofqvist, C., Aderman, C. M., Chen, J., Higuchi, A., Hong, S., Pravda, E. A., Majchrzak, S., Carper, D., Hellstrom, A., Kang, J. X., Chew, E. Y., Salem, N., Serhan, C. N., & Smith, L. E. H. (2007). Increased dietary intake of omega-3-polyunsaturated fatty acids reduces pathological retinal angiogenesis. *Nature Medicine, 13*(7), 868–873. https://doi.org/10.1038/nm1591

Dao, T., Green, A. E., Kim, Y. A., Bae, S. J., Ha, K. T., Gariani, K., Lee, M. R., Menzies, K. J., & Ryu, D. (2020). Sarcopenia and muscle aging: A brief overview. *Endocrinology and Metabolism, 35*(4), 716. https://doi.org/10.3803/ENM.2020.405

Dighriri, I. M., Alsubaie, A. M., Hakami, F. M., Hamithi, D. M., Alshekh, M. M., Khobrani, F. A., Dalak, F. E., et al. (2022). Effects of omega-3 polyunsaturated fatty acids on brain functions: A systematic review. *Cureus, 14*(10), e30091. https://doi.org/10.7759/CUREUS.30091

Drouin, G., Rioux, V., & Legrand, P. (2019). The n-3 docosapentaenoic acid (DPA): A new player in the n-3 long chain polyunsaturated fatty acid family. *Biochimie, 159*, 36–48. https://doi.org/10.1016/j.biochi.2019.01.022

Endo, J., & Arita, M. (2016). Cardioprotective mechanism of omega-3 polyunsaturated fatty acids. *Journal of Cardiology, 67*(1), 22–27. https://doi.org/10.1016/J.JJCC.2015.08.002

Folco, G., & Murphy, R. C. (2006). Eicosanoid transcellular biosynthesis: From cell-cell interactions to in vivo tissue responses. *Pharmacological Reviews, 58*(3), 375–388. https://doi.org/10.1124/pr.58.3.8

Frangioudakis, G., Garrard, J., Raddatz, K., Nadler, J. L., Mitchell, T. W., & Schmitz-Peiffer, C. (2010). Saturated- and n-6 polyunsaturated-fat diets each induce ceramide accumulation in mouse skeletal muscle: Reversal and improvement of glucose tolerance by lipid metabolism inhibitors. *Endocrinology, 151*(9), 4187–4196. https://doi.org/10.1210/en.2010-0250

Fuentes-Albero, M., Martínez-Martínez, M. I., & Cauli, O. (2019). Omega-3 long-chain polyunsaturated fatty acids intake in children with attention deficit and hyperactivity disorder. *Brain Sciences, 9*(5), 120. https://doi.org/10.3390/brainsci9050120

Gerster, H. (1998). Can adults adequately convert alpha-linolenic acid (18:3n-3) to eicosapentaenoic acid (20:5n-3) and docosahexaenoic acid (22:6n-3)? *International Journal for Vitamin and Nutrition Research. Internationale Zeitschrift Fur Vitamin- Und Ernahrungsforschung. Journal International De Vitaminologie Et De Nutrition, 68*(3), 159–173.

Gholami, Z., & Akhlaghi, M. (2021). The effect of flaxseed on physical and mental fatigue in children and adolescents with overweight/obesity: A randomised controlled trial. *British Journal of Nutrition, 126*(1), 151–159. https://doi.org/10.1017/S0007114520003888

Gregory, M. K., Gibson, R. A., Cook-Johnson, R. J., Cleland, L. G., & James, M. J. (2011). Elongase reactions as control points in long-chain polyunsaturated fatty acid synthesis. *PLoS One, 6*(12), e29662. https://doi.org/10.1371/journal.pone.0029662

Haidari, F., Banaei-Jahromi, N., Zakerkish, M., & Ahmadi, K. (2020). The effects of flaxseed supplementation on metabolic status in women with polycystic ovary syndrome: A randomized open-labeled controlled clinical trial. *Nutrition Journal, 19*(1), 1–11. https://doi.org/10.1186/S12937-020-0524-5/TABLES/6

Homroy, S., Chopra, R., Singh, P. K., Dhiman, A., Chand, M., & Talwar, B. (2024). Role of encapsulation on the bioavailability of omega-3 fatty acids. *Comprehensive Reviews in Food Science and Food Safety, 23*(1), 1–35. https://doi.org/10.1111/1541-4337.13272

ICMR. (2024). *Short summary report of nutrient requirements for Indians, Recommended Dietary Allowance (RDA) and Estimated Average Requirements (EAR)* (Revised short summary report –2024, ICMR-NIN Expert Group on Nutrient Requirements for Indians, Recommended Dietary Allowance (RDA) and Estimated Average Requirements (EAR)-2020) [Summary report]. ICMR-National Institute of Nutrition.

Jiang, H., Wang, L., Wang, D., Yan, N., Li, C., Wu, M., Wang, F., Mi, B., Chen, F., Jia, W., Liu, X., Lv, J., Liu, Y., Lin, J., & Ma, L. (2022). Omega-3 polyunsaturated fatty acid biomarkers and risk of type 2 diabetes, cardiovascular disease, cancer, and mortality. *Clinical Nutrition, 41*(8), 1798–1807. https://doi.org/10.1016/j.clnu.2022.06.034

Jin, J., Jin, Q., Wang, X., & Akoh, C. C. (2020). High Sn-2 docosahexaenoic acid lipids for brain benefits, and their enzymatic syntheses: A review. *Engineering, 6*(4), 424–431. https://doi.org/10.1016/j.eng.2020.02.009

Joffre, C. (2019). Polyunsaturated fatty acid metabolism in the brain and brain cells. In *Feed your mind-how does nutrition modulate brain function throughout life?* IntechOpen.

Judge, M. P., Harel, O., & Lammi-Keefe, C. J. (2007). A docosahexaenoic acid-functional food during pregnancy benefits infant visual acuity at four but not six months of age. *Lipids, 42*, 117–122. https://doi.org/10.1007/s11745-006-3007-3

Kalmijn, S., Launer, L. J., Ott, A., Witteman, J. C. M., Hofman, A., & Breteler, M. M. B. (1997). Dietary fat intake and the risk of incident dementia in the Rotterdam study. *Annals of Neurology, 42*(5), 776–782. https://doi.org/10.1002/ANA.410420514

Kendall, A. C., Kiezel-Tsugunova, M., Brownbridge, L. C., Harwood, J. L., & Nicolaou, A. (2017). Lipid functions in skin: Differential effects of n-3 polyunsaturated fatty acids on cutaneous ceramides, in a human skin organ culture model. *Biochimica et Biophysica Acta (BBA) – Biomembranes, 1859*(9), 1679–1689. https://doi.org/10.1016/j.bbamem.2017.03.016

Khalatbari Soltani, S., Jamaluddin, R., Tabibi, H., Mohd Yusof, B. N., Atabak, S., Loh, S., & Rahmani, L. (2013). Effects of flaxseed consumption on systemic inflammation and serum lipid profile in hemodialysis patients with lipid abnormalities. *Hemodialysis International, 17*(2), 275–281. https://doi.org/10.1111/j.1542-4758.2012.00754.x

Kouamé, K. J. E.-P., Bora, A. F. M., Li, X., Sun, Y., & Liu, L. (2021). Novel trends and opportunities for microencapsulation of flaxseed oil in foods: A review. *Journal of Functional Foods, 87*, 104812. https://doi.org/10.1016/j.jff.2021.104812

Lauritzen, L., Brambilla, P., Mazzocchi, A., Harsløf, L. B. S., Ciappolino, V., & Agostoni, C. (2016). DHA effects in brain development and function. *Nutrients, 8*(1). https://doi.org/10.3390/NU8010006

Layé, S., Nadjar, A., Joffre, C., & Bazinet, R. P. (2018). Anti-inflammatory effects of omega-3 fatty acids in the brain: Physiological mechanisms and relevance to pharmacology. *Pharmacological Reviews, 70*(1), 12–38. https://doi.org/10.1124/pr.117.014092

Le Floc'h, C., Cheniti, A., Connétable, S., Piccardi, N., Vincenzi, C., & Tosti, A. (2015). Effect of a nutritional supplement on hair loss in women. *Journal of Cosmetic Dermatology, 14*(1), 76–82. https://doi.org/10.1111/jocd.12127

Li, X., Bi, X., Wang, S., Zhang, Z., Li, F., & Zhao, A. Z. (2019). Therapeutic potential of ω-3 polyunsaturated fatty acids in human autoimmune diseases. *Frontiers in Immunology, 10*, 2241.

Lotfi, S., Esfahani, M., Ranjbar, A., & Mehri, F. (2023). Protective effect of flaxseed oil the on diazinon-induced hepatotoxicity in male rats. *Proceedings of the Indian National Science Academy, 89*(3), 655–663. https://doi.org/10.1007/s43538-023-00170-0

Lv, W., & Xu, D. (2022). Docosahexaenoic acid delivery systems, bioavailability, functionality, and applications: A review. *Foods, 11*(17), 2685. https://doi.org/10.3390/foods11172685

Manson, J. E., Cook, N. R., Lee, I.-M., Christen, W., Bassuk, S. S., Mora, S., Gibson, H., Albert, C. M., Gordon, D., Copeland, T., D'Agostino, D., Friedenberg, G., Ridge, C., Bubes,

V., Giovannucci, E. L., Willett, W. C., Buring, J. E., & VITAL Research Group. (2019). Marine n-3 fatty acids and prevention of cardiovascular disease and cancer. *The New England Journal of Medicine, 380*(1), 23–32. https://doi.org/10.1056/NEJMoa1811403

Mathias, R. A., Vergara, C., Gao, L., Rafaels, N., Hand, T., Campbell, M., Bickel, C., et al. (2010). FADS genetic variants and ω-6 polyunsaturated fatty acid metabolism in a homogeneous Island population. *Journal of Lipid Research, 51*(9), 2766–2774. https://doi.org/10.1194/JLR.M008359

McCloy, U., Ryan, M. A., Pencharz, P. B., Ross, R. J., & Cunnane, S. C. (2004). A comparison of the metabolism of eighteen-carbon 13C-unsaturated fatty acids in healthy women. *Journal of Lipid Research, 45*(3), 474–485. https://doi.org/10.1194/jlr.M300304-JLR200

Melo, L., Pessoa, D., de Araújo, L., De Oliveira, C., Guzen, F. P., de Moura Freire, M. A., & de Paiva Cavalcanti, J. R. L. (2019). Repercussions of linseed oil in morphofunctional mechanisms of the nervous system: A systematic Revie. *Research Journal of Pharmaceutical, Biological and Chemical Sciences, 7*, 147–156.

Miles, E. A., Childs, C. E., & Calder, P. C. (2021). Long-chain polyunsaturated fatty acids (LCPUFAs) and the developing immune system: A narrative review. *Nutrients, 13*(1), 247. https://doi.org/10.3390/nu13010247

Mirfatahi, M., Tabibi, H., Nasrollahi, A., Hedayati, M., & Taghizadeh, M. (2016). Effect of flaxseed oil on serum systemic and vascular inflammation markers and oxidative stress in hemodialysis patients: A randomized controlled trial. *International Urology and Nephrology, 48*(8), 1335–1341. https://doi.org/10.1007/s11255-016-1300-5

Morshedzadeh, N., Rahimlou, M., Shahrokh, S., Karimi, S., Mirmiran, P., & Zali, M. R. (2021a). The effects of flaxseed supplementation on metabolic syndrome parameters, insulin resistance and inflammation in ulcerative colitis patients: An open-labeled randomized controlled trial. *Phytotherapy Research, 35*(7), 3781–3791. https://doi.org/10.1002/ptr.7081

Morshedzadeh, N., Shahrokh, S., Chaleshi, V., Karimi, S., Mirmiran, P., & Zali, M. R. (2021b). The effects of flaxseed supplementation on gene expression and inflammation in ulcerative colitis patients: An open-labelled randomised controlled trial. *International Journal of Clinical Practice, 75*(5), e14035. https://doi.org/10.1111/ijcp.14035

Nakamura, M. T., & Nara, T. Y. (2004). STRUCTURE, FUNCTION, AND DIETARY REGULATION OF Δ6, Δ5, AND Δ9 DESATURASES. *Annual Review of Nutrition, 24*(1), 345–376. https://doi.org/10.1146/annurev.nutr.24.121803.063211

Neukam, K., De Spirt, S., Stahl, W., Bejot, M., Maurette, J.-M., Tronnier, H., & Heinrich, U. (2011). Supplementation of flaxseed oil diminishes skin sensitivity and improves skin barrier function and condition. *Skin Pharmacology and Physiology, 24*(2), 67–74. https://doi.org/10.1159/000321442

NIH. (2005). *National Instiutes of Health—Office of Dietary Supplements.* Dietary Supplement Fact Sheets – Omega-3 Fatty Acids. https://ods.od.nih.gov/factsheets/Omega3FattyAcids-HealthProfessional/

Ocaña-Sánchez, M. F., Soto-Ojeda, G. A., Cocotle-Ronzón, Y., Soria-Fregozo, C., Sánchez-Medina, A., García-Rodríguez, R. V., Rodríguez-Landa, J. F., Corro-Méndez, E. J., & Hernández-Lozano, M. (2023). Flaxseed oil (Linum usitatissimum) prevents cognitive and motor damage in rats with hyperammonemia. *Nutrients, 15*(21), 4550. https://doi.org/10.3390/nu15214550

Ogawa, T., Sawane, K., Ookoshi, K., & Kawashima, R. (2023). Supplementation with flaxseed oil rich in alpha-Linolenic acid improves verbal fluency in healthy older adults. *Nutrients, 15*(6), 1499. https://doi.org/10.3390/nu15061499

Oken, E., Radesky, J. S., Wright, R. O., Bellinger, D. C., Amarasiriwardena, C. J., Kleinman, K. P., Howard, H., & Gillman, M. W. (2008). Maternal fish intake during pregnancy, blood mercury levels, and child cognition at age 3 years in a US cohort. *American Journal of Epidemiology, 167*(10), 1171–1181. https://doi.org/10.1093/AJE/KWN034

Pal, P., Hales, K., Petrik, J., & Hales, D. B. (2019). Pro-apoptotic and anti-angiogenic actions of 2-methoxyestradiol and docosahexaenoic acid, the biologically derived active compounds from flaxseed diet, in preventing ovarian cancer. *Journal of Ovarian Research, 12*(1), 1–16. https://doi.org/10.1186/S13048-019-0523-3/TABLES/2

Panda, C., Varadharaj, S., & Voruganti, V. S. (2022). PUFA, genotypes and risk for cardiovascular disease. *Prostaglandins, Leukotrienes and Essential Fatty Acids, 176*, 102377. https://doi.org/10.1016/j.plefa.2021.102377

Pattanayak, C., Bahinipati, J., Srivastava, V., & Sarkar, S. (2021). Evaluation of hypolipidemic and hepatoprotective effects of Linum usitatissimum L. seeds on hypercholesterolemic rats. *Journal of Pharmaceutical Research International*, 85–93. https://doi.org/10.9734/jpri/2021/v33i53A33642

Plourde, M., & Cunnane, S. C. (2007). Extremely limited synthesis of long chain polyunsaturates in adults: Implications for their dietary essentiality and use as supplements. *Applied Physiology, Nutrition, and Metabolism, 32*(4), 619–634. https://doi.org/10.1139/H07-034

Poorbaferani, F., Rouhani, M. H., Heidari, Z., Poorbaferani, M., & Safavi, S. M. (2020). Flaxseed oil supplementation on severity of depression and brain-derived neurotrophic factor: A randomized, double blind placebo controlled clinical trial. *International Journal of Food Properties, 23*(1), 1518–1526. https://doi.org/10.1080/10942912.2020.1812639

Prasad, K. (2005). Hypocholesterolemic and antiatherosclerotic effect of flax lignan complex isolated from flaxseed. *Atherosclerosis, 179*(2), 269–275. https://doi.org/10.1016/j.atherosclerosis.2004.11.012

Roth, G. A., Mensah, G. A., Johnson, C. O., Addolorato, G., Ammirati, E., Baddour, L. M., Barengo, N. C., Beaton, A. Z., Benjamin, E. J., Benziger, C. P., Bonny, A., Brauer, M., Brodmann, M., Cahill, T. J., Carapetis, J., Catapano, A. L., Chugh, S. S., Cooper, L. T., Coresh, J., et al. (2020). Global burden of cardiovascular diseases and risk factors, 1990-2019: Update from the GBD 2019 study. *Journal of the American College of Cardiology, 76*(25), 2982–3021. https://doi.org/10.1016/j.jacc.2020.11.010

Sadat Masjedi, M., Mohammadi Pour, P., Shokoohinia, Y., & Asgary, S. (2022). Effects of flaxseed on blood lipids in healthy and dyslipidemic subjects: A systematic review and meta-analysis of randomized controlled trials. *Current Problems in Cardiology, 47*(7), 100931. https://doi.org/10.1016/j.cpcardiol.2021.100931

Saini, R. K., Prasad, P., Sreedhar, R. V., Akhilender Naidu, K., Shang, X., & Keum, Y.-S. (2021). Omega−3 polyunsaturated fatty acids (PUFAs): Emerging plant and microbial sources, oxidative stability, bioavailability, and health benefits—A review. *Antioxidants, 10*(10), 1627. https://doi.org/10.3390/antiox10101627

SanGiovanni, J. P., & Chew, E. Y. (2005). The role of omega-3 long-chain polyunsaturated fatty acids in health and disease of the retina. *Progress in Retinal and Eye Research, 24*(1), 87–138. https://doi.org/10.1016/j.preteyeres.2004.06.002

Scorletti, E., & Byrne, C. D. (2013). Omega-3 fatty acids, hepatic lipid metabolism, and nonalcoholic fatty liver disease. *Annual Review of Nutrition, 33*(1), 231–248. https://doi.org/10.1146/annurev-nutr-071812-161230

Serhan, C. N., & Levy, B. D. (2018). Resolvins in inflammation: Emergence of the pro-resolving superfamily of mediators. *Journal of Clinical Investigation, 128*(7), 2657–2669. https://doi.org/10.1172/JCI97943

Shang, T., Liu, L., Zhou, J., Zhang, M., Hu, Q., Fang, M., Wu, Y., Yao, P., & Gong, Z. (2017). Protective effects of various ratios of DHA/EPA supplementation on high-fat diet-induced liver damage in mice. *Lipids in Health and Disease, 16*(1), 65. https://doi.org/10.1186/s12944-017-0461-2

Sharma, M., & Lokesh, B. R. (2013). Modification of serum and tissue lipids in rats fed with blended and interesterified oils containing groundnut oil with linseed oil. *Journal of Food Biochemistry, 37*(2), 220–230.

Simopoulos, A. P. (2006). Evolutionary aspects of diet, the omega-6/omega-3 ratio and genetic variation: Nutritional implications for chronic diseases. *Biomedicine & Pharmacotherapy = Biomedecine & Pharmacotherapie, 60*(9), 502–507. https://doi.org/10.1016/j.biopha.2006.07.080

Sirotkin, A. V. (2023). Influence of flaxseed (Linum Usitatissimum) on female reproduction. *Planta Medica, 89*(06), 608–615. https://doi.org/10.1055/A-2013-2966

Soleimani, Z., Hashemdokht, F., Bahmani, F., Taghizadeh, M., Memarzadeh, M. R., & Asemi, Z. (2017). Clinical and metabolic response to flaxseed oil omega-3 fatty acids supplementation in patients with diabetic foot ulcer: A randomized, double-blind, placebo-controlled trial. *Journal of Diabetes and its Complications, 31*(9), 1394–1400. https://doi.org/10.1016/j.jdiacomp.2017.06.010

Stulnig, T. M. (2003). Immunomodulation by polyunsaturated fatty acids: Mechanisms and effects. *International Archives of Allergy and Immunology, 132*(4), 310–321. https://doi.org/10.1159/000074898

Taheri, M., Chilibeck, P. D., & Cornish, S. M. (2023). A brief narrative review of the underlying mechanisms whereby omega-3 fatty acids may influence skeletal muscle: From cell culture to human interventions. *Nutrients, 15*(13), 2926.

Tezze, C., Sandri, M., & Tessari, P. (2023). Anabolic resistance in the pathogenesis of sarcopenia in the elderly: Role of nutrition and exercise in young and old people. *Nutrients, 15*(18), 4073. https://doi.org/10.3390/NU15184073

Tou, J. C. L., Chen, J., & Thompson, L. U. (1999). Dose, timing, and duration of flaxseed exposure affect reproductive indices and sex hormone levels in rats. *Journal of Toxicology and Environmental Health, Part A, 56*(8), 555–570. https://doi.org/10.1080/009841099093501 77

Toulabi, T., Yarahmadi, M., Goudarzi, F., Ebrahimzadeh, F., Momenizadeh, A., & Yarahmadi, S. (2022). Effects of flaxseed on blood pressure, body mass index, and total cholesterol in hypertensive patients: A randomized clinical trial. *EXPLORE, 18*(4), 438–445. https://doi.org/10.1016/j.explore.2021.05.003

Valenzuela, R., Echeverria, F., Ortiz, M., Rincón-Cervera, M. Á., Espinosa, A., Hernandez-Rodas, M. C., Illesca, P., Valenzuela, A., & Videla, L. A. (2017). Hydroxytyrosol prevents reduction in liver activity of Δ-5 and Δ-6 desaturases, oxidative stress, and depletion in long chain polyunsaturated fatty acid content in different tissues of high-fat diet fed mice. *Lipids in Health and Disease, 16*(1), 64. https://doi.org/10.1186/s12944-017-0450-5

Valenzuela, R., Metherel, A. H., Cisbani, G., Smith, M. E., Chouinard-Watkins, R., Klievik, B. J., Videla, L. A., & Bazinet, R. P. (2023). Protein concentrations and activities of fatty acid desaturase and elongase enzymes in liver, brain, testicle, and kidney from mice: Substrate dependency. *BioFactors, 50*, 89. https://doi.org/10.1002/biof.1992

Venugopalan, V. K., Gopakumar, L. R., Kumaran, A. K., Chatterjee, N. S., Soman, V., Peeralil, S., Mathew, S., McClements, D. J., & Nagarajarao, R. C. (2021). Encapsulation and protection of omega-3-rich fish oils using food-grade delivery systems. *Foods, 10*(7), 1566. https://doi.org/10.3390/foods10071566

Videla, L. A., Hernandez-Rodas, M. C., Metherel, A. H., & Valenzuela, R. (2022). Influence of the nutritional status and oxidative stress in the desaturation and elongation of n-3 and n-6 polyunsaturated fatty acids: Impact on non-alcoholic fatty liver disease. *Prostaglandins, Leukotrienes, and Essential Fatty Acids, 181*, 102441. https://doi.org/10.1016/j.plefa.2022.102441

Walker, C. G., Browning, L. M., Mander, A. P., Madden, J., West, A. L., Calder, P. C., & Jebb, S. A. (2014). Age and sex differences in the incorporation of EPA and DHA into plasma fractions, cells and adipose tissue in humans. *British Journal of Nutrition, 111*(4), 679–689. https://doi.org/10.1017/S0007114513002985

Wang, J., Han, L., Wang, D., Sun, Y., Huang, J., & Shahidi, F. (2021a). Stability and stabilization of omega-3 oils: A review. *Trends in Food Science & Technology, 118*, 17–35. https://doi.org/10.1016/j.tifs.2021.09.018

Wang, B., Wu, L., Chen, J., Dong, L., Chen, C., Zheng, W., Hu, J., Fleming, I., & Wang, D. W. (2021b). Metabolism pathways of arachidonic acids: Mechanisms and potential therapeutic targets. *Signal Transduction and Targeted Therapy, 6*(1), 1–30. https://doi.org/10.1038/s41392-020-00443-w

Wang, J., Ossemond, J., Jardin, J., Briard-Bion, V., Henry, G., Le Gouar, Y., Ménard, O., Lê, S., Madadlou, A., Dupont, D., & Pédrono, F. (2022a). Encapsulation of DHA oil with heat-denatured whey protein in Pickering emulsion improves its bioaccessibility. *Food Research International, 162*, 112112. https://doi.org/10.1016/j.foodres.2022.112112

Wang, J., Ossemond, J., Le Gouar, Y., Boissel, F., Dupont, D., & Pédrono, F. (2022b). Encapsulation of docosahexaenoic acid oil substantially improves the oxylipin profile of rat tissues. *Frontiers in Nutrition, 8*, 812119. https://doi.org/10.3389/fnut.2021.812119

Weisberg, S. P., McCann, D., Desai, M., Rosenbaum, M., Leibel, R. L., & Ferrante, A. W. (2003). Obesity is associated with macrophage accumulation in adipose tissue. *Journal of Clinical Investigation, 112*(12), 1796–1808. https://doi.org/10.1172/JCI200319246

Williard, D. E., Nwankwo, J. O., Kaduce, T. L., Harmon, S. D., Irons, M., Moser, H. W., Raymond, G. V., & Spector, A. A. (2001). Identification of a fatty acid Δ6-desaturase deficiency in human skin fibroblasts. *Journal of Lipid Research, 42*(4), 501–508. https://doi.org/10.1016/S0022-2275(20)31158-5

Yang, L., Yang, C., Song, Z. X., Wan, M., Xia, H., Xu, D., Pan, D., Wang, S. K., Shu, G., & Sun, G. (2022). Effects of blended oils with different n-6/n-3 polyunsaturated fatty acid ratios on high-fat diet-induced metabolic disorders and hepatic steatosis in rats. *Food Science and Technology, 42*, e81322. https://doi.org/10.1590/fst.81322

Industrial Application of Linseed Oil

Aishwarya Dhiman and Prabodh Halde

Abstract

Linseeds constitute about 35–45% oil, which is used for both edible and non-edible industrial applications. The unique fatty acid profile of the oil serves as a major reason for its diverse applicability. The oil is a rich source of polyunsaturated fatty acids (PUFA), namely, α-linolenic acid and linoleic acid, which make it a nutritionally rich supplement for use as a nutraceutical. However, this reduces its stability and hence applicability as an edible oil. Techniques like blending, interesterification, and encapsulation have been studied to improve its stability, functionality, and implementation as a cooking oil, bakery fat, or nutraceutical. The high PUFA content is also responsible for its auto-oxidation, which serves as a primary basis for its utilization as a non-edible oil. It is classified as a drying oil and is thus used as a major ingredient in products such as paints, linoleum, furniture, lubricants, and so forth. The consumer awareness toward eco-friendly fuels has also contributed toward the increased interest in utilization of vegetable oil as biofuels. Linseed oil as an underutilized oil has also garnered attention due to the widening gap between the demand and availability of oils. This chapter delves into the wide-ranging applications of linseed oil, highlighting its potential in various industries.

Keywords

Culinary application · Nutraceutical · Biodiesel · Linoleun

A. Dhiman
Department of Food Science and Technology, National Institute of Food Technology Entrepreneurship and Management, Kundli, Haryana, India

P. Halde (✉)
Head Global Regulatory, Marico Ltd., Mumbai, India
e-mail: prabodh.halde@marico.com

© The Author(s), under exclusive license to Springer Nature Singapore Pte Ltd. 2025

R. Chopra et al. (eds.), *Dynamics of Linseed and its Valorization*,
https://doi.org/10.1007/978-981-96-8927-9_9

1 Introduction

The composition and health benefits of linseeds are well addressed in most of the chapters of this book. This chapter delves into the industrial use of its most economical product, i.e., linseed oil. The name "*L.usitatissimum*" itself means "extremely beneficial" or "very useful" in Latin (Özcan & Uslu, 2022; Shahada et al., 2024). Linseeds constitute about 35–45% oil, which is used for both edible and nonedible industrial applications. Linseed oil has very distinct properties that make it suitable for industrial applications. The oil has color ranging from golden yellow to brown to amber, and constitutes the highest amount of α-linolenic acid as compared to other plant-based oils. The unique fatty acid profile of the oil serves as a major reason for its diverse applicability. Depending on the variety of seeds, the oil is composed of 6–7% palmitic acid, 5–9% stearic acid, 22–28% oleic acid, 40–55% alpha-linolenic acid (ALA), and 10–13% linoleic acid (LA) (Beema et al., 2022). Thus, the oil is a rich source of polyunsaturated fatty acids (PUFA), namely, ALA and LA, which are also are essential fatty acids (EFAs), i.e., they need to be consumed via food sources and cannot be produced by the body itself (Djuricic & Calder, 2021). Studies have revealed these fatty acids to exhibit cardioprotective, anti-inflammatory, and anticancer properties. They are essential for overall well-being of an individual; however, their consumption has been reported to reduce with changing lifestyles and eating habits, leading to their deficiency in the population (Barnes et al., 2021; Bird et al., 2021; Shen et al., 2022). Thus, the oil is used as a cooking oil, as well as a nutritional supplement to address this deficiency. However, the very cause making this oil nutritionally rich is also responsible for its low food-grade application. The high PUFA content makes it susceptible to oxidation, thus reducing its stability and increasing its tendency to become rancid. This can be prevented by the addition of natural and synthetic antioxidants. Techniques like blending, interesterification, and encapsulation have also been used to enhance its food-based applications as cooking oil or nutraceuticals (Du et al., 2022; Su et al., 2023).

Linseed oil is also utilized for several nonfood applications. It is a type of unsaturated fatty oil that is classified as a drying oil. When such oils are spread on a surface as a thin layer and exposed to air, they solidify, and become elastic and tough. Drying oils are frequently employed as carriers in paints, varnishes, and printing inks because of this characteristic. The oil dries slowly and uniformly, which makes it an ideal drying agent for use in products like paint formula and wood finishes. It also imparts a glow to wooden surfaces, making them appear fresh for a longer duration. The oil also possesses water-resistant properties, i.e., it can keep the materials safe from water damage. This aids in preventing the metal surfaces from corrosion and furniture from damage by moisture. In recent years, it has also found application in development of additives that not only enhance and protect the durability of concrete structures but also prevent surface cracking and abrasion (Shahada et al., 2024). Additionally, it has excellent binding properties, which helps in development of a smooth and rich emulsion when several different ingredients are blended together. Linseed oil has been used for generations in wood-based furniture and linoleum floor coverings. Chia, camelina, and perilla oils are other underutilized oilseeds that are high in ALA and have potential uses similar to linseed. It has recently become a potential sustainable alternative to petroleum-based products and is also used for industrial application as a biodiesel, and lubricant. The growing interest of the consumers toward environmentally friendly products has contributed toward the increased nonfood applications of vegetable oils (İşeri-Çağlar et al., 2014). They have upsides of biodegradability along with low toxicity, price, and high availability. The use of oilseeds in nonfood products was quite popular up to the 1900s, after which fossil fuels or petroleum replaced seed oils as the primary source of such products. Nevertheless, the interest of researchers and industrialists is bouncing back to the traditional source, oilseeds. This is because fossil fuel use is linked to higher atmospheric CO_2 levels and other greenhouse gases, which contribute to climate change. Moreover, the long-term availability of fossil fuels for future generations is uncertain (Bahadorian et al., 2023). These industrial applications enhance the economic value of this versatile crop, making it a profitable endeavor for farmers. The oil is underutilized and hence can aid in narrowing the gap between the demand and availability. However, realizing the potential application of flaxseed in a multitude of industries comes with its own set of difficulties. For instance, incorporating flaxseed oil to food products includes concerns related to integration and formulation (Drozłowska et al., 2020).

2 Oleochemical Characterization and Oleochemistry

As discussed, linseed oil is a powerhouse of PUFAs, especially ALA. This distinct fatty acid profile makes it stand out as an ideal industrial oil among other vegetable oils. The most prominent PUFAs present in the oil include ALA and LA, of which the former represents about 50–65% of the total fatty acids, while the latter constitutes about 15% (Chand et al., 2024). They have been associated with several health benefits such as cardioprotective, anti-inflammatory, and anti-cancer properties and are essential for the overall well-being of the individuals (Dhiman et al., 2023). The nutritional profile makes them highly desirable for use as an edible oil. However, the high PUFA content also renders linseed oil susceptible to auto-oxidation. Thus, for use as an edible oil, it is either used as a blend or is incorporated with several natural or synthetic antioxidants. Techniques like microencapsulation have also been studied for its use as a nutraceutical and to protect its essential fatty acids from degradation, also leading to increased bioavailability of omega-3 FAs (Homroy et al., 2023). Contrary to this, auto-oxidation is also the technique that imparts it with its characteristic properties for application in film formation by oxidative drying, and yellowing caused by the homo-conjuene systems of polyene FAs. Products derived from linseed oil have a tendency to oxidize and polymerize because of the strong reactivity of the double-bond systems with oxygen, which is explained by the bisallyl positions in linoleic acid and particularly in linolenic acid. Because of this characteristic, linseed oil has long been valued as a raw material for paints, printing inks, and linoleum. The characteristic features of linseed oil are mostly due to the high chemical reactivity of the double-bond systems in linoleic and linolenic acids. However, this reactivity also presents synthetic potential for this domestic vegetable raw material's oleochemical utilization. Alkyl chains can be further developed chemically by using base chemicals, such as methyl ester of linseed oil. The olefinic reaction center of linolenic acid, whose high abundance in the triglyceride is the most distinctive characteristic of the raw material linseed oil compared to other industrially manufactured triglycerides, is the focus of the chemical derivatizations for manufacture of several industrial products (Knörr et al., 1995).

3 Linseed (Flaxseed) Production and Standards in India

Linseed, also known as flax (*Linum usitatissimum L.*), is one of the oldest cultivated crops, grown in approximately 47 countries for its seed oil and fiber. In countries like South West Asia and Canada, linseed is primarily cultivated for oil production, while in Russia, Egypt, and northwestern European countries, it is grown mainly for high-quality fiber used in making linen fabrics and other products. Globally, linseed occupies 32.23 lakh hectares, producing 30.68 lakh tonnes with an average productivity of 952 kg/ha. In India, linseed is grown on 1.7 lakh hectares, yielding about 1 lakh tonnes with an average productivity of 574 kg/ha. India ranks fifth in area and sixth in production globally.

The major linseed growing states in India include Madhya Pradesh, Chhattisgarh, Uttar Pradesh, Maharashtra, Bihar, Odisha, Jharkhand, West Bengal, Nagaland, and Assam, accounting for about 97% of the country's total area. Despite some improvement in productivity, India's yield is still lower than potential and experimental yields, highlighting the need for enhanced production practices and policy support.

3.1 FSSAI Standards for Linseed Oil

Linseed oil, known as "Tisi ka Tel" in India, is obtained by expressing clean and sound linseed. According to FSSAI standards, linseed oil must meet the following criteria:

- Butyro-refractometer Reading at 40 °C: 69.5–74.3 OR Refractive Index at 40 °C: 1.4720–1.4750
- Saponification Value: 188–195
- Iodine Value: Not less than 170
- Unsaponifiable Matter: Not more than 1.5%
- Acid Value: Not more than 4.0
- Test for Argemone Oil: Must be negative

The oil should be clear and free from rancidity, suspended or foreign matter, separated water, added coloring or flavoring substances, and mineral oil. It may contain permitted food additives as per the regulations and appendices.

These standards ensure the quality and safety of linseed oil, making it a crucial agricultural product in India. High-yielding varieties resistant to biotic and abiotic stresses, coupled with good agronomic practices and policy support, can significantly boost linseed production in India. This crop not only contributes to the nutritional security of the population through its omega-3 fatty acids but also provides economic benefits to Indian farmers. Long-term investment in research, development, and favorable policies is essential for achieving self-sufficiency in linseed production.

4 Linseed Oil Market

The global linseed oil production has observed a rising trend in the past decade. The world production of linseed oil is graphically represented in Fig. 1a and b in accordance with the quantity and regions, respectively (FAOSTAT). The demand for linseed oil is anticipated to be driven by its growing use in a variety of industries, including food, cosmetics, and medicines. The market's dynamics have changed recently, with a wide range of end-use industries generating sizable demand. While Canada has achieved a remarkable recovery into the mainstream market following a large fall in exports for several years running, Europe has been attempting to increase its production. Apart from its commercial applications, linseed oil is also consumed for its nutritional benefits and is becoming more and more popular in certain markets. A vast array of items, such as putty, paints, gilding, wood treatments, flooring, dietary supplements, linoleum, and food processing, are made using linseed oil. Linseed oil plays a crucial role in the production of linoleum, impregnators, and varnish for a wide range of industrial uses when mixed with different resins and solvents. Studies have shown that linseed oil may lower the risk of cardiovascular and cancer disorders, which has led to a rise in the use of this oil in nutritional supplement production (Langyan et al., 2023). Furthermore, linseed oil's ability to polymerize—that is, to change form and mix with different solvents and resins—improves its use in paints and coatings. Its adaptability is anticipated to fuel market expansion in these industries. The oil is a rich source of omega-3 fatty acids, which rises its application in pharmaceuticals, cosmetics, and food products. The oil mostly used in healthy and nutritious food and bakery formulations and its share of consumption is rising over the globe.

5 Industrial Applications

The industrial applications of linseed oil are very diverse due to its unique characteristics. The oil is used in an array of applications summed up together in the following sections and Fig. 2.

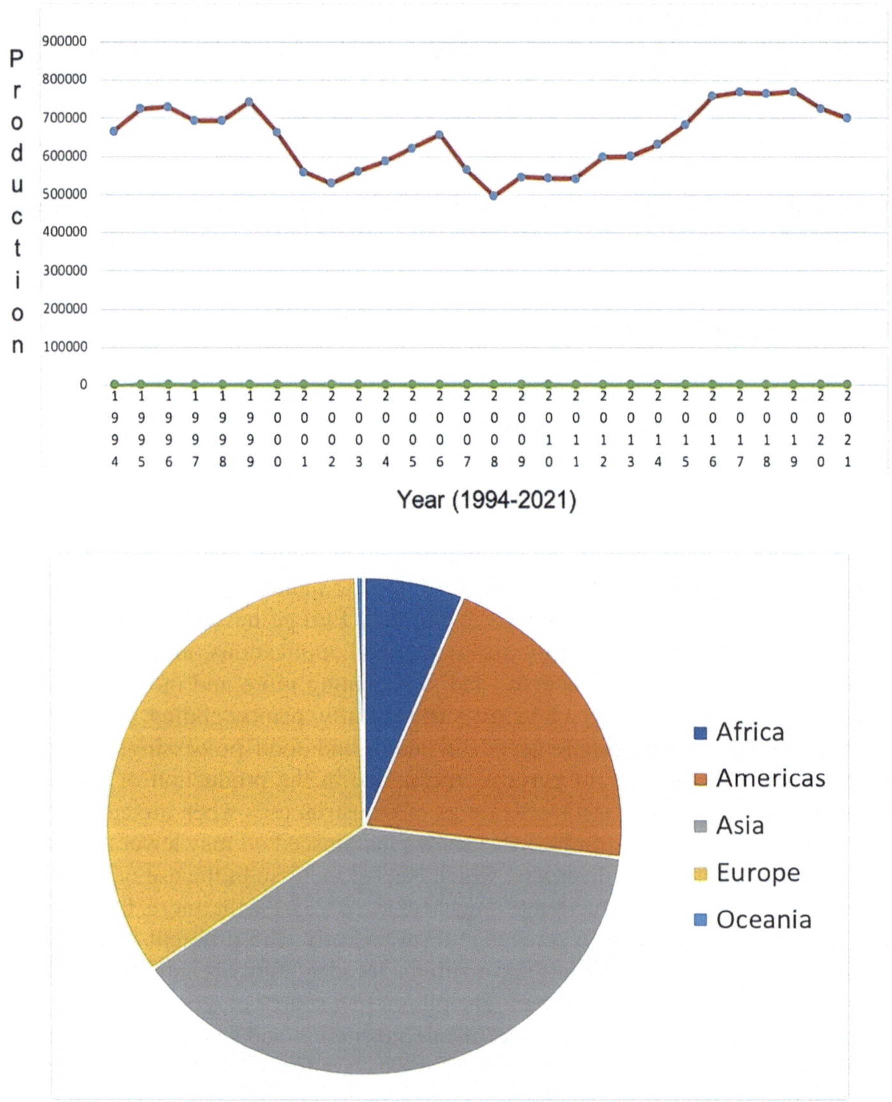

Fig. 1 (**a**) World production of linseed oil (1994–2021). (**b**) Region shares of linseed oil production

5.1 Food Industry

The use of linseed as a functional food is regaining awareness after its worldwide use in natural medicine. Every part of it from the stem(fiber), seeds, or leaves is utilized commercially. Since ancient times, linseed has been used in ayurvedic medicines and therapies but from the last two decades, linseed has grown in popularity

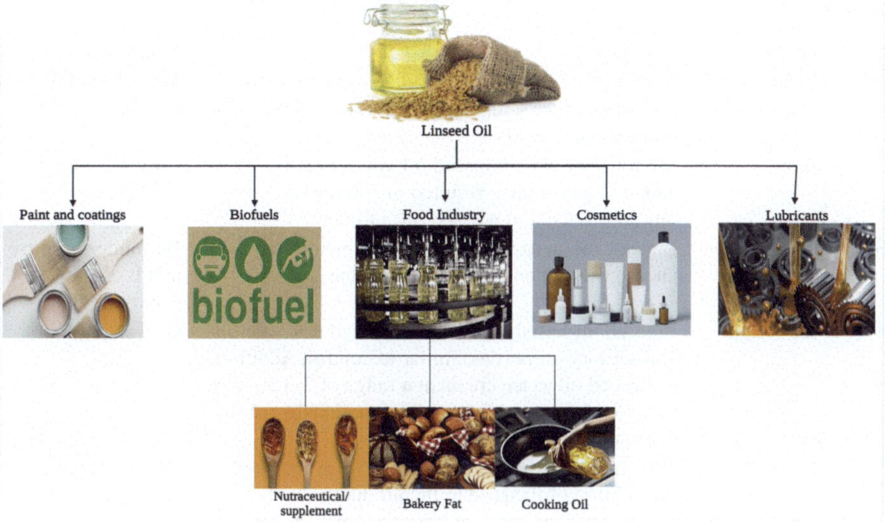

Fig. 2 Industrial applications of linseed oil

in the food industry due to its high nutritional value. It is considered as functional food as it provides specific health benefits along with good nutritional value. Linseed oil can be used in several food products as a neat oil, nano or microencapsulated powder, and a stable emulsion (Goyal et al., 2014). Linseed oil has now been used in various edible products such as cheese, bakery, ice cream, neat oils, stable emulsions and micro- and nano-encapsulated powder for nutritional, functional, and sensory properties. A few applications of linseed oil in food industry have been tabulated in Table 1.

5.1.1 Cooking Oil

Linseed oil has excellent nutritional profile with high content of omega-3 fatty acids. However, the very nutritional profile serves it as a limitation for use as a cooking oil. These PUFAs are highly susceptible to thermal and oxidative degradation (Singh et al., 2024a). Thus, it is used as a blend with other edible oils to increase it applicability. Also, recently a new genotype seed variety, TL99, developed by ICAR has 5% less ALA and the cold pressed oil has been found suitable for development of items such as banana chips, papad, crackers, fryums, and other fried items (Rathnakumar & Ambati, 2023). Linseed oil was used to replace the animal-based fat in chicken frankfurters. The replacement up to a 50% level was observed to be similar to control in terms of functional and sensory properties. However, further increase to 100% linseed oil impaired the sensory characteristics (Stajić et al., 2018). The cold press extracted oil can however be used as such in salad dressing and for applications where minimal heat is required.

Table 1 Use of linseed oil in food industry

S. No.	Product	Linseed oil	Reference
1.	Cake	Nano-encapsulated linseed oil (6%) was used to formulate cakes with high antioxidant potential and omega-3 fatty acids	Murugkar et al. (2021)
2	Juice	Microencapsulated linseed oil via freeze drying added to guava juice resulted in 300 mg of omega-3 fatty acid per 100 mL of juice	Correa et al. (2024)
3	Cheese	Linseed oil up to 5.2 mg/g was retained in the cheese without any implication on the shelf life	Bermúdez-Aguirre and Barbosa-Cánovas (2012)
4	Ice cream	Linseed oil-based ice cream exhibited flocculation and sensory properties similar to control. Addition of linseed oil to ice cream at a range of 2–12% w/w was done without affecting the functionality of the final product	Goh et al. (2006)
5	Bread	No effects on sensorial properties were observed on addition of flaxseed to the product	Gökmen et al. (2011)
6.	Biscuits and shortening	Biscuits were developed by substituting the shortening with linseed oil-based fat with sensory and functional properties comparable to control	Hassan et al. (2012)
7	Emulsions	Stable linseed oil emulsions in carrot juice were developed via ultrasonication without the addition of external stabilizers and emulsifiers	Shanmugam and Ashokkumar (2015)

5.1.2 Bakery Fat

The rising trend in consumption of bakery products daily due to changing lifestyles makes them ideal for fortification with EFAs. The conventionally used bakery fats are developed by partial hydrogenation of vegetable oils, a process resulting in formation of trans-fatty acids. These trans-fatty acids have various negative implications on health of consumers. They are a major cause of cardiovascular disorders and strokes (Li et al., 2018; Nagpal et al., 2021). Additionally, they are also rich in saturated fatty acids and there are several studies linking the consumption of these FAs to the prevalence of atherosclerosis, obesity, cardiovascular disorders, cancer, and hyperlipidemia (Mei et al., 2024; Patel et al., 2020). Since the last two decades, the composition of bakery fats has significantly evolved by reduction in total fat and SFA content and an increase in PUFAs. Refined linseed oil is used as a blend with other edible oils in the development of margarine and spreads. Significant levels of omega-3 fatty acids are found in margarines containing linseed oil, ranging from 3 g to 7 g per 100 g, depending on the bakery fat composition (Renault, 2015). Furthermore, the linseed oil incorporation to such products not only leads to an improved uptake of the essential fatty acids, but also, aids in balancing the ratio of omega-3 and omega-6 fatty acids. A healthy ratio closer to 5:1 can be attained by consuming margarine with a low omega-6 to omega-3 ratio, which naturally lowers the intake of omega-6 while preserving omega-3 levels. An imbalance in this ratio might result in a state of the body that is favorable to inflammation and associated illnesses, like heart disease. Linseed oil has high viscosity but due to its high PUFA content and low techno-functional properties, cannot be used as such in baked goods. It is thus used by blending with saturated fats to balance the fatty acid ratio and to improve the applicability. However, blending lacks uniformity and leads to phase separation. Thus, techniques like interesterification are being studied to further enhance its functional properties. Interesterification is the rearrangement of fatty acids among the triglycerides to produce a better and uniform product. Linseed oil interesterified with cottonseed oil and palm stearin was used to develop plastic fats with balanced omega-6 and omega-3 ratio using lipase enzyme (Su et al., 2023). The fats were produced as alternatives to shortenings and had zero trans fats and were low in saturated fatty acids. The similar technology has also been used for flaxseed oil with rapeseed oil and grapeseed oil (Ilyasoglu, 2017; Wirkowska-Wojdyła et al., 2021). The stability of these fats can be enhanced by addition of natural or synthetic antioxidants. Linseed oil is also incorporated into bakery items in the form of encapsulated powders. For instance, linseed oil encapsulated via spray drying using soy protein isolate and Gum Arabic was used to formulate eggless cakes. The cake was reported to constitute high-antioxidant activity and essential omega-3 fatty acids (Murugkar et al., 2021). Encapsulating edible oils with powder particles made of carbohydrates or proteins is a scientific process used to protect polyunsaturated oils from oxidation. This method helps preserve the flavors and aroma of the oils and allows bioactive oils to be transported in easily managed dried solids for food supplementation (Bordón et al., 2020). The most recent technology of addition of linseed oil to bakery products is by its conversion to oleogels. Oleogels formulated using different ratios of linseed oil and sunflower oil were studied for potential application as shortening replacer on cakes (Roufegarinejad et al., 2024). The most suitable formulation was found with 50:50 ratio of both the oils. They exhibited comparable thermal properties and enhanced morphological characteristics along with an improved nutritional profile.

5.1.3 Nutraceuticals

Nutraceuticals are the products developed by isolating or purifying ingredients from food, required for the overall development, maintenance, and growth of an individual (Kaur et al., 2024). These can be derived from various biologically active compounds. A few of them present in linseed include ALA, LA, lignans, vitamins, phenolics, polysaccharides, minerals, and so forth. Most of the products from linseed, i.e., whole seed, defatted seed cake, oil, hulls, extracts from seedcake, oil, and mucilage are used as nutraceuticals owing to their health benefits. Flaxseed supplementation was assessed in 15 studies and significant reduction in systolic as well as diastolic blood pressure was observed in after the treatment as compared to control (Ursoniu et al., 2016). In another meta-analysis, the effect of supplementing flaxseed oil on inflammation and oxidative stress was studied in population suffering from metabolic syndrome and related ailments (Tamtaji et al., 2020). The study reported a decrease in interleukin and malondialdehyde levels, along with an increased antioxidant capacity. It was suggested that the oil supplementation led to improvement in metabolic disorder symptoms. A significant reduction in LDL, cholesterol, triglycerides, and LDL cholesterol to HDL cholesterol ratio was also reported in another analysis on flaxseed oil supplementation. The lipid profile of the patients was significantly ameliorated (Moridpour et al., 2024). Linseed oil is one the best sources of alpha-linolenic acid. n-3 LCPUFA and other bio-converted metabolites of ALA have the ability to activate proliferator-activated receptor-γ (PPARγ). In order to control insulin action and lipid metabolism, PPARγ is essential (Marion-Letellier et al., 2016).

5.2 Biodiesel

The rising depletion of fossil fuels and environment degradation has led to an increased demand for eco-friendly, renewable fuels. Vegetable oils can be used as an alternative to conventional fuels, as they are not only renewable and environment friendly, but can also be produced on a large scale. Linseed oil has an excellent potential for application as a biodiesel. However, they cannot be used as such in diesel engines for their several limitations. For instance, linseed oil has a high viscosity and low volatility, which are the major problems for its application as a biodiesel. The most common issues with its use are improper combustion, high pumping power, and low atomization of the fuel particles. Thus, they need to be converted into high-capacity fuels like biodiesel (Kumar et al., 2013). Vegetable oils can be converted to engine fuel by four primary methods, i.e., micro-emulsification, pyrolysis, blending, and transesterification. In case of linseed, the most widely used method is transesterification. In this process, an alkali catalyst (potassium hydroxide or sodium hydroxide) is used along with an alcohol (methanol or ethanol) to produce methyl esters from linseed oil (Bahadorian et al., 2023). The process comprises of a series of three reversible reactions occurring consecutively. The triglycerides are converted to diglycerides, which are further converted to monoglycerides, and these are finally converted to glycerol. Thus, one mole of mono-alkyl ester is formed at the expense of three moles of alcohol, while glycerol is obtained as a by-product. The reaction is influenced by several parameters, namely, ratio of oil to alcohol, reaction temperature, presence of water, type of catalyst, amount of free fatty acids, and amount of catalyst (Singh et al., 2024b). The viscosity of the biodiesel is significantly reduced by this process and the properties of linseed biodiesel are very similar to those of traditional diesel fuel (Nabi & Hoque, 2008). The process of production of biodiesel from vegetable oils is diagrammatically presented in Fig. 3. Apart from base-catalyzed, or chemically induced transesterification, the process can also be carried out enzymatically by the use of lipase in the presence of methanol. In contrast to the chemical approach, it has several upsides such as, easier product separation, glycerol recovery, and absence of any side reactions (Dixit et al., 2012). Oxidation stability is a critical quality parameter for biodiesel. During storage, fatty acid methyl esters (FAME) undergo auto-oxidation, initially forming peroxides and hydroperoxides. This is followed by the formation of aldehydes and ketones, and finally, resins during the polymerization process. FAMEs are more prone to oxidative degradation compared to conventional diesel fuel due to their high concentration of unsaturated fatty acids, which are characteristic of vegetable

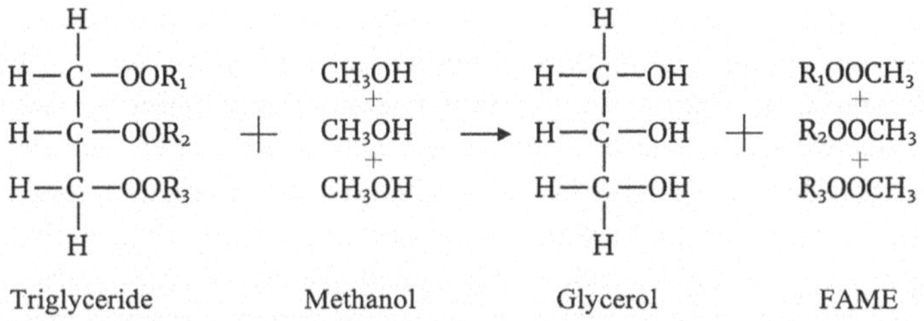

Fig. 3 Transesterification mechanism of vegetable oils and fats

oil esters. The oxidation rate of FAMEs depends on the nature of the fatty acids in the feed oil, temperature, reaction catalysts, and inhibitors present in the fats. Linseed oil, which is rich in unsaturated fatty acids, exhibits high reactivity and lower oxidative stability. However, linseed oil esters have been found to offer better stability in terms of free fatty acid (FFA) increase. Antioxidants, which can inhibit the oxidation process, contribute to the stabilization of lipid samples. In vegetable oils and their esters, antioxidants can be either natural or synthetic. The oxidation stability of FAMEs derived from linseed oil can be enhanced using synthetic antioxidants. Tocopherols, which are phenolic compounds naturally occurring in vegetable oils, are optimized for their antioxidant capabilities. The fatty acid composition and natural antioxidant content present in FAMEs of linseed oil play a crucial role in determining their oxidation stability. Thermal efficiency measures how effectively the chemical energy from fuel is converted into useful work. Studies have shown that increasing the concentration of biodiesel in fuel blends improves the engine's thermal efficiency. Notably, all biodiesel blends exhibit higher thermal efficiency than conventional diesel. Specifically, a 25% blend of linseed oil with diesel achieves thermal efficiency comparable to diesel fuel, while a 50% blend of linseed oil has been reported to be even more thermally efficient (Agarwal et al., 2008; Sriharikota et al., 2021). Research indicates that the thermal efficiency of engines using different biodiesel blends is almost equivalent to that of diesel. The improved thermal efficiency is likely due to more complete combustion of biodiesel and its superior lubricity, attributed to the higher oxygen content in biodiesel.

5.3 Linoleum

Linoleum is a smooth-surfaced floor covering developed by the blending of linseed oil to resins, gums, and other substances. This mixture is generally applied to a canvas backing or a felt. The traditional process of manufacturing linoleum involved the deliberate oxidation of linseed oil to a thin film. The oil was applied continuously onto the oxidized film surface as the oxidation process mainly occurs on the surface. This was then exposed for weeks, during which the thickness of the film increased to an inch or more after which the film was fused to a natural resin (Choi, 2021). This oxidized oil and resin was further mixed with corks and other fillers.

This process had the drawback of longer duration, and was thus replaced by a faster technique in large cylindrical kettles employed at high temperature to deliberately oxidize the oil to a stage until the oil barely flows at the reaction temperature. This oil is then mixed with the natural resins in the same kettles at an elevated temperature and this blend is subjected to hot air. The pigments, fillers, and binders are then added to the mixture and molded into sheets by passing them through rollers and applied to the canvas or felt saturated with asphalt. Modern technologies are utilized to develop linoleum with plain, inlaid, or decorative patterns. For instance, the inlaid patterns are synthesized by dividing the squares of two distinctly colored sheets and adhering them to one backing material. Linoleum is very resilient and is generally not affected by the floor temperatures and is also satisfactorily resistant to combustion (Rosso et al., 2020). It is resistant to damage from grease and oils, along with organic solvents and is specially hardened to protect itself from indentation. However, the prolonged attack from alkalis and moisture affects it.

5.4 Paint

Linseed oil has a major application in the paint industry. It has many distinctive properties, which make it desirable for use in several paints. Linseed oil possess drying qualities, which make it perfect for use in oil-based paints (Yasmeen et al., 2018). Flaxseed or linseed oil upon exposure to air, forms a tough protective layer by the process of polymerization. This film results in the increased endurance and protection of the painted surface (Azhar et al., 2020). Additionally, the oil has negligible toxicity, which further makes it an ideal ingredient for paint making. It serves as a sustainable and natural alternate to synthetic binders, which are well-known to include hazardous chemicals, which have implications on both the environment and health of consumers (Sharma et al., 2019). Apart from this, flaxseed oil has excellent color retention properties, which contribute to the enhancement of color and the paints' vitality. Thus, flaxseed oil is widely used by producers aiming for a long-lasting and high-quality paint due to its characteristic chemical nature. Another beneficial feature of using flaxseed oil is its ability to improve the leveling and flow behavior of the paint (Tasneem et al., 2022). The oil's viscosity makes it readily spreadable uniformly on the surface. It facilitates the painters to get a smooth and uniform finish. Another application of linseed oil is in wood finishes and varnishes (Shahada et al., 2024). It has excellent penetration properties, which allow its varnishes to offer protection to wood. Finishes made with flaxseed oil are renowned for their longevity and ability to endure adverse weather conditions (Debnath, 2021).

5.5 Other Applications

Linseed oil has excellent moisturizing and anti-inflammatory properties due to which it finds its application in the cosmetic industry. It is used as a major ingredient in skin creams, body lotions, hair conditioners, etc. The oil is also used in the treatment of dry and sensitive skin due to its high ALA and LA content. The oil is used in medical products such as anti-inflammatory supplements and topical treatments for skin conditions (Ebrahimi et al., 2021). It is also used for protection of wood surfaces. Linseed oil is widely used in wood preservation due to its ability to penetrate deep into the wood and provide a protective barrier against moisture. The auto-oxidation property of the oil is used to keep the wood surfaces safe from degradation for a longer duration. The lubricant industry is one of the fastest growing markets, dominated by the motor and gear oils, accounting for about 60% of the total consumption. This industry was mostly dependent on the use of animal or plant-based oils and fats before the development of the petrochemical. Linseed oil, owing to its desirable viscosity and lubrication properties is a potential alternative for such products.

6 Environment Impact and Sustainability

The global demand for fats and oils is continuously rising on an annual basis, driven by various factors including population growth, dietary changes, and industrial requirements. Oilseeds play a significant role in meeting this demand, serving both culinary and industrial markets. Among these, linseed is one of the underutilized oilseeds that requires more exposure and research for increased application in various industries (Woodfield & Harwood, 2017). Linseed oil is rich in alpha-linolenic acid (ALA), an essential omega-3 fatty acid. This makes it valuable not only in the culinary sector for its nutritional benefits but also in the industrial sector for its unique chemical properties. The whole linseed plant has diverse applications. Beyond the oil, its byproducts, such as seedcake, shives, and fibers, are nutritionally rich and have potential applications in both food and nonfood industries. For instance, seedcake can be used as animal feed due to its high protein content, while the fibers can be utilized in textile manufacturing and biocomposites. The overutilization of fossil fuels has resulted in significant environmental degradation and rapid depletion of these nonrenewable resources. This poses a serious threat to future generations as the availability of fossil fuels becomes increasingly uncertain. Addressing this energy crisis requires the exploration and utilization of underutilized vegetable oils, such as linseed oil, to narrow the gap between energy demand and supply. Biodiesel, derived from vegetable oils like linseed oil, has garnered significant attention in recent years as a renewable and sustainable fuel source for diesel engines. Biodiesel offers numerous environmental benefits, including lower emissions of pollutants such as carbon monoxide, particulate matter, and unburned hydrocarbons compared to conventional diesel. This makes it an attractive alternative in the quest to reduce greenhouse gas emissions and combat climate change. India, in particular, faces a dual challenge of environmental degradation and financial strain due to its heavy reliance on imported petroleum products and crude oil from Gulf nations. Indian scientists and policymakers have been actively seeking diesel fuel substitutes to protect both the environment and the economy. Linseed oil, with its high unsaturated fatty acid content and favorable properties for biodiesel production, presents a viable option. Research and development efforts are essential to enhance the properties of linseed oil for various applications. This includes improving its oxidative stability, which is crucial for both its use in food products and its performance as biodiesel. Advances in plant genomics, catalysis, and biotechnological processes can lead to the development of new linseed varieties with enhanced characteristics. For example, the introduction of the TL 99 variety has shown promise in terms of stability and quality, paving the way for broader use. Furthermore, linseed oil's polymerization property, which allows it to change form and blend with various solvents and resins, is advantageous for industrial applications such as paints, varnishes, and linoleum. Its natural composition and biodegradability make it a safer and more sustainable alternative to synthetic chemicals traditionally used in these industries. Linseed oil, an underutilized yet highly beneficial oilseed, has the potential to play a significant role in both the culinary and industrial sectors. By addressing the current challenges through targeted research and development, linseed oil can become a more versatile and valuable resource. Its adoption can help mitigate the environmental impact of fossil fuels, contribute to energy security, and provide numerous benefits across various industries.

7 Conclusion

Oilseeds play a crucial role in meeting the demand for both culinary and industrial applications, with linseed oil being a significant contributor due to its high nutritional value and versatility. However, despite its many benefits, linseed oil faces challenges such as susceptibility to oxidation and relatively slow drying times. These issues limit its widespread use and effectiveness in various applications. The fatty acid profile of linseed oil can be improved through further research and the introduction of new seed varieties. Continued exploration in this direction is essential to develop new varieties that can be used directly for culinary purposes, enhancing the usability and appeal of linseed oil in the food industry. Future research is focused on not only improving the fatty acid profile and oxidative stability of linseed oil but also expanding its industrial applications. By enhancing its properties, linseed oil can become a more viable option for a wider range of products, including paints, varnishes, and bio-based materials. Moreover, improving its drying times and resistance to oxidation can make it more competitive with other oils used in similar applications. Thus, while linseed oil has numerous benefits, addressing its current challenges through targeted research and development is crucial. By doing so, its properties can be enhanced, making it a more versatile and valuable resource for both culinary and industrial markets. Plant-based oils and their derivatives have a multitude of food and nonfood-based applications. They are used as a major ingredient in the paint and coating industry, and have applications as lubricants, biofuels, surfactants, cosmetics, and forth more. As an edible source, linseed oil offers an array of health benefits owing to its fatty acid profile, which has an abundance of omega-3 fatty acids. The oil is also a good source of several bioactive compounds, which aid in imparting beneficial effects, both as an edible and nonedible source.

The oil has unique characteristics, which enable it to be an ideal ingredient in paint, cosmetic, and food industry. The demand for oleochemicals is further expected to surge in the forthcoming years, due to growing interest of the population toward bio-based products caused by rising awareness of the consumers toward sustainable alternatives for conventional fossil-fuel-derived products. Underutilized oils such as linseed oil itself are a major contributing factor for narrowing this gap between the availability and demand of oleo-based biodegradable products. Advancements in plant genomics, biocatalysis, heterogeneous catalysis, artificial intelligence, and biomolecular engineering are expected to enhance the economic feasibility of oleochemical products and expand the range of products that can be developed.

References

Agarwal, D., Kumar, L., & Agarwal, A. K. (2008). Performance evaluation of a vegetable oil fuelled compression ignition engine. *Renewable Energy, 33*(6), 1147–1156. https://doi.org/10.1016/j.renene.2007.06.017

Azhar, S. W., Xu, F., Zhang, Y., & Qiu, Y. (2020). Fabrication and mechanical properties of flaxseed fiber bundle-reinforced polybutylene succinate composites. *Journal of Industrial Textiles, 50*(1), 98–113. https://doi.org/10.1177/1528083718821876

Bahadorian, A., Sadrameli, S. M., Pahlavanzadeh, H., & Ilani Kashkouli, M. N. (2023). Optimization study of linseed biodiesel production via in-situ transesterification and slow pyrolysis of obtained linseed residue. *Renewable Energy, 203*, 10–19. https://doi.org/10.1016/j.renene.2022.12.043

Barnes, S., Chowdhury, S., Gatto, N. M., Fraser, G. E., & Lee, G. J. (2021). Omega-3 fatty acids are associated with blood-brain barrier integrity in a healthy aging population. *Brain and Behavior, 11*(8), e2273. https://doi.org/10.1002/brb3.2273

Beema, N., Mukkamula, N., Mothuku, S., Thumu, R., Azmeera, T., & Biman, K. K. (2022). Comparative analysis of physico-chemical properties and fatty acid composition of linseed (Linum usitatissimum L.) oils of Indian accessions. *Journal of Applied Biology & Biotechnology*. https://doi.org/10.7324/JABB.2023.110112

Bermúdez-Aguirre, D., & Barbosa-Cánovas, G. V. (2012). Fortification of *queso fresco*, cheddar and mozzarella cheese using selected sources of omega-3 and some nonthermal approaches. *Food Chemistry, 133*(3), 787–797. https://doi.org/10.1016/j.foodchem.2012.01.093

Bird, J. K., Troesch, B., Warnke, I., & Calder, P. C. (2021). The effect of long chain omega-3 polyunsaturated fatty acids on muscle mass and function in sarcopenia: A scoping systematic review and meta-analysis. *Clinical Nutrition ESPEN, 46*, 73–86. https://doi.org/10.1016/j.clnesp.2021.10.011

Bordón, M. G., Barrera, G. N., Penci, M. C., Bori, A., Caballero, V., Ribotta, P., & Martínez, M. L. (2020). Microencapsulation of chia seed oil (Salvia hispanica L.) in spray and freeze-dried Whey Protein Concentrate/Soy Protein Isolate/Gum Arabic (WPC/SPI/GA) matrices. *Proceedings, 53*(1), 1. https://doi.org/10.3390/proceedings2020053022

Chand, M., Chopra, R., Talwar, B., Homroy, S., Singh, P. K., Dhiman, A., & Payyunni, A. W. (2024). Unveiling the potential of linseed mucilage, its health benefits, and applications in food packaging. *Frontiers in Nutrition, 11*, 1334247. https://doi.org/10.3389/fnut.2024.1334247

Choi, J. (2021). A study on the linoleum of the Deoksugung and Changdeokgung palaces in the early 20th century: Focusing on its manufacturing process, characteristics, and usage. *Korean Journal of Heritage: History & Science, 54*(1), 18–31. https://doi.org/10.22755/kjchs.2021.54.1.18

Correa, L. G., Kato, T., Giuliangeli, V. C., Torquato, A. S., & Shirai, M. A. (2024). Fruit juice fortification with omega-3 by adding chia and linseed oil microcapsules. *Food Chemistry Advances, 4*, 100649. https://doi.org/10.1016/j.focha.2024.100649

Debnath, S. (2021). *Flax fibre extraction to textiles and sustainability: A holistic approach* (pp. 73–85). https://doi.org/10.1007/978-981-16-1850-5_4

Dhiman, A., Chopra, R., Singh, P., Homroy, S., Chand, M., & Talwar, B. (2023). Amelioration of nutritional properties of bakery fat using omega-3 fatty acid rich edible oils- A review. *Journal of the Science of Food and Agriculture, 104*, 3175. https://doi.org/10.1002/jsfa.13225

Drozłowska, E., Bartkowiak, A., & Łopusiewicz, Ł. (2020). Characterization of Flaxseed Oil Bimodal Emulsions Prepared with Flaxseed Oil Cake Extract Applied as a Natural Emulsifying Agent. *Polymers, 12*(10), Article 10. https://doi.org/10.3390/polym12102207

Dixit, S., Kanakraj, S., & Rehman, A. (2012). Linseed oil as a potential resource for bio-diesel: A review. *Renewable and Sustainable Energy Reviews, 16*(7), 4415–4421. https://doi.org/10.1016/j.rser.2012.04.042

Djuricic, I., & Calder, P. C. (2021). Beneficial outcomes of omega-6 and omega-3 polyunsaturated fatty acids on human health: An update for 2021. *Nutrients, 13*(7), 2421. https://doi.org/10.3390/nu13072421

Du, Q., Zhou, L., Li, M., Lyu, F., Liu, J., & Ding, Y. (2022). Omega-3 polyunsaturated fatty acid encapsulation system: Physical and oxidative stability, and medical applications. *Food Frontiers, 3*(2), 239–255. https://doi.org/10.1002/fft2.134

Ebrahimi, B., Nazmara, Z., Hassanzadeh, N., Yarahmadi, A., Ghaffari, N., Hassani, F., Liaghat, A., Noori, L., & Hasanzadeh, G. (2021). Biomedical features of flaxseed against different pathologic situations: A narrative review. *Iranian Journal of Basic Medical Sciences, 24*(5), 551–560. https://doi.org/10.22038/ijbms.2021.49821.11378

Goh, K. K. T., Pinder, D. N., Hall, C. E., & Hemar, Y. (2006). Rheological and light scattering properties of flaxseed polysaccharide aqueous solutions. *Biomacromolecules, 7*(11), 3098–3103. https://doi.org/10.1021/bm060577u

Gökmen, V., Mogol, B. A., Lumaga, R. B., Fogliano, V., Kaplun, Z., & Shimoni, E. (2011). Development of functional bread containing nanoencapsulated omega-3 fatty acids. *Journal of Food Engineering, 105*(4), 585–591. https://doi.org/10.1016/j.jfoodeng.2011.03.021

Goyal, A., Sharma, V., Upadhyay, N., Gill, S., & Sihag, M. (2014). Flax and flaxseed oil: An ancient medicine & modern functional food. *Journal of Food Science and Technology, 51*(9), 1633–1653. https://doi.org/10.1007/s13197-013-1247-9

Hassan, A., Rasmy, N., & Bahgaat, W. (2012). Production of functional biscuits for lowering blood lipids. *World Journal of Dairy & Food Sciences, 7*, 01–20.

Homroy, S., Chopra, R., Singh, P., Dhiman, A., & chand, monika, & Talwar, B. (2023). Role of encapsulation on the bioavailability of omega-3 fatty acids. *Comprehensive Reviews in Food Science and Food Safety, 23*, 1–35. https://doi.org/10.1111/1541-4337.13272

Ilyasoglu, H. (2017). Production of structured lipid with a low omega-6/omega-3 fatty acids ratio by enzymatic interesterification. *Grasas y Aceites, 68*(2), 191. https://doi.org/10.3989/gya.0565161

İşeri-Çağlar, D., Baştürk, E., Oktay, B., & Kahraman, M. V. (2014). Preparation and evaluation of linseed oil based alkyd paints. *Progress in Organic Coatings, 77*(1), 81–86. https://doi.org/10.1016/j.porgcoat.2013.08.005

Kaur, S., Seem, K., Ali, A., Jaiswal, S., Gumachanamardi, P., Kaur, G., Singh, N., Touthang, L., Singh, S. K., Bhardwaj, R., Singh, B. K., Mishra, V. K., & Riar, A. (2024). A comprehensive review on nutritional, nutraceutical, and industrial perspectives of perilla (Perilla frutscens L.) seeds—An orphan oilseed crop. *Heliyon, 10*(12), e33281. https://doi.org/10.1016/j.heliyon.2024.e33281

Knörr, W., Daute, P., Grützmacher, R., & Höfer, R. (1995). Development of new fields of application for linseed oil. *Lipid / Fett, 97*(5), 165–169. https://doi.org/10.1002/lipi.19950970502

Kumar, R., Tiwari, P., & Garg, S. (2013). Alkali transesterification of linseed oil for biodiesel production. *Fuel, 104*, 553–560. https://doi.org/10.1016/j.fuel.2012.05.002

Langyan, S., Yadava, P., Khan, F. N., Sharma, S., Singh, R., Bana, R. S., Singh, N., Kaur, V., Kalia, S., & Kumar, A. (2023). Trends and advances in pre- and post-harvest processing of linseed oil for quality food and health products. *Critical Reviews in Food Science and Nutrition, 1–24*, 746. https://doi.org/10.1080/10408398.2023.2280768

Li, Y., Zhao, J., Xie, X., Zhang, Z., Zhang, N., & Wang, Y. (2018). A low trans margarine fat analog to beef tallow for healthier formulations: Optimization of enzymatic interesterification using soybean oil and fully hydrogenated palm oil. *Food Chemistry, 255*, 405–413. https://doi.org/10.1016/j.foodchem.2018.02.086

Marion-Letellier, R., Savoye, G., & Ghosh, S. (2016). Fatty acids, eicosanoids and PPAR gamma. *European Journal of Pharmacology, 785*, 44–49. https://doi.org/10.1016/j.ejphar.2015.11.004

Mei, J., Qian, M., Hou, Y., Liang, M., Chen, Y., Wang, C., & Zhang, J. (2024). Association of saturated fatty acids with cancer risk: A systematic review and meta-analysis. *Lipids in Health and Disease, 23*(1), 32. https://doi.org/10.1186/s12944-024-02025-z

Moridpour, A. H., Goodarzi, M., Kavyani, Z., Nademi, N., Daneshvar, M., Musazadeh, V., & Faghfouri, A. H. (2024). Application of flaxseed as an effective approach for improving lipid profile parameters: An updated systematic review and meta-analysis of randomized controlled trials. *PharmaNutrition, 27*, 100366. https://doi.org/10.1016/j.phanu.2023.100366

Murugkar, D. A., Zanwar, A. A., & Shrivastava, A. (2021). Effect of nano-encapsulation of flaxseed oil on the stability, characterization and incorporation on the quality of eggless cake. *Applied Food Research, 1*(2), 100025. https://doi.org/10.1016/j.afres.2021.100025

Nabi, M. N., & Hoque, S. N. (2008). Biodiesel production from linseed oil and performance study of a diesel engine with diesel bio-diesel. *Journal of Mechanical Engineering, 39*(1), 40. https://doi.org/10.3329/jme.v39i1.1832

Nagpal, T., Sahu, J. K., Khare, S. K., Bashir, K., & Jan, K. (2021). Trans fatty acids in food: A review on dietary intake, health impact, regulations and alternatives. *Journal of Food Science, 86*(12), 5159–5174. https://doi.org/10.1111/1750-3841.15977

Özcan, M. M., & Uslu, N. (2022). Investigation of changes in some chemical properties, bioactive compounds, antioxidant activity, phenolic and fatty acid profiles of flaxseed and oils. *Journal of Food Processing and Preservation, 46*(11), e17091. https://doi.org/10.1111/jfpp.17091

Patel, A. R., Nicholson, R. A., & Marangoni, A. G. (2020). Applications of fat mimetics for the replacement of saturated and hydrogenated fat in food products. *Current Opinion in Food Science, 33*, 61–68. https://doi.org/10.1016/j.cofs.2019.12.008

Rathnakumar, A. L., & Ambati, D. (2023). A perspective on linseed breeding and varietal development in India. *Journal of Oilseeds Research, 40*(Specialissue)., https://doi.org/10.56739/hvjv2x10

Renault, A. (2015). Margarines with linseed oil: Nutritional interests, specificities and development. *OCL, 22*(6), D609. https://doi.org/10.1051/ocl/2015024

Rosso, F., Pisello, A. L., Pigliautile, I., Cavalaglio, G., & Coccia, V. (2020). Natural, bio-based, colored linoleum: Design, preparation, characteristics and preliminary life cycle assessment. *Journal of Cleaner Production, 267*, 122202. https://doi.org/10.1016/j.jclepro.2020.122202

Roufegarinejad, L., Dehghani, S., Bakhshi, S., Toker, O. S., Pirouzian, H. R., & Khiabani, A. H. (2024). Oleogelation of sunflower-linseed oils with carnauba wax as an innovative strategy for shortening substitution in cakes. *Food Chemistry, 437*, 137745. https://doi.org/10.1016/j.foodchem.2023.137745

Shahada, C., Morya, S., & Awuchi, C. G. (2024). A narrative review on nutraceutical, food and industrial applications of flaxseed (*Linum usitatissimum*. L). *Cogent Food & Agriculture, 10*(1), 2306017. https://doi.org/10.1080/23311932.2024.2306017

Sharma, S., Cheng, S.-F., Bhattacharya, B., & Chakkaravarthi, S. (2019). Efficacy of free and encapsulated natural antioxidants in oxidative stability of edible oil: Special emphasis on nanoemulsion-based encapsulation. *Trends in Food Science & Technology, 91*, 305–318. https://doi.org/10.1016/j.tifs.2019.07.030

Shanmugam, A., & Ashokkumar, M. (2015). Characterization of Ultrasonically Prepared Flaxseed oil Enriched Beverage/Carrot Juice Emulsions and Process-Induced Changes to the Functional

Properties of Carrot Juice Food and Bioprocess Technology, *8*(6), 1258–1266. https://doi.org/10.1007/s11947-015-1492-1

Shen, S., Gong, C., Jin, K., Zhou, L., Xiao, Y., & Ma, L. (2022). Omega-3 fatty acid supplementation and coronary heart disease risks: A meta-analysis of randomized controlled clinical trials. *Frontiers in Nutrition, 9*, 809311. https://doi.org/10.3389/fnut.2022.809311

Singh, P. K., Chopra, R., Garg, M., Chauhan, K., & Agarwal, A. (2024a). Stability of perilla seed oil based PUFA-rich structured lipids using enzymatic interesterification: A thermo-oxidative kinetic study. *Industrial Crops and Products, 209*, 118029. https://doi.org/10.1016/j.indcrop.2024.118029

Singh, N., Saluja, R. K., Rao, H. J., Kaushal, R., Gahlot, N. K., Suyambulingam, I., Sanjay, M. R., Divakaran, D., & Siengchin, S. (2024b). Progress and facts on biodiesel generations, production methods, influencing factors, and reactors: A comprehensive review from 2000 to 2023. *Energy Conversion and Management, 302*, 118157. https://doi.org/10.1016/j.enconman.2024.118157

Sriharikota, C. S., Karuppasamy, K., Nagarajan, V., Sathyamurthy, R., Ramani, B., Muthu, V., & Karuppiah, S. (2021). Experimental investigation of the emission and performance characteristics of a DI diesel engine fueled with the Vachellia nilotica seed oil methyl ester and diesel blends. *ACS Omega, 6*(22), 14068–14077. https://doi.org/10.1021/acsomega.1c00437

Stajić, S., Stanišić, N., Tomasevic, I., Djekic, I., Ivanović, N., & Živković, D. (2018). Use of linseed oil in improving the quality of chicken frankfurters. *Journal of Food Processing and Preservation, 42*(2), e13529. https://doi.org/10.1111/jfpp.13529

Su, R., Liu, X., Sun-Waterhouse, D., Wang, W., & Wang, Y. (2023). Enzymatic interesterification of palm stearin, flaxseed oil and cottonseed stearin to produce stable plastic fat with balanced omega-6 and omega-3 fatty acids. *Journal of Oleo Science, 72*(8), 799–810. https://doi.org/10.5650/jos.ess23034

Tamtaji, O. R., Milajerdi, A., Reiner, Ž., Dadgostar, E., Amirani, E., Asemi, Z., Mirsafaei, L., Mansournia, M. A., Dana, P. M., Sadoughi, F., & Hallajzadeh, J. (2020). Effects of flaxseed oil supplementation on biomarkers of inflammation and oxidative stress in patients with metabolic syndrome and related disorders: A systematic review and meta-analysis of randomized controlled trials. *Clinical Nutrition ESPEN, 40*, 27–33. https://doi.org/10.1016/j.clnesp.2020.09.017

Tasneem, R., Khan, H. M. S., Rasool, F., Khan, K.-U.-R., Umair, M., Esatbeyoglu, T., & Korma, S. A. (2022). Development of phytocosmeceutical microemulgel containing flaxseed extract and its in vitro and in vivo characterization. *Pharmaceutics, 14*(8), 1656. https://doi.org/10.3390/pharmaceutics14081656

Ursoniu, S., Sahebkar, A., Andrica, F., Serban, C., & Banach, M. (2016). Effects of flaxseed supplements on blood pressure: A systematic review and meta-analysis of controlled clinical trial. *Clinical Nutrition, 35*(3), 615–625. https://doi.org/10.1016/j.clnu.2015.05.012

Wirkowska-Wojdyła, M., Chmiel, M., Ostrowska-Ligęza, E., Górska, A., Bryś, J., Słowiński, M., & Czerniszewska, A. (2021). The influence of interesterification on the thermal and technological properties of milkfat-rapeseed oil mixture and its potential use in incorporation of model meat batters. *Applied Sciences, 11*(1), 1. https://doi.org/10.3390/app11010350

Woodfield, H. K., & Harwood, J. L. (2017). Oilseed crops: Linseed, rapeseed, soybean, and sunflower. In B. Thomas, B. G. Murray, D. J. Murphy (Eds.), *Encyclopedia of applied plant sciences* (2nd ed., pp. 34–38). Academic Press. https://doi.org/10.1016/B978-0-12-394807-6.00212-4

Yasmeen, M. Nisar, S. Tavallali, V. Khalid, T. (2018). A review of phytochemicals and uses of flaxseed. *Int. J. Chem. Biochem. Sci, 13*, 70–75.

Utilizing By-Products from the Linseed Processing Industry: Opportunities and Challenges

Binanshu Talwar, Rajni Chopra, and Neetu Kumra Taneja

Abstract

The linseed oil extraction industry generates significant by-products including oil cake, mucilage, and hulls each having its potential for valorization. Linseed oilcake is a by-product that consists of protein and fiber, making it a suitable raw material to be incorporated into different food formulations. However, various antinutrients in linseed oil cake such as cyanogenic glycosides and phytic acid pose challenges in its direct consumption. Various methods of removal of antinutrients include thermal treatments (boiling, steaming, and autoclaving) along with extrusion and enzymatic treatments. Innovative methods of detoxification include microbial fermentation, which enhances the nutritional quality and functional properties. Linseed mucilage is characterized by the polysaccharide composition, which offers various functional properties such as gelling, thickening, and emulsification, thereby being used as an additive in the food industry. Linseed hulls are another by-product that is rich in dietary fibers and lignans. These possess a potential application in developing functional foods. This chapter provides insights into the nutritional profile of by-products of the linseed oil extraction industry emphasizing the need for different detoxification methods. By effectively utilizing these by-products, sustainability can be enhanced contributing to the circular bioeconomy. This exploration emphasizes on the future of linseed by-products and its application to enhance it health benefits.

B. Talwar · R. Chopra
Department of Food Science and Technology, National Institute of Food Technology Entrepreneurship and Management, Kundli, Haryana, India

N. K. Taneja (✉)
Department of Interdisciplinary Science, National Institute of Food Technology Entrepreneurship and Management, Kundli, Haryana, India

© The Author(s), under exclusive license to Springer Nature Singapore Pte Ltd. 2025

R. Chopra et al. (eds.), *Dynamics of Linseed and its Valorization*,
https://doi.org/10.1007/978-981-96-8927-9_10

Keywords

By-product · Oilseed cake · Linseed · Omega-3

1 Introduction

India has been known to contribute 6.5% of the oilseeds produced worldwide. In India, oilseeds, which include nine annual crops including groundnut, soybean, rapeseed, linseed, sesame, sunflower, safflower mustard, and castor are cultivated in both the rainy (Kharif) and winter (rabi) seasons (Chauhan et al., 2021). After oil extraction, oilseed cake (OSC) is produced as a by-product. The production of oil-cake is believed to reach 386 million tonnes by the year 2025 (Kaur et al., 2021). OSC is known to be a rich source of protein, carbohydrates, various minerals, dietary fiber, and residual lipids. OSC has also found potential applications in developing functional and nutraceutical foods. Valorization of OSC for developing value-added products are now emerging owing to various bioactive components with health benefits (Kaur et al., 2021). The cake that is produced when oil is extracted using the cold press technique has significant concentrations of soluble fibers, protein, and lignans (Poreda, 2017). The quality of the cake is also defined by milling conditions such as relative temperature and humidity (Ogunronbi et al., 2011). Oil cakes contain proteins and other bioactive components, which makes the cake potential to be used for either food for humans or as animal feed (Zhang et al., 2023a, b).

Linseed *(Linum usitatissimum)*, an oilseed, is used to expel oil that contains PUFA (polyunsaturated fatty acid), MUFA (monounsaturated fatty acid), and SFA (saturated fatty acid). After the oil is expelled, a substantial volume of by-products, i.e., oil cake, is produced; disposing of these byproducts is troublesome because of associated negative environmental effects (Mannucci et al., 2019). Also, oilseed cakes of linseed, along with soybean, groundnut, rapeseed, and cottonseed, are primarily used as animal feed if not disposed of (Stodolak et al., 2017).

In the intricate world of different oilseed crops, the linseed plant emerges not only for its oil that is rich in omega 3 fatty acids but also for oil cake. The terms cake and meal are generally interchanged but are different based on the process by which these are produced. The term "cake" is used when oilseed is expelled by mechanical pressing without using heat like cold-press whereas the term "meal" is used when extraction is done using various organic solvents such as hexane (Woyengo et al., 2016). Linseed oil cake (LSC) is generally used for feed for the livestock of ruminants. It is also fed to alter the fatty acid composition of meat and egg products, which changes it profile (Oomah, 2020). The nutritional profile of LSC comprises protein, fiber, residual oil, and minerals, which makes it a potential raw material for different food products (Teh & Birch, 2014). However, LSC finds limited food application due to the antinutrients, which may bind with the minerals and decrease its bioavailability and protein digestibility (Imran et al., 2014). Antinutrients present in LSC are cyanogenic glycosides, phytic acid, and tannins. Cyanogenic glycoside being the major antinutrient gets converted into hydrogen cyanide (HCN) upon ingestion. Using several treatments, linseed oil cake can be detoxified and its nutritional content and market value increased (Bekhit et al., 2018). The LSC is considered to have higher digestibility when compared to whole seeds (Stodolak et al., 2017). Additionally, it is reported that antinutritional factors such as cyanogenic compounds contribute to the profile of linseed oil cake (Woyengo et al., 2017). This book chapter explores the by-products of the linseed oil industry, including their nutritional profile and the antinutrients present in LSC. It also discusses strategies to reduce these antinutrients and highlights the potential applications of LSC and other by products in the food industry.

2 By-Products of Linseed Processing

2.1 Linseed Oil Cake

Linseed oil cake comprises a high proportion of protein, fiber, antioxidants, and residual oil. Polyphenols, flavonoids, and antioxidants are among the several bioactive compounds found in LSC, which adds up to its rich nutritional profile (Kajla et al., 2017). Since LSC is rich in protein and carbohydrates, it exhibits different functional properties, namely, water-holding capacity, oil-holding capacity, emulsification capacity, and activity (Bekhit et al., 2013). However, the presence of antinutrients such as cyanogenic glucosides and phytic acid restricts the usage of LSC directly after oil extraction. These antinutrients can be removed partially or completely by subjecting LSC to different physical and biological methods, which include boiling, soaking, steaming, and fermentation (Safdar et al., 2020), (Zhai et al., 2019). Processed linseed oil cake (LSC) can be integrated into various food products, improving both their nutritional and functional properties (Bekhit et al., 2013). The geographical position of the crop's cultivation and seed processing determines the oil cake's composition (Russo & Reggiani, 2016). LSC has high-profile protein, residual oil, dietary fibers, and minerals, which are given in detail below. The subsequent section presents detailed nutritional and antinutritional characteristics of linseed oil cake.

2.2 Linseed Mucilage

The carbohydrate part of linseed comprises of both soluble and insoluble fiber. Mucilage is the soluble part, which is found in the outermost layer of the linseed hull. Once moisture is provided to the linseed, the mucilage, a thick viscous layer, leaches out. Mucilage accounts for 2–7.5% of the seed, which is the major part of the five distinctive layers of the linseed coat (Chand et al., 2024). Mucilage is obtained from aqueous extraction, which is a mixture of polysaccharides namely, xylose, and glucose, along with galactose, arabinose, rhamnose, fucose, and galacturonic acid, 75% of which is neutral whereas there are two acid fractions.

Galacto-arabino-xylan is the neutral fraction which is of high molecular weight while the acid fraction is rhamno-galacturan. Mucilage, which is obtained from linseed cake, shows similar emulsifying properties to gum arabic and guar gum in terms of water-binding capacity (Gutiérrez et al., 2010), (Coşkuner & Karababa, 2007). The insoluble part is made up of cellulose and lignin, which are non-starch polysaccharides. Linseed mucilage has xylose as its major component followed by galacturonic acid, rhamnose, arabinose, galactose, and then glucose. Mucilage has two acidic fractions: acidic fraction 1 and acidic fraction 2. Rhamnose, fucose, galactose, and galacturonic acid make up the acidic part whereas xylose, arabinose, and galactose make the neutral part of mucilage (Chand et al., 2024).

2.3 Linseed Hulls

Linseed hull is a coproduct of linseed processing that is rich in hulls and consequently in (+)-secoisolariciresinol (SECO). Lignans and phenolic compounds make up the major profile of linseed hulls (Christophe Hano et al., 2012). Oil extracted from linseed hull yields approximately 18.2% oil with a profile made up of 92.5% neutral lipids and a small quantity of free fatty acids (2.1%) along with phospholipids (3.1%) and acidic lipids (2.4%) (Oomah, 2020).

3 Chemical Composition of By-Products of Linseed Oilcake and Linseed Mucilage

3.1 Protein

Linseed cake, the major residue left after oil extraction industry, has the major protein (Oomah, 2001). LSC contains approximately 36% protein of which 85% is known to be digestible (Singh et al., 2022). The globulin content in linseed is high, i.e., 18.6% and 17.7% of a protein, which is similar to albumin. The linseed proteins comprise arginine, aspartic acid, and glutamic acid whereas lysine, methionine, and cysteine are limiting amino acid (Chung et al., 2005). The protein present in linseed is divided into two fractions, namely, high molecular and low molecular fraction based on the size exclusion chromatography named as linin and conlinin, respectively. These are made up of five (bonded by either hydrophobic, hydrogen, or electrostatic bonds) and single polypeptide subunits, respectively (Waszkowiak & Mikołajczak, 2020), (Bekhit et al., 2018). Linin is a high molecular weight fraction that makes up to 64–66% of total linseed protein. The linin protein is made up of 17% nitrogen and the range of its molecular weight is estimated to be 252–298 kDa. Colinin is a low molecular fraction of protein, which makes up 42% of total linseed protein with a molecular weight of 16–7 kDa (Bekhit et al., 2018). Two types of storage proteins are also present, which are either salt or water-soluble (Mueller et al., 2010). The amino acids that make up the linseed proteins are lysine, leucine, arginine, aspartic acid, and glutamic acid (Bekhit et al., 2013).

3.2 Lipids

Linseed oil comprises low concentrations of saturated, moderate concentrations of monounsaturated, and high concentrations of polyunsaturated fatty acids. Also, linseed oil has approximately 58% of linolenic acid (Gutte et al., 2015). Linseed oil is recognized as one of the richest sources of omega-3 fatty acids, ALA (alpha-linolenic acid). LSC contains 7–10% residual oil, which further depends upon the type of extraction method used (Singh et al., 2022).

3.3 Fiber

Linseed cake is not only a protein-rich, by-product by also a source of fiber fractions that are water soluble and have high lignin content (Oomah & Mazza, 1993), (Hyvärinen et al., 2006). It is speculated that lignans, in particular secoisolariciresinol diglucoside (SDG), might effectively lower the risk of cardiovascular conditions and may also effectively prevent the onset of diabetes (Westcott & Muir, 2003). LSC contains insoluble dietary fibers, which include lignin, cellulose, and hemicellulose (Basiri et al., 2018).

3.4 Polyphenols

Polyphenols are found in the vacuoles, lipoprotein bilayers, lignins, hull, and cell wall (Gutiérrez et al., 2010). Various polyphenols present in LSC are chlorogenic acid, ferulic acid, coumaric acid, and p-hydroxybenzoic acid. Other minor phenolic acids are cinnamic acid, caffeic acid, hydrocinnamic acid glucosides, and 4-hydroxybenzoic acid (Ganorkar et al., 2016), (Teh & Birch, 2014). These polyphenols can be extracted from LSC by using different extraction methods, which define the efficiency as well as the concentration of the extract (Sanmartin et al., 2020). The significant quantity of phenolics found in LSC allows it to have antioxidant potential (Hao et al., 2020). Free phenolics present in LSC (defatted) are 784.78 mg/g whereas esterified phenolics are 1522.69 mg/g (Özkaynak Kanmaz, 2017).

3.5 Flavonoids

Plant phenolics are classified as flavonoids which are made up of two aromatic rings joined in a heterocyclic configuration by a three-carbon bridge (Oomah et al., 1996a, b). The flavonoid content is found to be higher in pressed cakes when compared to the solvent-extracted meals. Flavonoids are polar in nature, due to which they are retained in oilcake (Sanmartin et al., 2020). These flavonoids include flavanols, flavones, and flavanones. These substances function as potent reactive species scavengers and signaling molecules as barriers against infections. The flavonoid content

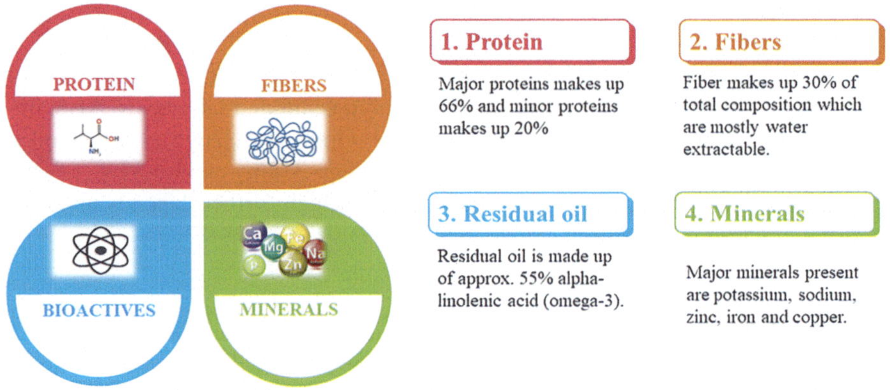

Fig. 1 Nutritional profile of linseed oil cake

gets concentrated in the cake. The methanolic extract of linseed contains 1.7 mg/g of flavonoid whereas linseed cake accounts for 2.8 mg/g (Quezada & Cherian, 2012).

3.6 Lignans

Lignans, which are phytoestrogens, are minor components responsible for plant cell development. They consist of two phenylpropane units (Prasad, 1997). The major polyphenols present in defatted linseed meal are lignans (Teh & Birch, 2014). Lignans are made up of monomeric units SDG (secoisolariciresinol diglucoside), which possess biological activity. In LSC, lignans occur as oligomers which are formed through ester links between 3-hydroxy-3-methylglutaric acid (HMGA) and glycosidic bonds with phenolic compounds (Tavarini et al., 2021). Linseed as well as LSC are known to be a rich plant source of SDG (Rudra et al., 2021). Lignans exhibit various health-promoting properties, such as anticarcinogenic and antioxidant effects. Lignans possess antioxidant properties by scavenging the free radicals (Prasad, 1997). Figure 1 depicts the nutritional profile of linseed oil cake. The chemical composition of linseed oil cake is tabulated in Table 1.

4 Antinutrients in Linseed Oil Cake

4.1 Cyanogenic Glycosides (CGs)

Cyanogenic compounds are nitrogen-containing secondary metabolites found in plants that come from the amino acids valine and isoleucine, which can cause chronic effects if consumed in large amounts. Cyanogenic glycosides are known to be made up of a sugar component and α-hydroxy nitrile-type aglycon. The major antinutrient present in linseed are CGs. A toxic compound, HCN, is formed when

Table 1 Chemical composition of linseed oil cake

S.No.	Component	Concentration %	References
1.	Carbohydrate	34–40	Singh et al. (2011)
2	Protein	32.2–35.9	Gutiérrez et al. (2010), Ogunronbi et al. (2011), Tirgar et al. (2017), and Zamindar et al. (2017)
3	Fat	11.5–21.4	Gutiérrez et al. (2010), Ogunronbi et al. (2011), and Hady and Elsorady (2020)
4	Ash	4.9–5.9	Gutiérrez et al. (2010), Ogunronbi et al. (2011), and Tirgar et al. (2017)
5	Fiber	10–35	Gutiérrez et al. (2010), Ogunronbi et al. (2011), and Ganorkar et al. (2016)
6	Moisture	6–10	Gutiérrez et al. (2010), and Tirgar et al. (2017)

cyanogenic glycosides are ingested by humans (Russo & Reggiani, 2014). When CGs are ingested, the intestinal β-glucosidase activity causes cyanogenic glycosides to release HCN, which is known to harm the neurological, endocrine, and respiratory systems (Zhai et al., 2019). The advantages of linseed are hindered by the presence of cyanogenic glycosides, which are concentrated in the meal after the oil is extracted (Bekhit et al., 2018). The binding of CGs with different minerals, such as iron and manganese, causes hindrances in their availability for human body (Imran et al., 2013).

4.2 Phytic Acid

Phytic acid, an organic phosphate that is the calcium-magnesium salt of myoinositol, is known to be the primary form of storing phosphorus in plants (Ali et al., 2010). An insoluble complex is formed by phytic acid with metals such as iron, magnesium, copper, and calcium (Zhang et al., 2023a, b). Due to the formation of these complexes, bioavailability of these metals is hindered in the human body. 70% of the total phosphorus is found to be in the form of phytic acid (Oomah et al. 1996a, b). In addition to minerals, phytic acid may interact with proteins and carbohydrates, potentially decreasing the solubility and digestibility (Salem, 2020).

4.3 Tannins

Tannins are found in vacuoles that can bind with proteins to form either soluble or insoluble tannin-protein complexes, which are water-soluble. Tannins are categorized into two types, namely, condensed and hydrolyzable tannins. Tannins are one of the compounds in linseed, which leads to its limited use. These compounds hinder the bioavailability of micronutrients and protein digestibility (Imran et al., 2014).

5 Approaches to Reduce Antinutrients in Linseed Oil Cake and Enhancing Nutritional Profile

It is experimentally shown that to produce LSC fit for human consumption, the antinutrients present must be removed by appropriate processing procedures (Bekhit et al., 2018). Several methods, which include microwave heating, boiling, steaming, enzymatic treatment, and fermentation, can be used to eliminate these chemical components (Russo & Reggiani, 2014). Table 2 includes the studies of processing methods used to decrease antinutrients and enhance nutritional values. Heating methods such as roasting, boiling, and microwave treatments reduces the antinutritional factors as well as nutritional values of oil cakes (Xu et al., 2022). In oilcakes such as soybean, canola, and cottonseed, high temperature-short time combination by extrusion has been applied to reduce antinutrients (Imran et al., 2013).

Fermentation has been known to be a biotechnological approach that can be applied to reduce antinutritional content and enhance the nutritional profile (Zhai et al., 2019). Oilseed cake can be processed by using solid-state fermentation (SSF), which is a biotechnological process where microorganisms, a solid substrate with no free liquid, are used as a substrate (Pandey et al., 2016). During the SSF process, complex molecules, such as fibers and lignocellulose, are converted to simple molecules. This conversion leads to the release of nutrients (Shrestha et al., 2008). The steps of SSF initiate with choosing the substrate and pretreating the substrate by

Table 2 Processing methods to decrease antinutrients in linseed cake

Processing methods	Treatment	Findings	References
Physical treatment	Heating at 90 °C for an hour	Reduction of HCN (94.05%) due to deactivation of glycoside due to hydrolysis	Safdar et al. (2020)
	Boiling for up to 30 min	HCN removal (48.2%) was observed	
	Soaking for up to 48 h	62.6% HCN reduction	
Fermentation	Inoculum used—*Aspergillus niger* and *Candida utilis* for 72 h	60 h of fermentation decreased 73.35% HCN content by 73.35%	Zhai et al. (2019)
Enzyme treatment	Enzymatic treatment with 0.1 M sodium citrate	Complete removal of cyanogenic compounds	Yamashita et al. (2007)
Extrusion	Extrusion at 80^0 C at 40% moisture	Up to 61.27% tannin reduction	Mukhopadhyay et al. (2007)
Solvent treatment	Multistage extraction using methanol-ammonia-water hexane solvent	Up to 90% removal of CG. Methanol was found to be the optimal solvent for removal of CGs. Linustatin and neolinustatin were observed to be removed up to 80%	Wanasundara et al. (1993)

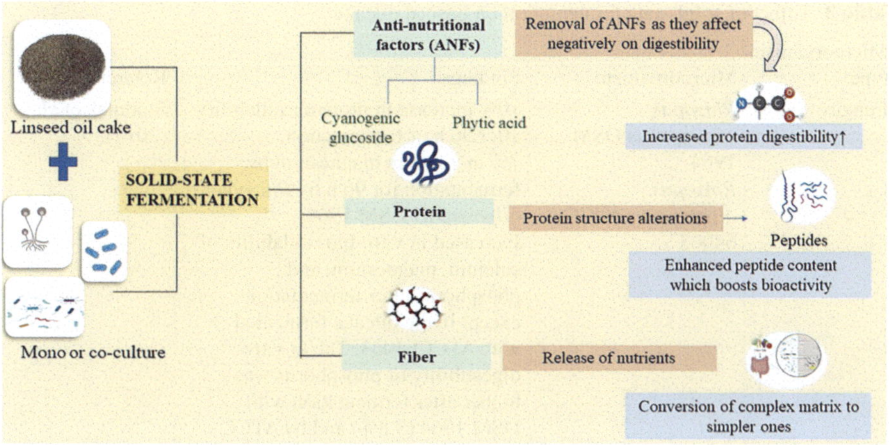

Fig. 2 Effect of solid-state fermentation on various components of linseed oil cake

chemical, mechanical, or any biochemical method to micronize the particle size, which also improves nutrient availability. This process is followed by fermentation and then downstream processes used to purify and measure the end products (Sadh et al., 2018a, b). Figure 2 depicts the alterations in different components of linseed oil cake.

SSF can be done using a single type (monoculture) of microorganism as well as consortia (co-culture) (Sadh et al., 2018a). The yield of metabolite is affected by some factors, which include inoculum size, inoculum type, incubation temperature and time, moisture content, aeration, and agitation (Nema et al., 2019; Lonsane et al., 1985, and Yadav, 1988). Table 3 includes the studies that include SSF of linseed oil cake.

6 Functional Properties

Given the increasing cost of animal proteins and their limited supply, research on the nutritional properties and other aspects of protein from low-cost, underutilized oilseeds and legumes (high-protein) has taken importance. Flours, which are protein-rich, derived from distinct sources must exhibit the necessary properties to interact with different food ingredients to make it easier to incorporate them into different food matrix (Khattab & Arntfield, 2009). The solubility of nitrogen in different proteins acts as an indicator of the functional properties. The functional qualities of the meal are majorly impacted by the different solvents employed to extract it. In a study, the hexane-extracted meal exhibited a 9.7-fold increase in water adsorption compared to its weight. Additionally, it was shown that meals extracted using methanol, ammonia, and water enhanced the ability of the meal to adsorb fat by 3.2 times, whereas meals removed using hexane absorbed soybean oil 2.6 times greater than their initial weight (Wanasundara & Shahidi, 1994). Water holding

Table 3 Effect of solid-state fermentation on linseed oilcake

Microorganism type	Microorganism	Findings	References
Fungus	*Rhizopus oligosporus* DSM 1964 *Rhizopus oligosporus* ATCC 64063	10% increase in protein availability after 96 h of fermentation 7% increase in magnesium by fermentation for 96 h by *Rhizopus oligosporus* DSM 1964 Increased in vitro bioavailability of calcium, magnesium, and phosphorus after fermentation except in the oilcake fermented with ATCC64063. The in vitro digestibility of phosphorus was higher after fermentation with DSM 1964 (3.8%) and by ATCC 64063 (1.6%)	Stodolak et al. (2017)
Fungi and bacteria	*Rhizopus oligosporus: Lactobacillus plantarum*	Increase in antioxidant potential of grass pea tempeh (with added LSC) by 67% and 87% due to addition of seed oil cake (by 10% and 20%, respectively)	Tempe and Starzy (2020)
Mold	*Aspergillus oryzae* (koji mold*): Neurospora intermedia (*oncom mold*)*	Up to 92% increase in antiradical activity and 71% increase in radical scavenging activity of oil cake fermented by *Aspergillus oryzae.* Up to 42% increase in protein digestibility of fermented oil cake. Protein digestibility increased by 47% of oil cake fermented by *N. intermedia.* Cheese paste incorporated with LSC had 41% increase in digestibility	Stodolak et al. (2020)
Fungi	*Penicillium camemberti, Geotrichum candidum*, Lactic acid bacteria	Excellent survivability of consortium of fungus-bacteria combination. Development of cheese analogue with higher total phenols, flavonoids, and antioxidant activities	Łopusiewicz, Drozłowska, Tarnowiecka-Kuca, et al. (2020b)
Fungi	*Rhizopus oligosporus tempeh mold (DSM 1964): Rhizopus oligosporus (ATCC 64063)*	Increase in phenolics and protein by 18 and 9%, respectively	Stodolak et al. (2017)
Fungi	*Mortierella alpina* Peyronel (MUM 9412)	Lipids content increased by 49.9%. Particularly, PUFA content increased by 32.8%. Synthesis of gamma-linolenic acid and docosahexaenoic acid by SSF	Ferreira et al. (2020)

capacity depends upon the plant variety, cultivation geography, and temperature along with the extraction method whereas oil holding capacity depends on hydrophilic and hydrophobic bonds. Bulk density is influenced by intermolecular forces, which play a critical role in determining the physical properties of materials and, consequently, impact the development of innovative products. The quantity and type of soluble proteins affect the foaming capacity. Compared to soybean and mustard oil cake, linseed cake has a moderate foaming capacity. Linseed oil cake showed the highest emulsion capacity when compared to soybean and mustard oil cake (Bárta et al., 2021), (Bekhit et al., 2013). Different processing methods, such as microwaves, heat treatment, fermentation, and solvent treatment affect the functional properties. Also, defatting of oil cake increases the water due to the availability of hydrophilic components (Safdar et al., 2020).

7 Utilization of Linseed By-Products

7.1 Linseed Oil Cake

Given the growing awareness regarding health issues, the demand for nutraceuticals has been increased. Along with this, an inclination toward plant-based foods has also been observed. The fact is that plant-based foods are rich in antioxidants, vitamins, fibers, and minerals is well known. Due to the rich nutrient profile and different functional properties of linseed oil cake, it can be utilized as a raw material to be incorporated to develop different functional food products (Łopusiewicz et al., 2020a, b). Antinutrients like cyanogenic glucosides, phytic acid, and tannins should be considered. However, there are several ways to remove them. Linseed oil cake can be used to develop into various products, for innovation in bakery items, beverages, and extruded products.

- *Bread:* Linseed oil cake incorporated bread was developed. The incorporation levels were 0–10%. Bread with no linseed oil cake served as control. The major findings included an increase in α-linolenic acid, total phenols, and flavonoids with increasing levels of LSC. A significant increase in free fatty acid and α-linolenic was observed on increase in LSC, whereas an inverse relationship between n-6/n-3 ratio was observed (Taglieri et al., 2020).
- *Bread (incorporated with LSC extract):* Gluten-free bread was developed by replacing 100% water with LSC extract. Increase in SDG from undetectable to 526 μg/100 g as water was replaced by SDG extract. Textural changes were noted in the gluten-free bread, as incorporation decreased the softness due to the presence of mucilage and gums in the LSC extract. The bread made with 50% replacement was found to be comparable to the control bread (Łopusiewicz et al., 2023).
- *Pita bread:* Functional bread was made using LSC and incorporation levels were from 5% to 20%. Major findings include an increase in protein (40%), fibers (6%), and ash (8.63%) in the bread incorporated with LSC. A significant increase

in the various minerals, namely, phosphorus (21%), magnesium (48%), and potassium (29%) was also noted. A twofold increase in calcium content was observed on incorporation of LSC in pita bread (Khattab et al., 2012).

- *Toast:* Development of toast by incorporation of LSC from levels 5–15%. The mineral content in toast with a 5% substitution of linseed cake showed significant increases: potassium by 30%, magnesium by 27%, phosphorus by 14%, and calcium by 21%. This enhancement suggests that linseed cake can be a valuable ingredient for boosting the nutritional profile of bakery products (Hamid Selim et al., 2019).
- *Puff:* Puffs were developed by incorporating linseed cake at levels ranging from 7% to 20%. The addition of linseed cake not only enhanced the nutritional value of the puffs but also imparted a unique flavor and texture. This demonstrates the potential of linseed cake as a versatile ingredient in snack food production. The inclusion of linseed cake at concentrations between 7.5% and 20% resulted in increased breaking strength. The fiber in defatted linseed cake contributes to structural integrity through its interaction with proteins, thereby significantly increasing breaking strength. As the percentage of defatted linseed cake increased, there was a decrease in the expansion ratio and overall acceptability, attributed to the accumulation of protein molecules (Ganorkar et al., 2016).
- *Corn puffs:* Corn puffs enriched with linseed oil cake were developed, resulting in final products with lignan content ranging from 0% to 15%. However, the extrusion process caused a decrease in lignan content, ranging from 25% to 52%. It was also observed that an increased level of substitution led to the development of dark-colored products with harder textures (Puff et al., 2006).
- *Grass-pea tempeh:* Tempeh, a solid-state fermentation of soybeans originated in Indonesia, which is a popular technique for processing legumes. Tempeh products have interesting organoleptic properties and a high nutritional value. Grass-pea tempeh was developed by the inclusion of LSC ranging from 5% to 35%. The fat level was found to be three times higher with 35% linseed cake substitution.
- *Yogurt-like plant milk:* By heating LSC followed by fermentation using a commercial starting culture, yogurt-like plant milk was developed. The chemical composition was altered with respect to the levels of incorporation as well as days of storage. An increase in linseed cake content increased in total phenolics and flavonoid content of the final product. High antioxidant levels were exhibited by yogurt-like plant milk made using LSC (Łopusiewicz et al., 2020a, b). Figure 3 depicts the by-products of linseed oil industry, antinutrients, and application in food industry.

7.2 Linseed Mucilage (LM)

Linseed mucilage has such chemical composition and features that it acts as an excellent fat replacer and exhibits gelling and thickening properties. It also exhibits emulsifying and binding properties. Along with this, LM is a potential antioxidant

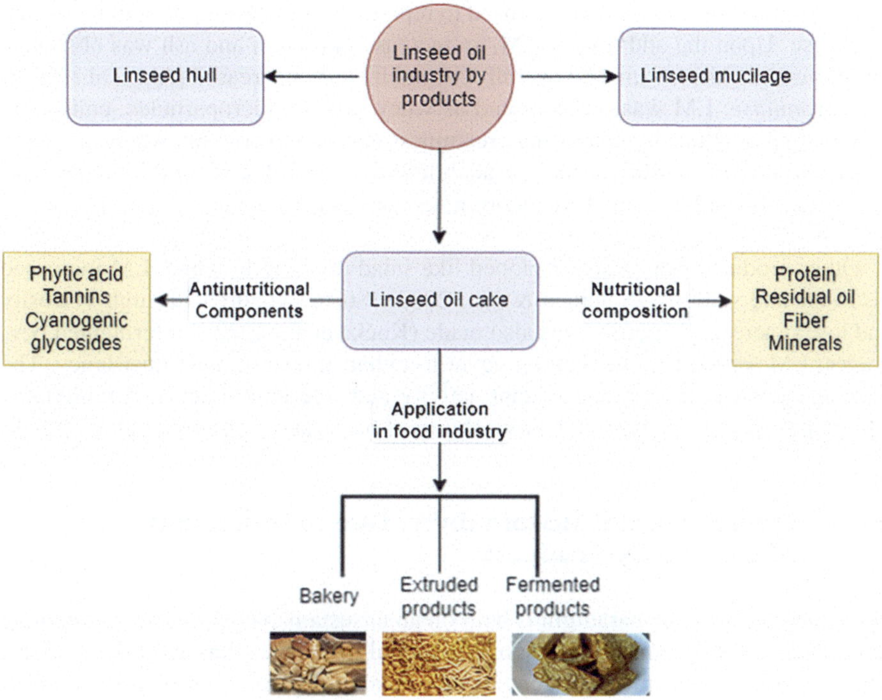

Fig. 3 Linseed by-products—nutritional aspects, antinutrients, and applications

and possesses bioactive compounds. LM is considered as a hydrocolloid, which is known to enhance the strength of materials, as it contains the ability to retain water due to cross-linking, which leads to the formation of consistent emulsion and high viscosity (25,159). The gelling strength of LM is affected by various physical factors such as temperature, Ph, and salt concentration. LM can be incorporated in various food products to enhance their nutritional and functional properties.

- *Gluten-free bread*: LM was used in developing gluten-free bread to assess and study the effect of LM on rheological characteristics; minor impact on the texture and crumb of the bread was found. The sensory acceptance was enhanced by the addition of 1.8 and 2.4% of LM to bread (Korus et al., 2015).
- *Cookies*: LM was used as a butter replacer in cookies to develop low-calorie cookies. When LM was added, it increased the antioxidant capacity and overall acceptability (30%). The cookies incorporated with 20% LM contained the lowest fat. Low-calorie cake was made by substituting butter with LM and the major findings indicated that the substitution of LM up to 60% was best in terms of sensorial, textural, and nutritional values. Also, a decrease in elasticity, specific volume, and hardness was observed (Mohtarami et al., 2022).

- *Fat-free cream cheese:* LM was used to replace fat and develop functional cream cheese. Upon the addition of LM, an increase in protein and ash was observed. Along with this, texture and overall acceptability also increased (Akl et al., 2020).
- *Mayonnaise*: LM was incorporated as whey protein microparticles, enhancing sensorial qualities by increasing creaminess and mouth coating, whereas factors such as fluidity, hardness, and spreadability decreased. The shear thinning behavior was shown by all the LM-incorporated products (Yang et al., 2023).

Other products were also developed like salad dressing in which LM increased viscosity and stability (Smetana & Jan, 2022). Stirred yogurt with high viscosity and low syneresis properties was also made (Kučka et al., 2022). In fermented beverages, LM served as a thickening agent to enhance texture and consistency. The beverage possessed high antioxidant activity and free amino acids. Additionally, LM enhanced the viscosity and survivability of bacteria (Łopusiewicz et al., 2019).

8 Environmental Sustainability Due to Utilization of Linseed By-Products

The existing economic paradigm is built on an unsustainable approach. An increase in human activity produces postindustrial global challenges that harm the ecology. These issues include mismanagement of available resources, overexploitation of natural resources, and unsustainable consumption practices. Adopting a circular economy approach by eliminating waste across the supply chain is crucial for sustainability and resource efficiency. Recycling and recirculating waste during processing to create a concept of using it is important (Borrello et al., 2017) (Pesce et al., 2020). According to FAO, one-third of the total food production is lost (20% from oilseed). It is estimated that food waste generates 8% of total greenhouse gas emissions, which then adds to increased environmental temperature globally (Vilariño et al., 2017). A solution to decrease the waste is processing the waste in such a way that bioactive molecules are extracted from the by-products (Ancuţa & Sonia, 2020). A holistic approach can be followed to strategically utilize LSC in the circular economy framework. This might include using a variety of processes and repurposing the oil cake into food items, which would not only reduce waste but also improve resource efficiency. The application of circular economy in the linseed oil extraction industry depicts the integration of environmental management, economic viability, and innovation, emphasizing the potential for sustainable development with little environmental impact.

9 Challenges and Future Trends

The use of by-products from the linseed oil industry faces various challenges. First is the variability in the composition of LSC, which complicates the standardization process. Second is the presence of antinutrients present, which necessitates effective detoxification strategies to ensure safety for consumption. Additionally, high fiber content limits its direct use in food industries. Overcoming the challenges associated with linseed oil by-product utilization requires a multifaceted approach. Advances in biotechnological techniques such as microbial fermentation and enzymatic treatments offer promising avenues for enhancing nutritional profile and functional properties.

By addressing such challenges, significant economic and environmental benefits can be unlocked by transforming its by-products from waste to wealth, contributing to a more sustainable and efficient use of by-products.

10 Conclusion

In conclusion, using linseed oil industry by-products such as linseed oil cake, linseed hulls, and mucilage gives substantial opportunities for augmenting the nutritional profile of food products while advancing sustainable practices. The rich nutritional profile of these by-products renders valuable components to the human diet. Nevertheless, the presence of antinutrients necessitates effective removal strategies to ensure safety and optimize maximum nutritional benefits. Different processing methodologies, such as thermal treatments, fermentation, and enzymatic interventions, have shown efficacy in mitigating antinutrient levels. The incorporation of these by-products facilitates the development of innovative functional foods. The potential application of linseed oil cake lies in bakery and extruded products, whereas mucilage finds its uses as a thickening and stabilizing agent. The linseed oil industry can significantly contribute to advancing food innovation and fostering a sustainable system. As research and development continue to the progress, the full potential of linseed by-products in food industry will be actualized, which can promote healthier diets and environmental sustainability.

References

Akl, E. M., Abdelhamid, S. M., Wagdy, S. M., & Salama, H. H. (2020). Manufacture of functional fat-free cream cheese fortified with probiotic bacteria and flaxseed mucilage as a fat replacing agent. *Current Nutrition & Food Science, 16*(9), 1393–1403.

Ali, F., Ippersiel, D., Lamarche, F., & Mondor, M. (2010). Characterization of low-phytate soy protein isolates produced by membrane technologies. *Innovative Food Science and Emerging Technologies, 11*(1), 162–168. https://doi.org/10.1016/j.ifset.2009.08.004

Ancuţa, P., & Sonia, A. (2020). Oil press-cakes and meals valorization through circular economy approaches: A review. *Applied Sciences (Switzerland), 10*(21), 1–31. https://doi.org/10.3390/app10217432

Bárta, J., Bártová, V., Jarošová, M., Švajner, J., Smetana, P., Kadlec, J., Filip, V., Kyselka, J., Berčíková, M., Zdráhal, Z., Bjelková, M., & Kozak, M. (2021). Oilseed cake flour composition, functional properties and antioxidant potential as effects of sieving and species differences. *Food, 10*(11), 1–17. https://doi.org/10.3390/foods10112766

Basiri, S., Haidary, N., Shekarforoush, S. S., & Niakousari, M. (2018). Flaxseed mucilage: A natural stabilizer in stirred yogurt. *Carbohydrate Polymers, 187*(January), 59–65. https://doi.org/10.1016/j.carbpol.2018.01.049

Bekhit, S. T. A. E., Carne, A., & Birch, J. (2013). Effect of the defatting process, acid and alkali extraction on the physicochemical and functional properties of hemp, flax and canola seed cake protein isolates. *Journal of Food Measurement and Characterization, 8*, 92–104. https://doi.org/10.1007/s11694-013-9168-x

Bekhit, A. E. D. A., Shavandi, A., Jodjaja, T., Birch, J., Teh, S., Mohamed Ahmed, I. A., Al-Juhaimi, F. Y., Saeedi, P., & Bekhit, A. A. (2018). Flaxseed: Composition, detoxification, utilization, and opportunities. *Biocatalysis and Agricultural Biotechnology, 13*(December 2017), 129–152. https://doi.org/10.1016/j.bcab.2017.11.017

Borrello, M., Caracciolo, F., Lombardi, A., Pascucci, S., & Cembalo, L. (2017). Consumers' perspective on circular economy strategy for reducing food waste. *Sustainability (Switzerland), 9*(1), 141. https://doi.org/10.3390/su9010141

Chand, M., Chopra, R., Talwar, B., Homroy, S., Singh, P. K., Dhiman, A., & Payyunni, A. W. (2024). Unveiling the potential of linseed mucilage, its health benefits, and applications in food packaging. *Frontiers in Nutrition, 11*(February), 1–20. https://doi.org/10.3389/fnut.2024.1334247

Chauhan, J. S., Choudhary, P. R., & Singh, K. (2021). Oilseeds: Current scenario and future prospects. *Journal of Oilseeds Research, 38*(1).

Christophe Hano, A., Corbin, C., Drouet, S., Quéro, A., Rombaut, N., Savoire, R., Molinié, R., Thomasset, B., Mesnard, F., & Lainé, E. (2012). The lignan (+)-secoisolariciresinol extracted from flax hulls is an effective protectant of linseed oil and its emulsion against oxidative damage. *European Journal of Lipid Science and Technology, 119*(8), 1–31.

Chung, M. W. Y., Lei, B., & Li-Chan, E. C. Y. (2005). Isolation and structural characterization of the major protein fraction from NorMan flaxseed (Linum usitatissimum L.). *Food Chemistry, 90*(1–2), 271–279. https://doi.org/10.1016/j.foodchem.2003.07.038

Coşkuner, Y., & Karababa, E. (2007). Some physical properties of flaxseed (Linum usitatissimum L.). *Journal of Food Engineering, 78*(3), 1067–1073. https://doi.org/10.1016/j.jfoodeng.2005.12.017

Ferreira, M., Fernandes, H., Peres, H., Oliva-teles, A., Belo, I., & Salgado, M. (2020, May). Bio-enrichment of oilseed cakes by Mortierella alpina under solid-state fermentation. *LWT, 134*, 109981. https://doi.org/10.1016/j.lwt.2020.109981

Ganorkar, P. M., Patel, J. M., Shah, V., & Rangrej, V. V. (2016). Defatted flaxseed meal incorporated corn-rice flour blend based extruded product by response surface methodology. *Journal of Food Science and Technology, 53*(April), 1867–1877. https://doi.org/10.1007/s13197-015-2134-3

Gutiérrez, C., Rubilar, M., Jara, C., Verdugo, M., Sineiro, J., & Shene, C. (2010). Flaxseed and flaxseed cake as a source of compounds for food industry. *Journal of Soil Science and Plant Nutrition, 10*(4), 454–463. https://doi.org/10.4067/S0718-95162010000200006

Gutte, K. B., Sahoo, A. K., & Ranveer, R. C. (2015). Effect of ultrasonic treatment on extraction and fatty acid profile of flaxseed oil. *OCL – Oilseeds and Fats, 22*(6), D606. https://doi.org/10.1051/ocl/2015038

Hady, M. A. M. A.-E., & Elsorady, M. E. I. (2020). Effect of sprouting on chemical, fatty acid composition, antioxidants and Antinutrients of flaxseeds. *Asian Food Science Journal, 19*(1), 40–51. https://doi.org/10.9734/afsj/2020/v19i130231

Hamid Selim, K. A., Kamal Mostafa, M., Tawab Mahmoud, A. A., & Afifi Ali, R. (2019). Effect of bioactive compounds of defatted flaxseed meal on rheological and sensorial properties of toast and cake. *SDRP Journal of Food Science & Technology, 4*(4), 707–719. https://doi.org/10.25177/jfst.4.4.ra.479

Hao, X. Y., Yu, S. C., Mu, C. T., Wu, X. D., Zhang, C. X., Zhao, J. X., & Zhang, J. X. (2020). Replacing soybean meal with flax seed meal: Effects on nutrient digestibility, rumen microbial protein synthesis and growth performance in sheep. *Animal, 14*(9), 1841–1848. https://doi.org/10.1017/S1751731120000397

Hyvärinen, H., Pihlava, J.-M., Hiidenhovi, J., Hietaniemi, V., Korhonen, H. J. T., Ryhänen, E.-L. (2006). Effect of processing and storage on the stability of flaxseed lignan added to bakery products. *J. Agric. Food Chem, 54*, 48–53.

Imran, M., Anjum, F. M., Butt, M. S., Siddiq, M., & Sheikh, M. A. (2013). Reduction of cyanogenic compounds in flaxseed (Linum usitatissimum L.) meal using thermal treatment. *International Journal of Food Properties, 16*(8), 1809–1818. https://doi.org/10.1080/10942912.2011.608914

Imran, M., Anjum, F. M., Butt, M. S., & Sheikh, M. A. (2014). Influence of extrusion processing on tannin reduction and oil loss in flaxseed (Linum Usitatissimum L.) Meal. *Journal of Food Processing and Preservation, 38*(1), 622–629. https://doi.org/10.1111/jfpp.12012

Kajla, P. S., Sharma, A., & Sood, D. R. (2017). Effect of germination on proximate principles, minerals and antinutrients of flaxseeds. *Asian Journal of Dairy and Food Research, 36*(1), 52–57. https://doi.org/10.18805/ajdfr.v36i01.7459

Kaur, M., Singh, B., Kaur, A., & Singh, N. (2021). Proximate, mineral, amino acid composition, phenolic profile, antioxidant and functional properties of oilseed cakes. *International Journal of Food Science and Technology, 56*(12), 6732–6741. https://doi.org/10.1111/ijfs.15386

Khattab, R. Y., & Arntfield, S. D. (2009). Functional properties of raw and processed canola meal. *Lwt, 42*(6), 1119–1124. https://doi.org/10.1016/j.lwt.2009.02.009

Khattab, R., Zeitoun, M., & Barbary, O. M. (2012). Evaluation of Pita bread fortified with defatted flaxseed flour. *Current Nutrition & Food Science, 8*(2), 91–101.

Korus, J., Witczak, T., Ziobro, R., & Juszczak, L. (2015). Linseed (Linum usitatissimum L.) mucilage as a novel structure forming agent in gluten-free bread. *Lwt, 62*(1), 257–264. https://doi.org/10.1016/j.lwt.2015.01.040

Kučka, M., Ražná, K., Harenčár, Ľ., & Kolarovičová, T. (2022). Plant seed mucilage—Great potential for sticky matter. *Nutraceuticals, 2*(4), 253–269. https://doi.org/10.3390/nutraceuticals2040019

Lonsane, B. K., Ghildyal, N. P., Budiatman, S., & Ramakrishna, S. V. (1985). Engineering aspects of solid state fermentation. *Enzyme and Microbial Technology, 7*(6), 258–265. https://doi.org/10.1016/0141-0229(85)90083-3

Łopusiewicz, Ł., Drozłowska, E., Siedlecka, P., Bartkowiak, A., & Sienkiewicz, M. Z. (2019). Non-dairy kefir-like fermented beverage based on flaxseed oil cake. *Foods, 8*(11), 544.

Łopusiewicz, Ł., Drozłowska, E., Siedlecka, P., Mężyńska, M., & Bartkowiak, A. (2020a). Preparation and characterization of novel flaxseed oil cake yogurt-like plant milk fortified with inulin. *Journal of Food and Nutrition Research, 59*(1), 61–70.

Łopusiewicz, Ł., Drozłowska, E., Tarnowiecka-Kuca, A., Bartkowiak, A., Mazurkiewicz-Zapałowicz, K., & Salachna, P. (2020b). Biotransformation of flaxseed oil cake into bioactive camembert-analogue using lactic acid bacteria, penicillium camemberti and geotrichum candidum. *Microorganisms, 8*(9), 1–16. https://doi.org/10.3390/microorganisms8091266

Łopusiewicz, Ł., Kowalczewski, P. Ł., Baranowska, H. M., Masewicz, Ł., Amarowicz, R., & Krupa-Kozak, U. (2023). Effect of flaxseed oil cake extract on the microbial quality, texture and shelf life of gluten-free bread. *Food, 12*(3), 1–15. https://doi.org/10.3390/foods12030595

Mannucci, A., Castagna, A., Santin, M., Serra, A., Mele, M., & Ranieri, A. (2019). Quality of flaxseed oil cake under different storage conditions. *Lwt, 104*(January), 84–90. https://doi.org/10.1016/j.lwt.2019.01.035

Mohtarami, F., Rashidi, Z., & Pirsa, S. (2022). Extraction of flaxseed and Plantago Psyllium mucilage: Investigation of rheological properties and efficiency as a fat substitute for the production of low-calorie cookies. *Journal of Food Processing and Preservation, 46*(11), 1–15. https://doi.org/10.1111/jfpp.16964

Mueller, K., Eisner, P., Yoshie-stark, Y., Nakada, R., & Kirchhoff, E. (2010). Functional properties and chemical composition of fractionated brown and yellow linseed meal (Linum usitatissimum L.). *Journal of Food Engineering, 98*(4), 453–460. https://doi.org/10.1016/j.jfoodeng.2010.01.028

Mukhopadhyay, N., Sarkar, S., & Bandyopadhyay, S. (2007). Effect of extrusion cooking on anti-nutritional factor tannin in linseed (Linum usitatissimum) meal. *International Journal of Food Sciences and Nutrition, 58*(8), 588–594. https://doi.org/10.1080/09637480701343952

Nema, A., Patnala, S. H., Mandari, V., Kota, S., & Devarai, S. K. (2019). Production and optimization of lipase using Aspergillus Niger MTCC 872 by solid-state fermentation. *Bulletin of the National Research Centre, 43*(1), 82. https://doi.org/10.1186/s42269-019-0125-7

Ogunronbi, O., Jooste, P. J., Abu, J. O., & Van Der Merwe, B. (2011). Chemical composition, storage stability and effect of cold-pressed flaxseed oil cake inclusion on bread quality. *Journal of Food Processing and Preservation, 35*(1), 64–79. https://doi.org/10.1111/j.1745-4549.2009.00452.x

Oomah, B. D. (2001). Flaxseed as a functional food source. *Journal of the Science of Food and Agriculture, 81*(9), 889–894. https://doi.org/10.1002/jsfa.898

Oomah, B. D. (2020, January). Flaxseed by-products. *Food Wastes and By-products, 2020*, 267–289. https://doi.org/10.1002/9781119534167.ch9

Oomah, B. D., & Mazza, G. (1993). Flaxseed proteins-a review. *Food Chemistry, 48*(2), 109–114. https://doi.org/10.1016/0308-8146(93)90043-F

Oomah, B. D., Kenaschuk, E. O., & Mazza, G. (1996a). Phytic acid content of flaxseed as influenced by cultivar. *Growing Season, and Location., 44*, 2663–2666.

Oomah, B. D., Mazza, G., & Kenaschuk, E. O. (1996b). Flavonoid content of flaxseed. Influence of cultivar and environment. *Euphytica, 90*(2), 163–167. https://doi.org/10.1007/bf00023854

Özkaynak Kanmaz, E. (2017). The effect of roasting process on fatty acid composition and phenolic content of whole flaxseed, flaxseed flour and flaxseed meal flour. *Gida/the Journal of Food, 42*(4), 382–391. https://doi.org/10.15237/gida.gd16081

Pandey, A. K., Edgard, G., & Negi, S. (2016). Optimization of concomitant production of cellulase and xylanase from Rhizopus oryzae SN5 through EVOP-factorial design technique and application in sorghum Stover based bioethanol production. *Renewable Energy, 98*, 51–56. https://doi.org/10.1016/j.renene.2016.05.071

Pesce, M., Tamai, I., Guo, D., Critto, A., Brombal, D., Wang, X., Cheng, H., & Marcomini, A. (2020). Circular economy in China: Translating principles into practice. *Sustainability (Switzerland), 12*(3), 1–31. https://doi.org/10.3390/su12030832

Poreda, A. (2017). Solid-state fermentation reduces Phytic acid level. *Improves the Profile of Myo-Inositol Phosphates and Enhances the Availability of Selected Minerals in Flaxseed Oil Cake., 55*(3), 413–419.

Prasad, K. (1997). Hydroxyl radical-scavenging property of secoisolariciresinol diglucoside (SDG) isolated from flax-seed. *Molecular and Cellular Biochemistry, 168*(1–2), 117–123. https://doi.org/10.1023/A:1006847310741

Puff, F., Wu, W., Huff, H. E., & Hsieh, F. (2006). Processing and properties of extruded flaxseed-corn puff. *Journal of Food Processing and Preservation, 31*(2007), 211–226.

Quezada, N., & Cherian, G. (2012). Lipid characterization and antioxidant status of the seeds and meals of Camelina sativa and flax. *European Journal of Lipid Science and Technology, 114*(8), 974–982. https://doi.org/10.1002/ejlt.201100298

Rudra, A., Arvind, I., & Mehra, R. (2021). Polyphenols: Types, sources and therapeutic applications. *International Journal of Home Science, 7*(3), 69–75. https://doi.org/10.22271/23957476.2021.v7.i3a.1182

Russo, R., & Reggiani, R. (2014). Variation in the content of cyanogenic glycosides in flaxseed meal from twenty-one varieties. *Food and Nutrition Sciences, 05*(15), 1456–1462. https://doi.org/10.4236/fns.2014.515159

Russo, R., & Reggiani, R. (2016). Evaluation of protein and antinutritional compounds content in meal from seven flax varieties. *Journal of Global Agriculture and Ecology, 6*(3), 182–188. www.camfeed.it/en

Sadh, P. K., Chawla, P., Bhandari, L., & Duhan, J. S. (2018a). Bio-enrichment of functional properties of peanut oil cakes by solid state fermentation using aspergillus oryzae. *Journal of Food Measurement and Characterization, 12*(1), 622–633. https://doi.org/10.1007/s11694-017-9675-2

Sadh, P. K., Duhan, S., & Duhan, J. S. (2018b). Agro-industrial wastes and their utilization using solid state fermentation: A review. *Bioresources and Bioprocessing, 5*(1), 1–15. https://doi.org/10.1186/s40643-017-0187-z

Safdar, B., Pang, Z., Liu, X., Rashid, M. T., & Jatoi, M. A. (2020). Structural and functional properties of raw and defatted flaxseed flour and degradation of cynogenic contents using different processing methods. *Journal of Food Process Engineering, 43*(6), 1–13. https://doi.org/10.1111/jfpe.13406

Salem, R. (2020, March). Evaluation of chemical composition and nutrition value of two varieties of flaxseed meal and oil.

Sanmartin, C., Taglieri, I., Venturi, F., Macaluso, M., Zinnai, A., Tavarini, S., Botto, A., Serra, A., Conte, G., Flamini, G., & Angelini, L. G. (2020). Flaxseed cake as a tool for the improvement of nutraceutical and sensorial features of sourdough bread. *Foods, 9*(2), *204*.

Shrestha, P., Rasmussen, M., Khanal, S. K., Pometto, A. L., & Van Leeuwen, J. (2008). Solid-substrate fermentation of corn fiber by Phanerochaete chrysosporium and subsequent fermentation of hydrolysate into ethanol. *Journal of Agricultural and Food Chemistry, 56*(11), 3918–3924. https://doi.org/10.1021/jf0728404

Singh, K. K., Mridula, D., Rehal, J., & Barnwal, P. (2011). Flaxseed: A potential source of food, feed and fiber. *Critical Reviews in Food Science and Nutrition, 51*(3), 210–222. https://doi.org/10.1080/10408390903537241

Singh, R., Langyan, S., Sangwan, S., Rohtagi, B., Khandelwal, A., & Shrivastava, M. (2022). Protein for human consumption from oilseed cakes: A review. *Frontiers in Sustainable Food Systems, 6*(March), 1–12. https://doi.org/10.3389/fsufs.2022.856401

Smetana, P., & Jan, B. (2022). Flaxseed hydrocolloids and their application. 1–24.

Stodolak, B., Starzyńska-Janiszewska, A., Wywrocka-Gurgul, A., & Wikiera, A. (2017). Solid-state fermented flaxseed oil cake of improved antioxidant capacity as potential food additive. *Journal of Food Processing and Preservation, 41*(2), 1–9. https://doi.org/10.1111/jfpp.12855

Stodolak, B., Starzyńska-Janiszewska, A., & Bączkowicz, M. (2020). Aspergillus oryzae (Koji Mold) and Neurospora intermedia (Oncom Mold) application for flaxseed oil cake processing. *Lwt, 131*(May), 109651. https://doi.org/10.1016/j.lwt.2020.109651

Taglieri, I., Sanmartin, C., Venturi, F., Macaluso, M., Zinnai, A., Tavarini, S., Serra, A., Conte, G., Flamini, G., & Angelini, L. G. (2020). Effect of the leavening agent on the compositional and sensorial characteristics of bread fortified with flaxseed cake. *Applied Sciences (Switzerland), 10*(15), 5235. https://doi.org/10.3390/APP10155235

Tavarini, S., De Leo, M., Matteo, R., Lazzeri, L., Braca, A., & Angelini, L. G. (2021). Flaxseed and camelina meals as potential sources of health-beneficial compounds. *Plants, 10*(1), 1–17. https://doi.org/10.3390/plants10010156

Teh, S. S., & Birch, E. J. (2014). Effect of ultrasonic treatment on the polyphenol content and antioxidant capacity of extract from defatted hemp, flax and canola seed cakes. *Ultrasonics Sonochemistry, 21*(1), 346–353. https://doi.org/10.1016/j.ultsonch.2013.08.002

Tempe, O., & Starzy, A. (2020). Co-fermentation as a tool for increasing the antioxidant potential of grass pea and flaxseed.

Tirgar, M., Silcock, P., Carne, A., & Birch, E. J. (2017). Effect of extraction method on functional properties of flaxseed protein concentrates. *Food Chemistry, 215*, 417–424. https://doi.org/10.1016/j.foodchem.2016.08.002

Vilariño, M. V., Franco, C., & Quarrington, C. (2017). Food loss and waste reduction as an integral part of a circular economy. *Frontiers in Environmental Science, 5*, 21. https://doi.org/10.3389/fenvs.2017.00021

Wanasundara, J. P. D., & Shahidi, F. (1994). Functional properties and amino-acid composition of solvent-extracted flaxseed meals. *Food Chemistry, 49*(1), 45–51. https://doi.org/10.1016/0308-8146(94)90231-3

Wanasundara, P. K. J. P. D., Amarowicz, R., Kara, M. T., & Shahidi, F. (1993). Removal of cyanogenic glycosides of flaxseed meal. *Food Chemistry, 48*(3), 263–266. https://doi.org/10.1016/0308-8146(93)90138-6

Waszkowiak, K., & Mikołajczak, B. (2020). The effect of roasting on the protein profile and antiradical capacity of flaxseed meal. *Food, 9*(10), 1383. https://doi.org/10.3390/foods9101383

Westcott, N. D., & Muir, A. D. (2003). Flax seed lignan in disease prevention and health promotion. *Phytochemistry Reviews, 2*(3), 401–417. https://doi.org/10.1023/B:PHYT.0000046174.97809.b6

Woyengo, T. A., Sánchez, J. E., Yáñez, J., Beltranena, E., Cervantes, M., Morales, A., & Zijlstra, R. T. (2016). Nutrient digestibility of canola co-products for grower pigs. *Animal Feed Science and Technology, 222*, 7–16. https://doi.org/10.1016/j.anifeedsci.2016.09.009

Woyengo, T. A., Beltranena, E., & Zijlstra, R. T. (2017). Effect of anti-nutritional factors of oilseed co-products on feed intake of pigs and poultry. *Animal Feed Science and Technology, 233*, 76–86. https://doi.org/10.1016/j.anifeedsci.2016.05.006

Xu, L., Wei, Z., Guo, B., Bai, R., Liu, J., Li, Y., Sun, W., Jiang, X., Li, X., & Pi, Y. (2022). Flaxseed meal and its application in animal husbandry: A review. *Agriculture (Switzerland), 12*(12), 1–16. https://doi.org/10.3390/agriculture12122027

Yadav, J. S. (1988). SSF of wheat straw with alcaliphilic Coprinus. *Biotechnology and Bioengineering, 31*(5), 414–417. https://doi.org/10.1002/bit.260310504

Yamashita, T., Sano, T., Hashimoto, T., & Kanazawa, K. (2007). Original article development of a method to remove cyanogen glycosides from flaxseed meal. *International Journal of Food Science & Technology, 42*, 70–75. https://doi.org/10.1111/j.1365-2621.2006.01212.x

Yang, J., Choi Y,J., Hahn, J. (2023) Development of flaxseed gum/konjac glucomannan with agar as gelling agents with enhanced elastic properties. *Food Sci Biotechnol, 32*, 181–92. https://doi.org/10.1007/s10068-022-01179-9

Zamindar, N., Bashash, M., Khorshidi, F., Serjouie, A., Shirvani, M. A., Abbasi, H., & Sedaghatdoost, A. (2017). Antioxidant efficacy of soybean cake extracts in soy oil protection. *Journal of Food Science and Technology, 54*(7), 2077–2084. https://doi.org/10.1007/s13197-017-2646-0

Zhai, S. S., Zhou, T., Li, M. M., Zhu, Y. W., Li, M. C., Feng, P. S., Zhang, X. F., Ye, H., Wang, W. C., & Yang, L. (2019). Fermentation of flaxseed cake increases its nutritional value and utilization in ducklings. *Poultry Science, 98*, 5636–5647. https://doi.org/10.3382/ps/pez326

Zhang, S., Chen, Y., McClements, D. J., Hou, T., Geng, F., Chen, P., Chen, H., Xie, B., Sun, Z., Tang, H., Pei, Y., Quan, S., Yu, X., & Deng, Q. (2023a). Composition, processing, and quality control of whole flaxseed products used to fortify foods. *Comprehensive Reviews in Food Science and Food Safety, 22*(1), 587–614. https://doi.org/10.1111/1541-4337.13086

Zhang, T., Zhang, Z., & Wang, X. (2023b). Composition and antioxidant ability of extract from different flaxseed cakes and its application in flaxseed oil. *Journal of Oleo Science, 72*(1), 59–67. https://doi.org/10.5650/jos.ess22181

Recent Marketing Trends and Future Perspective of Linseed and Its Products

Rashim Kumari, Arshia Prashar, and Anju Kapoor

Abstract

Linseed, also known as flaxseed (*Linum usitatissimum L.*), is one of the world's earliest domesticated crops. Its unique properties and wide range of uses have been acknowledged through both archaeological discoveries and historical texts. Linseed has a long history of being utilized for food, textile fiber, animal feed, and medicine. The term "linseed" originated from the practice of making fine linen cloth from the plant's stems. The species name "*usitatissimum*" signifies the plant's extensive value due to its diverse applications. While "flaxseed" can also refer to the plant's unspun fibers, its potential as a multiuse crop is being increasingly recognized and explored on both the national and international levels. Flourishing usage of flaxseed in human consumption, animal feed, industrial products, and growing demand for fiber and protein-rich foods are leading to the growth of the linseed market in the present era. In the recent times of microplastic pollution and climate change, linseed also offers hope in terms of Phytoremediation practices. To meet the future growing linseed market demands, new breeding and biotechnological approaches should be used to improve the quality and production of linseed globally and in the country.

Keywords

Linseed · Multiuse · Phytoremediation · Biotechnological · Breeding

R. Kumari
Department of Agriculture, Guru Nanak Dev University, Amritsar, Punjab, India

A. Prashar · A. Kapoor (✉)
Chaudhary Sarwan Kumar Himachal Pradesh Krishi Vishvavidyalaya,
Palampur, Himachal Pradesh, India

© The Author(s), under exclusive license to Springer Nature Singapore Pte Ltd. 2025

R. Chopra et al. (eds.), *Dynamics of Linseed and its Valorization*,
https://doi.org/10.1007/978-981-96-8927-9_11

1 Introduction

Linseed, also known as flaxseed, is one of the oldest crops cultivated for its fiber and oil. It belongs to the genus *Linum* and the family Linaceae. The botanical name *Linum usitatissimum* was assigned by Carl Linnaeus in his work *Species Plantarum* in 1753. Flaxseed is an herbaceous plant that produces blue flowers and small, flat seeds that range in color from golden yellow to reddish brown. These seeds have a rich nutty flavor and a crisp, chewy texture. It has a spherically shaped fruit capsule containing two seeds in each of its five compartments. The seeds are flat and oval in shape with a pointed tip and a smooth glossy surface, varying from yellow to dark brown color. Flaxseed is often used to describe "flax" when consumed by humans while "linseed" represents its use specifically for industrial applications. Nearly all parts of the linseed plant are used for various purposes. Its seed contains oil which after refining is used for edible purposes whereas, the stem yields fiber possessing high strength and durability (Fig. 1).

Mediterranean and Southwest Asia have been reported to be the centers of origin of linseed with three geographic centers of diversification, i.e., Southern North America, the Mediterranean area, and all of Mexico and South America. Further evidence show that its cultivation started even thousands of years earlier, during the Neolithic Era of roughly 10,000 BC. Sometime between 4000 and 2000 BC, flax cultivation became common in countries bordering the Mediterranean Sea and in regions of the Middle East. In the beginning linseed was primarily grown for its textile fibers but was also used to produce seeds and oil for dietary, medical, and other purposes. However, in today's world, flaxseed is grown more for its oil content and nutritional value.

Linseed has been cultivated and consumed for thousands of years. Its production grew across countries like Africa, Europe, and North America over the ages. Each year, about 3 to four million tonnes of flaxseed are produced all around the world. The largest producers are Canada, the USA, Kazakhstan, Russia, and India. With yearly exports between CAN$150–180 million, Canada is the world's top linseed

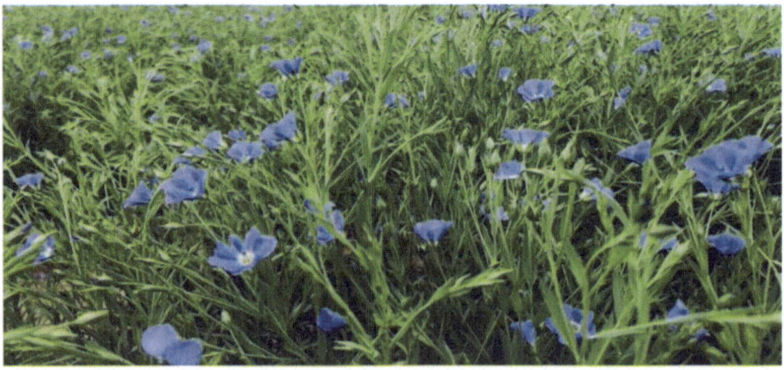

Fig. 1 Flaxseed, a fibrous and oilseed crop

producer and exporter, and 40% of all flax productions come from Canada. While, China, the USA, India, and Russia together account for 40% of the world linseed production. Flaxseed in Canada is grown within an area ranging from 300,000 to 700,000 hectares with an average yield per hectare of around 2000 kg. Meanwhile, India produces 0.127 million tonnes of flaxseed from an area of 0.2 million hectares with an average productivity of 0.635 tonnes per hectare (Golshenas, 2023).

Linseed has been utilized by human societies for a variety of purposes. It is considered a dual-purpose plant, providing both seeds and fiber. The fiber obtained from linseed stems is known for its high strength and durability. The seeds are valued for their oil, which is rich in omega-3 fatty acids, accounting for more than half of its fatty acid composition. Linseed oil is approximately 40% oil by weight, containing about 53% alpha-linolenic acid (ALA), 17% linoleic acid, 19% oleic acid, 5% palmitic acid, and 3% stearic acid. It has a favorable omega-6 to omega-3 fatty acid ratio of 0.3:1 (Simopoulos, 2002). Additionally, linseed oil is rich in antioxidants and phytosterols, which are essential for maintaining good health. Linseed is also a good source of high-quality protein and contains phenolic compounds. Because of these attributes, linseed is regarded as an important oilseed crop for industrial uses, as well as a source of food, feed, and fiber.

2 Recent Marketing Trends

The growing use of linseed in linen manufacturing, its numerous health benefits, and the increasing demand for fiber and protein-rich foods are key factors driving the growth of the linseed market today. However, climate change, supply chain disruptions, and restrictions related to virus mutations could negatively impact overall market growth. The linseed market can be divided into several application categories, including food, cosmetics, pharmaceuticals, animal feed, linen manufacturing, and paints and varnishes. The food sector currently holds the largest share in the global market, largely due to the increasing popularity of linseed as a superfood. Refined linseed and its products are often classified as vegan food, which is boosting demand as the vegan population grows. Linseed's antioxidant properties and high fiber content help combat health issues such as obesity, diabetes, cancer, and heart disease. It has become a staple in various food products, including wholegrain bread, pasta, cereals, and snacks.

Additionally, linseed is considered a natural alternative to hormone replacement therapy for managing menopause symptoms in aging women. The food, pharmaceutical, and linen sectors are projected to be the fastest-growing segments, with a compound annual growth rate (CAGR) of 4.2% from 2022 to 2027. This growth is attributed to the increasing use of linseed in linen products such as bed sheets and table linens, which are valued for their durability and moisture absorption. The expanding market for linseed capsules and tablets for pharmaceutical uses also offers growth opportunities and supports the overall market expansion for linseed (Fig. 2).

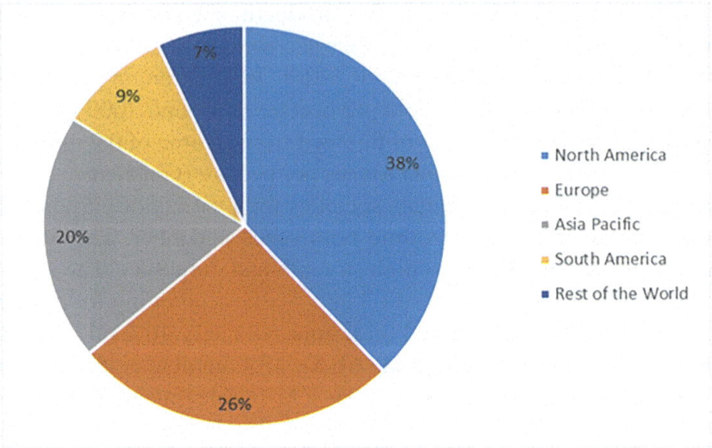

Fig. 2 Linseed market by geography in 2023. (Source: www.Statistica.com)

The global linseed market encompasses North America, Asia-Pacific, Europe, South America, and other regions. North America holds the largest market share, accounting for 38% of the global market. This growth is attributed to several factors, including the presence of major linseed-producing countries such as Canada, the USA, Russia, Poland, Belgium, Italy, and France, which collectively have the highest annual linseed production. These countries offer favorable low-temperature conditions essential for linseed cultivation. Additionally, high GDP per capita and health consciousness among consumers in these nations make linseed a preferred choice.

Looking ahead, the Asia-Pacific region is expected to experience the fastest growth from 2022 to 2027. This growth is driven by the increasing demand resulting from the region's large elderly population, which is among the largest globally. As the incidence of age-related diseases rises, linseed's health benefits become more appealing, leading to a significant increase in market demand.

- *Health and Wellness Boom:* Increasing consumer awareness of health and wellness has significantly increased the demand for linseed and its products. Linseed is rich in omega-3 fatty acids, lignans, and fiber, and is recognized for its potential benefits for heart health, cancer prevention, and digestive health. Studies have shown that regular consumption of linseed can help lower cholesterol levels and reduce inflammation, contributing to overall well-being. In particular, linseed is high in alpha-linolenic acid (ALA), an omega-3 fatty acid essential for cardiovascular health. ALA has been linked to a reduced risk of heart disease by lowering blood pressure, improving arterial function, and reducing blood clots (Brown, 2019a, b, c). Furthermore, lignans, a type of phytoestrogen found in abundance in linseed, have shown potential in reducing the risk of hormone-related cancers like breast and prostate cancer. The fiber content in linseed supports digestion by promoting regular bowel movements and preventing constipation. Additionally, linseed can help stabilize blood sugar levels, which is beneficial for managing diabetes (Smith, 2020a, b).

- *Organic and Non-GMO Movements:* As consumers become more health-conscious, there is a growing preference for organic and non-GMO products. Linseed, often grown without synthetic pesticides and fertilizers, fits well within this trend. The market for organic linseed is expanding as consumers seek products that are free from genetic modifications and chemicals, believing them to be safer and more nutritious. Organic linseed farming practices emphasize soil health, biodiversity, and sustainable agriculture, which appeal to environmentally conscious consumers (Green, 2018). The certification of linseed as organic involves rigorous standards and practices that ensure the absence of synthetic chemicals and genetically modified organisms (GMOs). This certification process reassures consumers about the purity and quality of the product. Additionally, non-GMO labeling on linseed products provides further assurance to consumers who are wary of the potential health risks associated with genetically modified foods. The demand for organic and non-GMO linseed is also driven by the perception that these products are more wholesome and environmentally friendly, contributing to a growing market segment that prioritizes health and sustainability (Davis, 2021).
- *Sustainability and Environmental Concerns:* Linseed's natural resistance to pests reduces the need for pesticides, making it a more sustainable option than other crops. However, some environmental concerns are associated with its production, particularly in areas where it may be cultivated intensively. Overcultivation can lead to soil degradation, water use concerns, and a reduction in biodiversity. To maximize sustainability, it's crucial to manage linseed production practices carefully, ensuring that cultivation methods are balanced and considerate of local ecosystems.
- *Eco-friendly Packaging:* Sustainability has become a critical concern for both consumers and manufacturers. The push toward eco-friendly packaging is a direct response to environmental concerns. Linseed products are increasingly being packaged in biodegradable and recyclable materials, reducing the environmental footprint and appealing to eco-conscious consumers. This trend is part of a broader movement toward reducing plastic waste and promoting a circular economy. Manufacturers are investing in innovative packaging solutions such as compostable bags, recyclable containers, and minimalistic designs that use fewer resources. Eco-friendly packaging reduces the impact on landfills and aligns with consumers' values, enhancing brand loyalty and marketability. Moreover, regulatory pressures and environmental standards are driving companies to adopt sustainable packaging practices, further accelerating this trend. The shift to eco-friendly packaging also involves educating consumers about proper disposal methods to ensure that the environmental benefits are fully realized (White, 2020).
- *Sustainable Farming Practices:* Sustainable farming practices are gaining traction in linseed cultivation. Practices such as crop rotation, reduced pesticide use, and organic farming not only help in maintaining soil health but also enhance biodiversity. These methods ensure that linseed production is environmentally

sustainable and economically viable in the long run. Crop rotation, for example, helps prevent soil depletion and reduces the buildup of pests and diseases, leading to healthier crops and higher yields. Reduced pesticide use minimizes the impact on nontarget species, including beneficial insects and pollinators, while organic farming eliminates the use of synthetic chemicals altogether. Sustainable farming practices also include water conservation techniques, such as drip irrigation and rainwater harvesting, which are crucial in regions facing water scarcity. Additionally, the use of cover crops and green manures can improve soil structure and fertility, further supporting sustainable production. By adopting these practices, linseed farmers can produce high-quality crops while preserving natural resources and protecting the environment (Brown, 2019a, b, c).

- *Innovative Product Development:* Linseed has become a focal point for innovative product development across various industries due to its versatile properties. In the food sector, linseed is being incorporated into functional foods, such as nutrient-rich snacks and fortified breads, to harness its high omega-3 fatty acid content and dietary fiber. The cosmetic industry is also exploring linseed oil as a key ingredient in skincare products, thanks to its moisturizing and anti-inflammatory properties. Moreover, in sustainable materials development, linseed is being utilized to create biodegradable composites and eco-friendly linoleum flooring, which offer alternatives to petroleum-based products. These innovations highlight linseed's potential to contribute to healthier lifestyles and more sustainable practices across multiple sectors.
- *Linseed Oil Derivatives:* The market for linseed oil and its derivatives is expanding, driven by their versatile applications in food, cosmetics, and industrial products. Innovations in processing techniques have led to the development of high-quality linseed oil products that retain their nutritional properties and offer enhanced stability and shelf life. Cold-pressed linseed oil, for instance, is valued for its purity and nutrient retention, making it a popular choice for culinary and dietary uses. In the cosmetics industry, linseed oil is prized for its moisturizing and anti-inflammatory properties, making it a key ingredient in skincare products such as lotions, creams, and serums. Industrial applications of linseed oil include its use as a drying oil in paints, varnishes, and linoleum production, where its ability to form a durable, protective film is highly beneficial. Furthermore, advancements in extraction and refinement processes have resulted in linseed oil derivatives with specific functional properties, such as improved oxidative stability and enhanced bioavailability of nutrients. These innovations are driving the growth of the linseed oil market by catering to diverse consumer needs and applications (Clark, 2018).
- *Plant-Based Diets:* The shift toward plant-based diets has also fueled the popularity of linseed. As a plant-based source of essential nutrients, linseed is being incorporated into a variety of foods such as breads, cereals, and snacks. Its inclusion in plant-based products not only enhances nutritional value but also meets the dietary preferences of vegans and vegetarians. Linseed is a rich source of plant-based omega-3 fatty acids, protein, and dietary fiber, making it a valuable addition to plant-based diets. It can be used as an egg substitute in baking, added

to smoothies for a nutritional boost, or sprinkled on salads and yogurt for added texture and flavor. The versatility of linseed in plant-based cooking and its compatibility with various dietary restrictions make it a popular choice among health-conscious consumers. Moreover, the growing trend of clean labeling and natural ingredients in the food industry further supports the use of linseed as a wholesome and functional ingredient in plant-based products (Smith, 2021).

- *Online Retail Expansion:* The online retail expansion of linseed products has opened new avenues for both consumers and producers, making this versatile crop more accessible than ever before. Through e-commerce platforms, a wider audience can now purchase linseed-based products, ranging from health supplements to natural skincare items, with just a few clicks. This growth in online availability has also allowed small and medium-sized businesses to reach global markets, driving innovation and competition. Furthermore, the convenience of online shopping has encouraged more consumers to explore linseed's health benefits, contributing to increased awareness and demand. This digital shift not only supports the growth of the linseed market but also promotes sustainable practices by reducing the need for physical retail space and associated environmental costs.
- *E-Commerce Platforms:* The rise of e-commerce has greatly affected the distribution and accessibility of linseed products. Online platforms provide consumers with a convenient way to purchase a variety of linseed products, including whole seeds, oils, and supplements. This trend has allowed manufacturers to reach a wider audience and has driven the growth of the linseed market. E-commerce platforms offer detailed product information, customer reviews, and competitive pricing, enabling consumers to make well-informed purchasing decisions. The convenience of shopping from home, along with the option of home delivery, makes online shopping an attractive choice for many consumers. Additionally, e-commerce platforms often feature subscription services and discounts, encouraging repeat purchases and building customer loyalty. The use of advanced technologies such as artificial intelligence and machine learning further enhances the shopping experience by providing personalized recommendations and targeted marketing (Johnson, 2019).
- *Direct-to-Consumer Models:* Direct-to-consumer (DTC) models are becoming increasingly popular in the linseed market. By bypassing traditional retail channels, manufacturers can offer their products directly to consumers, often at lower prices and with personalized marketing strategies. This model allows for better control over branding, customer relationships, and feedback, leading to increased consumer loyalty. DTC models also enable manufacturers to collect valuable consumer data, which can be used to optimize product offerings and marketing efforts. The ability to directly engage with customers through social media, email marketing, and other digital channels enhances brand visibility and fosters a sense of community. Moreover, DTC models provide flexibility in product launches and innovations, allowing manufacturers to quickly respond to market trends and consumer demands. The success of DTC models in the linseed market is also supported by the growing trend of online shopping and the preference for

unique, high-quality products that may not be available in traditional retail stores (Lee, 2020).

- *Future Perspectives:* The future perspectives of linseed are promising as its potential continues to be explored across various industries. With growing consumer interest in health and sustainability, linseed is likely to see increased demand for its nutritional and environmental benefits. In agriculture, advances in cultivation techniques may enhance yield and resilience, making linseed an even more viable crop in the face of climate change. The development of new linseed-based products, from biodegradable materials to plant-based nutrition, is expected to expand its applications further. Additionally, research into linseed's bioactive compounds could unlock new uses in medicine and health supplements. As these trends converge, linseed is poised to play a significant role in the future of sustainable agriculture, innovative product development, and global health.

2.1 Technological Advancements in Agriculture

Technological advancements are poised to revolutionize linseed cultivation. Innovations such as automated machinery, remote sensing, and data analytics can optimize planting, irrigation, and harvesting processes, thereby increasing efficiency and reducing costs. These technologies also enable farmers to monitor crop health and address issues promptly, ensuring higher yields and better quality. Automated machinery, including GPS-guided tractors and harvesters, can perform precise agricultural operations with minimal human intervention, reducing labor costs and increasing productivity. Remote sensing technologies, including satellite imagery and drones, offer real-time data on crop conditions, soil moisture levels, and pest infestations, enabling timely and precise interventions. Data analytics and machine learning algorithms can process large datasets to identify patterns and provide predictive recommendations, enhancing decision-making and resource management. These technological advancements boost the efficiency and profitability of linseed farming and promote sustainable agricultural practices by optimizing resource use and reducing environmental impact (Wilson, 2018).

2.2 Precision Farming

Precision farming technologies hold significant promise for linseed cultivation. By utilizing GPS, drones, and IoT devices, farmers can apply inputs like water, fertilizers, and pesticides with greater accuracy. This targeted approach not only improves the yield and quality of linseed but also reduces resource wastage and minimizes environmental impact. GPS technology enables precise field mapping and accurate input application, reducing overlaps and ensuring even coverage. Drones equipped with multispectral cameras capture high-resolution images of crops, providing detailed insights into plant health, nutrient status, and pest pressures. IoT devices, such as soil moisture sensors and weather stations, gather real-time data on environmental conditions, allowing farmers to make informed decisions regarding irrigation, fertilization, and pest control. The integration of these technologies in precision farming systems facilitates site-specific management, where inputs are applied only when and where needed, optimizing resource use and enhancing sustainability. Additionally, precision farming supports the adoption of conservation practices like reduced tillage and cover cropping, which improve soil health and resilience (Smith, 2020a, b).

2.3 Genetic Research

Advances in genetic research are expected to play a significant role in the future of linseed production. Genetic engineering and selective breeding can lead to the development of linseed varieties with improved traits such as higher oil content, disease resistance, and adaptability to different climatic conditions. These advancements will help in meeting the growing demand for linseed and its products while ensuring sustainability. Genetic research can identify and introduce specific genes responsible for desirable traits, enabling the creation of linseed varieties that are more productive and resilient. For example, genes associated with increased oil biosynthesis can be targeted to enhance the oil yield of linseed crops. Similarly, genes conferring resistance to common pests and diseases can be incorporated to reduce the reliance on chemical pesticides and improve crop health. Genetic research also enables the development of linseed varieties that can thrive in diverse environmental conditions, including drought and salinity, ensuring stable production in the face of climate change. The application of modern biotechnological tools, such as CRISPR-Cas9 gene editing, further accelerates the development of improved linseed varieties with precise and targeted modifications (Brown, 2019a, b, c).

- *Expansion into emerging markets:* Linseed is experiencing significant expansion into emerging markets, driven by increasing awareness of its health benefits and versatility. As economies in regions like Asia, Africa, and Latin America grow, so does the demand for nutrient-dense foods, natural health supplements, and sustainable products—areas where linseed excels. This expansion is supported by the rise of local production capabilities, reducing dependence on imports and making linseed more affordable and accessible to a broader population. Additionally, the versatility of linseed in various industries, from food to cosmetics and industrial applications, makes it an attractive option for markets looking to diversify their agricultural and manufacturing sectors. As these emerging markets continue to develop, linseed's presence is likely to strengthen, contributing to both local economic growth and global sustainability efforts.

2.4 Market Penetration

Market penetration for linseed involves strategies and tactics aimed at increasing the presence and consumption of linseed products within a specific market and requires the following steps to achieve it. The global linseed (*Linum usitatissimum*) market has seen significant growth due to its recognized health benefits and versatile applications. However, market penetration in emerging markets remains a key opportunity. Strategic approaches to penetrate these markets include tailored marketing strategies, understanding local consumer behavior, and aligning products with regional health trends. Linseed is rich in alpha-linolenic acid (ALA), a type of omega-3 fatty acid, as well as lignans, which are phytoestrogens with antioxidant properties. These components are linked to various health benefits, including cardiovascular health, anti-inflammatory effects, and potential cancer risk reduction. Targeting markets with rising lifestyle diseases such as cardiovascular diseases and diabetes can be particularly effective. For instance, a study highlighted that ALA intake is inversely associated with coronary heart disease, which can be a key message in health campaigns in these regions. Leveraging digital marketing and e-commerce platforms can help reach a broader audience, especially in countries with high internet penetration. For example, in India, where internet usage is rapidly growing, online platforms can be used to market linseed products. Collaborating with local influencers and nutritionists can enhance brand credibility and consumer trust, as their endorsements can significantly influence consumer behavior. Market penetration strategies should also consider pricing models that make linseed products accessible to a broader demographic. Offering smaller packaging options for cost-sensitive consumers or bulk packaging for health-conscious families and institutions can cater to different market segments. Promotional deals and discounts through both online and offline channels can stimulate initial interest and trial purchases (Smith & Doe, 2022).

2.5 Local Production: Encouraging Local Cultivation of Linseed

Encouraging local cultivation of linseed in emerging markets can reduce dependency on imports and ensure a steady supply chain. Initiatives can include government subsidies, training programs for farmers, and the introduction of high-yield linseed varieties. Local production not only supports the agricultural sector but also contributes to the economy by creating jobs and promoting sustainable farming practices. Government and agricultural organizations can provide farmers with high-quality seeds, modern farming equipment, and access to irrigation systems. For example, introducing drought-resistant linseed varieties can be crucial in regions with water scarcity. Educational programs focused on sustainable farming techniques, such as crop rotation and integrated pest management, can improve yield and soil health. Building local processing facilities can add value to the raw linseed, creating opportunities for producing linseed oil, flour, and other derivatives. This not only meets local demand but also opens up potential export markets. Partnerships with local universities and research institutions can drive innovation in cultivation techniques and product development, ensuring that the local linseed industry remains competitive on a global scale (Brown, 2021).

3 Collaboration and Innovation

Collaboration with different institutes and innovation in terms of breeding, biotechnology, and yield improvement are key drivers for advancing linseed production, improving efficiency, and expanding different market opportunities by increasing its utility. Biotechnology also offers opportunities for refining the nutritional profile of linseed, potentially increasing its omega-3 fatty acid content or reducing antinutritional factors, making it even more appealing to health-conscious consumers.

Moreover, these innovations open up new market opportunities by expanding linseed's applications in various industries, from food and nutraceuticals to sustainable materials and biofuels. Collaborative research can also lead to the development of more efficient and environmentally friendly farming practices, reducing the carbon footprint of linseed production and making it a more sustainable crop. As these innovations continue to unfold, the linseed industry is likely to see significant growth, driven by improved efficiency, greater utility, and a broader range of applications in both existing and emerging markets.

3.1 Industry Collaboration

Collaboration of farmers with different academic institutions and agricultural research centers help in exploring new linseed varieties, improving yield and enhancing disease resistance toward many diseases, which directly influences the market. Further, farmers and institute engagement with innovation labs using different new technologies being focused on plant breeding and genetic modification helps in developing advanced linseed strains with higher nutritional content or better adaptability, which additionally help in uplifting the linseed market nationally and internationally. Many national projects like the AICRP (All India coordinated Research Project) on linseed has been established since 1967, which collaborated different farmers and institutes together further providing new varieties to the market by use of systematic and intensive breeding programs. A total number of 87 improved varieties including ten dual purpose varieties suitable for different agro-climatic growing situations of the country have been developed under the project. While, during 2019–2020, seven varieties were recommended for general cultivation for farmers and market suitability. Collaboration of different institutes and use of new innovative technologies can help in doubling the income of farmers and improving the linseed produce in market. Collaboration between farmers, researchers, and companies can drive innovation in linseed product development and marketing strategies. By working together, these stakeholders can share knowledge, pool resources, and tackle common challenges more effectively. Farmers can provide valuable insights into cultivation practices and challenges, while researchers can develop new linseed varieties that are more resistant to pests and diseases. For instance, genetic studies on linseed have identified markers for traits like disease resistance and oil content, which can be used to breed improved varieties (Diederichsen & Fu, 2008). Companies can then use this information to create better products and marketing strategies that highlight the unique benefits of these new varieties. Industry collaboration can also facilitate the development of new linseed-based products. For instance, food companies can work with researchers to develop linseed-enriched foods that cater to specific dietary needs, such as gluten-free or high-protein diets. Collaborations can also explore the use of linseed in nonfood applications, such as biodegradable packaging materials or natural cosmetics. Research into linseed oil's potential as a bio-lubricant or in bioplastics is ongoing, highlighting its versatility (Green & White, 2023).

3.2 New Applications

These collaborations and innovations have expanded the applications of linseed into new areas. Recently, linseed oil has gained traction in the health and beauty industry due to its natural properties, making it a valuable ingredient in skincare and haircare products. Rich in omega-3 fatty acids and antioxidants, linseed oil offers numerous benefits for both skin and hair and is increasingly used in the cosmeceutical industry. Beyond its external benefits, linseed oil is also valuable as a nutritional supplement, providing a rich source of essential fatty acids, particularly omega-3 s. These fatty acids are vital for maintaining overall health and well-being. Nutraceuticals, which are purified products derived from food, play an important role in the proper development, growth, and maintenance of the body (Liu et al., 2020). Linseed contains a range of biologically active compounds, including linoleic and linolenic acids, polysaccharides, cyclo-linopeptides, lignans, alkaloids, cyclic peptides, phytic acid, selenium, cadmium, linatine, trypsin inhibitors, minerals, vitamins, phenolics, and cyanogenic glycosides. These components contribute to linseed's growing popularity in the nutraceutical and pharmaceutical industries.

Ongoing research is likely to reveal new applications for linseed in pharmaceuticals, nutraceuticals, and bio-based materials. Known for its health benefits such as reducing inflammation and improving heart health, linseed holds potential for additional uses. In the pharmaceutical sector, compounds from linseed are being explored for their potential to treat various conditions, including cancer and autoimmune diseases. For instance, lignans in linseed have shown potential in inhibiting the growth of certain cancer cells in laboratory studies. In the field of nutraceuticals, which are food-derived products offering health benefits beyond basic nutrition, linseed's high fiber content and omega-3 fatty acids make it an ideal ingredient for functional foods and dietary supplements. Additionally, the increasing interest in sustainable and eco-friendly materials has led to research into linseed's applications in bio-based products. Linseed oil can be used as a natural ingredient in paints, varnishes, and linoleum flooring, while the fibrous parts of the plant are utilized in creating biodegradable composites and textiles. Recent advancements in material science have demonstrated that linseed-based composites possess excellent mechanical properties, making them suitable for various industrial uses (Thompson & Cunnane, 2003).

4 Consumer Education and Engagement

Consumer education and engagement programs are important to teach consumers about the linseed industry (and its products) to encourage them to be larger participants in the linseed industry's economy and further contributing to the linseed market in larger areas (Grewal et al., 2022). Educational initiatives might include informative campaigns, workshops, and online resources that highlight how linseed contributes to a healthy diet, sustainable agriculture, and eco-friendly products. Additionally, engagement efforts such as community events, cooking demonstrations, and interactive platforms can create a more connected consumer base, encouraging them to explore and adopt linseed products in their daily lives. As consumers become more knowledgeable and engaged, their increased participation can drive demand, spur innovation, and ultimately contribute to the growth and resilience of the linseed market in broader regions. This approach not only benefits the industry but also aligns with broader goals of promoting sustainable consumption and supporting local economies.

4.1 Awareness Campaigns

Different educational campaigns should be conducted highlighting the health benefits of linseed, such as its omega-3 fatty acids, fiber, and antioxidant properties and including evidence-based research and practical tips. Visually appealing infographics should be made that summarize the nutritional benefits and uses of linseed. Infographics are easy to share and can quickly convey complex information to the consumers. Developing comprehensive recipe guides or e-books featuring linseed in various dishes, including breakfast options, snacks, and main courses showcasing its uses and importance should be made. Development of online tools that help users calculate the nutritional benefits of adding linseed to their diet is also a simple and effective way helping consumer gain knowledge about linseed and its products. By implementing these strategies, one can effectively educate consumers about the benefits of linseed, engage them with valuable content, and build a loyal customer base further helping in more market value and demand of the linseed crop.

Educational campaigns highlighting the health benefits and versatility of linseed can drive consumer interest and demand. By raising awareness about the nutritional value of linseed, such as its high omega-3 fatty acid content, rich fiber, and lignans, consumers can be encouraged to incorporate it into their diets. These campaigns can take various forms, including social media content, informational websites, and in-store promotions (Johnson, 2020). Collaborations with healthcare professionals, nutritionists, and influencers can amplify the message and reach a wider audience. For instance, nutritionists can host webinars or workshops on the health benefits of linseed, while influencers can share recipes and personal testimonials on social media platforms. AAA effective educational campaigns should also address common misconceptions about linseed, such as concerns about its taste or how to incorporate it into everyday meals. Providing easy-to-follow recipes and usage tips can help consumers see the practical benefits of adding linseed to their diet. For example, demonstrating how to use linseed oil in salad dressings or how to add ground linseed to smoothies can make it more approachable for consumers (Goyal et al., 2014).

4.2 Community Engagement

Community engagement is a powerful way to build relationships, enhance brand loyalty, and drive awareness about linseed among people. Engaging with the community can help educate consumers, foster a positive brand image, and create a sense of belonging among users for linseed. Establishing dedicated social media groups or forums (e.g., Facebook Groups, Reddit communities) focused on linseed where they can be used to share content, answer questions, and foster discussions can be helpful. Further engaging in existing online forums and platforms related to health, nutrition and cooking, sharing expertise on linseed, answering queries helps providing value to community members. By employing these community engagement approaches, one can create a strong, supportive network of consumers and advocates for linseed. Engaging with the community not only boosts awareness but also builds trust, loyalty, and advocacy for linseed and its products. Engaging with communities through social media and events can foster a loyal customer base and promote linseed's benefits. Social media platforms offer a direct way to interact with consumers, answer their questions, and share valuable content. Regular posts about linseed's health benefits, cooking tips, and success stories can keep the community engaged and informed. Hosting events such as cooking classes, health seminars, and farmer's markets can provide hands-on experiences for consumers to learn about linseed. These events can be organized in collaboration with local health clubs, schools, and community centers to reach a broader audience. Offering free samples and demonstrations can encourage trial and adoption of linseed products. Engaging with consumers through online forums, blogs, and newsletters can create a sense of community and loyalty. Encouraging consumers to share their experiences and recipes can build a user-generated content base that adds authenticity to marketing efforts. Recognizing and rewarding loyal customers through exclusive offers and promotions can further strengthen the brand–consumer relationship. By focusing on these strategies, the linseed industry can expand its market presence, drive innovation, and build strong consumer relationships. The future of linseed looks promising as it continues to gain recognition for its health benefits and versatile applications in various industries (Oomah, 2001).

5 Conclusion

Linseed (*Linum usitatissimum L.*), a versatile oilseed and fiber crop, has been utilized by humans for over 6000 years, making it one of the earliest domesticated plants. Its uses span a wide range of applications, including industrial, nutraceutical, biopharmaceutical, fiber, animal feed, and human food products. The growing demand for linseed is driven by the increasing cost of synthetic fibers and the numerous benefits offered by natural flax fiber. Advances in technology and new equipment for cultivating and harvesting flax further enhance its value, establishing linseed as a model plant in modern agriculture. Often referred to as the "Golden Elixir," linseed is praised for its potential to restore and enhance ecological balance. Its extensive applications and health benefits, including high omega-3 fatty acid content and antioxidant properties, are contributing to a rising market demand. This growing interest presents a challenge for countries to expand production and increase cultivation areas for linseed. To meet this demand and enhance global production, there is a need for new technologies and improved breeding methods. Innovations in crop management, genetic improvements, and sustainable farming practices will be crucial in increasing the quality and quantity of linseed production. Furthermore, continued research and development are essential to maximize the crop's potential and address the challenges faced by linseed cultivation worldwide.

References

All India Coordinated Research Project on Linseed, ICAR, Krishi Bhavan, Dr. Rajendra Prasad Road, New Delhi-110001.

Brown, A. (2019a). Omega-3 fatty acids and heart health. *Cardiovascular Review, 28*(1), 45–60.

Brown. (2019b). Sustainable agriculture practices for linseed cultivation. *Agricultural Sustainability Journal, 18*(3), 145–160.

Brown, P. (2019c). Genetic research in crop improvement. *Biotechnology Review, 8*(2), 75–90.

Brown, L. (2021). Local cultivation and its impact on the linseed market. *Agriculture Today, 12*(4), 89–102.

Clark, D. (2018). Advances in linseed oil processing. *Food Science and Technology, 12*(2), 95–110.

Davis, L. (2021). Non-GMO foods: Consumer preferences and market trends. *Food Industry Insights, 10*(4), 200–215.

Diederichsen, A., & Fu, Y. B. (2008). Flax genetic diversity as the raw material for future success. *Genus, 32*, 33.

Golshenas, P. (2023). The usage of flax as biodiesel and biomass. *The Canadian Science Fair Journal, 5*(1) www.Statistica.com

Goyal, A., Sharma, V., Upadhyay, N., Gill, S., & Sihag, M. (2014). Flax and flaxseed oil: An ancient medicine & modern functional food. *Journal of Food Science and Technology, 51*, 1633–1653.

Green, M. (2018). The organic movement: Trends and implications. *Organic Farming Journal, 22*(2), 88–102.

Green, P., & White, S. (2023). Innovations in linseed product development. *Food Science and Technology, 20*(2), 113–129.

Grewal, R., Meyer, R., & Mittal, V. (2022). Education and marketing: Decision making, spending, and consumption. *Journal of Marketing Research, 59, 1*.

Johnson, R. (2019). The rise of e-commerce in the food industry. *Retail Innovations, 14*(3), 155–170.
Johnson, M. (2020). Consumer education strategies in the health food sector. *Journal of Consumer Marketing, 18*(1), 77–90.
Lee, S. (2020). Direct-to-consumer models in the linseed market. *Market Trends Review, 7*(1), 90–105.
Liu, M., Tu, X., & Vorodi, A. M. (2020). A comparative study on the effects of linseed oil and shellac treatment on the hygroscopicity, dimensional stability, and color changes of Chinese ash wood. *BioResources, 15*(4), 8085–8092.
Oomah, B. D. (2001). Flaxseed as a functional food source. *Journal of the Science of Food and Agriculture, 81*(9), 889–894.
Simopoulos, A. P. (2002). The importance of the ratio of omega-6/omega-3 essential fatty acids. *Biomedicine & Pharmacotherapy, 56*(8), 365–379.
Smith, J. (2020a). Health benefits of linseed. *Journal of Nutrition, 15*(3), 120–135.
Smith, A. (2020b). Precision farming and its benefits. *Farming Technology Insights, 16*(3), 200–215.
Smith, E. (2021). Plant-based diets and linseed consumption. *Nutritional Science Journal, 19*(2), 215–230.
Smith, J., & Doe, A. (2022). Market trends in emerging economies: The case of linseed. *Journal of Agricultural Economics, 15*(3), 245–263.
Thompson, L. U., & Cunnane, S. C. (2003). *Flaxseed in human nutrition* (No. Ed. 2, pp. vi+-458).
White, P. (2020). Eco-friendly packaging innovations. *Sustainable Packaging Review, 5*(1), 30–45.
Wilson, T. (2018). Technological innovations in agriculture. *AgriTech Journal, 11*(2), 85–100.

Quality and Labeling Standards for Linseed and Its Products

Sakshi Singh, Ankur Ojha, Heena Yadav, Shreya Saran, Shweta Jaiswal, and Shumaila Jan

Abstract

Linseed (*Linum usitatissimum*), also known as flaxseed, is a nutrient-dense oilseed widely recognized for its health benefits and industrial uses. For consumer safety, legal compliance, and commercial acceptability, linseed and goods produced from it must be labeled with precision and high quality. This chapter provides an in-depth analysis of the quality and labeling standards associated with linseed and its products, beginning with an overview of its nutritional significance, industrial applications, and grading criteria based on physical and chemical properties such as moisture content, oil composition, and purity. It further examines the established quality and labeling requirements for raw and processed linseed products, including oil, flour, and supplements, alongside regulatory frameworks from international bodies like Codex Alimentarius and country-specific guidelines from key markets such as the USA and the European Union. Additionally, it discusses labeling elements, including nutritional declarations, allergen warnings, and organic certifications, to enhance consumer transparency and confidence. The chapter also addresses potential contaminants and adulterants, such as pesticide residues, heavy metals, and microbial impurities, which can affect the safety and overall quality of linseed products.

Keywords

Linseed · Regulatory framework · Labeling

S. Singh
Department of Food Technology, Jamia Hamdard, New Delhi, India

A. Ojha (✉) · H. Yadav · S. Saran · S. Jaiswal · S. Jan
Department of Food Science and Technology, National Institute of Food Technology and Entrepreneurship and Management, Kundli, India

© The Author(s), under exclusive license to Springer Nature Singapore Pte Ltd. 2025
R. Chopra et al. (eds.), *Dynamics of Linseed and its Valorization*,
https://doi.org/10.1007/978-981-96-8927-9_12

1 Introduction

Flaxseed or linseed (*Linum usitatissimum* L.) is one of the oldest oilseed crops, known for its diverse applications, as reflected in its Latin name. It is predominantly cultivated in the northern hemisphere, including Canada, the USA, Russia, China, and India, for both seed oil and stem fiber production (Farag et al., 2021). Flaxseed serves multiple purposes, ranging from nutritional and health benefits to industrial applications in textiles, paints, linoleum flooring, and bio-fibers, as well as being used as animal feed (Saleem et al., 2020). Canada, the leading global producer of flaxseed, exports approximately 150–180 million Canadian dollars' worth annually. Due to extensive domestication, flaxseed has developed into two primary morphotypes: fiber and oil. Fiber-type flaxseed is typically taller, with fewer branches, higher seed protein content, greater straw weight, and increased resistance to pathogens. In contrast, the oil-type flaxseed yields more seeds and exhibits resistance to powdery mildew. Linseed oil has been associated with various health benefits, including cholesterol reduction, anti-inflammatory, antioxidant, and anti-obesity effects (Shahidi et al., 2022). These benefits are likely attributed to its high content of alpha-linolenic acid (ALA), which serves as a precursor for the synthesis of docosahexaenoic acid (DHA) and eicosapentaenoic acid (EPA) in the human body (Yang et al., 2021).

2 Grading of Linseed

Grading of linseed *(Linum usitatissimum L.)* is a crucial process that ensures quality, market value, and industrial suitability by evaluating various physical, chemical, and biological parameters (Table 1). The grading criteria differ by country, with standards set by regulatory bodies such as the US Department of Agriculture (USDA), Canadian Grain Commission (CGC), and Food and Agriculture Organization (FAO). Physical parameters include seed purity (percentage of clean linseed free from foreign matter), seed size and weight (with larger, heavier seeds preferred for oil extraction), and color uniformity (golden or brown seeds without discoloration or damage). Moisture content, typically maintained below 10%, prevents fungal growth and rancidity, while oil content, ranging between 35% and 45%, is a key determinant of linseed's commercial value. Protein content, generally 18–24%, is critical for food and feed applications. Biological factors such as insect damage, mycotoxin contamination (e.g., aflatoxins and ochratoxins), and microbial load also influence grading. Standard grading classifications, such as those used in Canada and the USA, categorize linseed into Grade 1 (highest purity and oil content), Grade 2, and lower grades based on these criteria. International regulations, including Codex Alimentarius, emphasize food safety, pesticide residue limits, and labeling requirements to ensure global trade compliance. Proper grading enhances the efficiency of oil extraction, food processing, and industrial applications while maintaining consumer trust and market stability (Canadian Grain Commission, (2023), USDA, (2022), FAO, (2021)).

Table 1 Grading of different types of linseed oil by Agmark

Grade designation	Moisture and insoluble impurities present by weight (not more than)	Color on lovibond scale in ¼ inch cell expressed as Y + 10 (not deeper than)	Specific gravity at 30 °C	Refractive index at 40 °C	Saponification value	Iodine value (Wiji's method not less than)	Unsaponifiable matter percent by weight (not more than)	Acid value not more
Refined	0.10	10	0.923–0.926	1.4720–1.4750	188–195	170	1.5	0.5
Semirefined	0.10	10	0.923–0.928	1.4720–1.4750	188–195	170	1.5	0.5
Raw	0.25	35	0.923–0.928	1.4720–1.4750	188–195	170	1.5	4.0

3 Types and Grades of Linseed Oil

The material is of two types:

(a) Expressed:

- Alkali refined
- Acid refined
- Raw grade 1 and
- Raw grade 2

(b) Solvent-extracted:

- Semirefined and
- Raw

3.1 Alkali Refined or Semirefined Linseed Oil

Alkali-refined or semirefined linseed oil undergoes a purification process to enhance its quality, stability, and usability across various industries. Refining is essential for eliminating free fatty acids, phospholipids, pigments, and other impurities that could compromise its performance in both food and industrial applications (Belur et al., 2017). The alkali refining process includes neutralization, where free fatty acids react with an alkaline solution, typically sodium hydroxide (NaOH), forming soap stock, which is then removed from the oil (Dijkstra & Dijkstra, 2013). Following this, the bleaching process employs bleaching earth, activated carbon, or a combination of both to eliminate pigments, peroxides, and undesirable color compounds, thereby improving the oil's clarity and oxidative stability (Singh, 2021).

Prior to alkali refining, linseed oil may undergo acid treatment with mineral acids such as phosphoric or sulfuric acid to break down non-hydratable phospholipids and lower impurity levels (Dijkstra & Segers, 2007). This pretreatment step enhances the efficiency of subsequent refining stages, ensuring a higher-quality final product. Due to its improved color, minimized odor, and enhanced oxidative stability, alkali-refined linseed oil finds widespread use in coatings, paints, inks, and food-grade applications (Lusas et al., 2017).

3.2 Acid-Refined Linseed Oil

Acid-refined linseed oil undergoes a purification process that involves treatment with mineral acids to eliminate impurities such as phospholipids, gums, and trace metals, which can impact the oil's stability and performance (Dijkstra & Segers, 2007). This treatment, typically using phosphoric or sulfuric acid, breaks down non-hydratable phospholipids, transforming them into hydratable forms that can be efficiently removed through subsequent washing and separation steps. This process plays a key role in enhancing refining efficiency and ensuring a higher degree of purity in the final product. After acid treatment, the oil is subjected to a bleaching process using activated carbon, bleaching earth, or a combination of both. This stage helps eliminate unwanted pigments, oxidation by-products, and other impurities that contribute to discoloration and instability (Gharby, 2022). Activated carbon effectively adsorbs residual color compounds and contaminants, while bleaching earth reduces oxidative compounds and enhances the oil's transparency. Compared to crude linseed oil, acid-refined linseed oil offers superior oxidative stability, fewer impurities, and a lighter color, making it well-suited for applications in coatings, paints, varnishes, and certain food-related industries. Its enhanced clarity and purity also improve its effectiveness in industrial formulations where color consistency and stability are essential.

4 Quality and Labeling Standards for Linseed and Its Value-Added Products

The manufacture of linseed and its derivative articles of food must adhere to strict quality standards for several reasons. Initially, they guarantee the protection of the consumer by averting hazardous substances and stopping contamination. Preserving key elements like omega-3 fatty acids and guaranteeing a stable nutrient content are reasons alone for maintaining linseed's nutritional integrity. By fostering customer trust and satisfying the demands of global trade, quality standards improve marketability. By certifying the efficacy of linseed products and confirming its health advantages, they validate health claims.

5 Regulatory Frameworks for Linseed Oil

5.1 BIS

The Bureau of Indian Standards is the National Standard Body of India. The BIS standards as well as the rules and regulations enacted thereunder, regulate how the Standard Mark is used.

5.2 Requirement for Linseed Oil Under BIS

- The substance must be extracted either by solvent extraction from high-quality linseed cake or by expression method from sound, clean linseeds from *Linum usitatissimum* Linn., Linaceae.
- The substance must be transparent and free of added coloring and flavoring, adulterants, sediment, suspended particles, and other foreign materials.
- The filtered sample must be kept at 30 °C for 24 h to determine the material's clarity. Turbidity must not be present throughout this time.

The product shall not contain any of the toxic metals over the quantities prescribed in Table 2.

Table 2 Limits for toxic metals

Sl. No.	Characteristics	Requirement	Method of test
1	Lead, mg/kg, Max	5.0	IS 1699:1995
2	Arsenic, mg/kg, Max	0.5	"
3	Cadmium, mg/kg, Max	1.0	"
4	Mercury, mg/kg, Max	0.25	"

6 Food Safety and Standards Authority of India (FSSAI) Is the Statutory Regulatory Bo dy for Enforcing Indian Standards

6.1 FSSAI Standards for Linseed Oil

Refers to the oil that is produced by pressing healthy, clean flaxseed or linseed (*Linum usitatissimum*). It must be transparent, devoid of rancidity, suspended particles or other foreign objects, and separated water, mineral oil, additional flavoring, or coloring. It must meet the requirements listed below in Table 2.

6.2 Tanzania Bureau of Standards

The requirements, sample procedures, and testing protocols for linseed oil, which is made from the seeds of different farmed species of *Linum usitatissimum* and is meant for human use, are outlined in the Tanzanian standard. A comparison of linseed oil standards with Indian Standards is reported in Table 3.

7 Labeling Requirements for Linseed and Linseed Products

The packaging and labeling of linseed and its products are regulated by various laws and regulations from country to country. Some common points that are essential for Fair Packaging and Labeling are indicated below:

- *Fair Packaging and Labeling (FPL):* According to the FPL "All consumer commodities from Linseed including its oil" must have labels that reveal the net contents, the nature of the commodity, and the name, address, and phone number of the product's maker, packer, or distributor.
- *Food Labeling:* Linseed and all its food derivatives are required to adhere to the Food Labeling Regulations according to the country in which it is sold. According to these generic rules, the following details must be disclosed on the labels of all package of linseed and its derivatives:

Table 3 Comparison of standards for linseed oil

Regulatory body / Characteristics		AG-MARK	BIS	FSSAI	Tanzania-bureau of standards
Moisture and insoluble impurities present by weight (not more than		0.10	0.10	0.10	–
Color on Lovibond scale in ¼ inch cell expressed as Y + 10 (not deeper than)		10	10	10	–
Specific gravity at 30 °C		0.923–0.926	0.923–0.926	0.923–0.926	–
Refractive index at 40 °C		1.472–1.475	1.472–1.475	1.472–1.475	1.472–1.475
Saponification value, mg KOH/g oil		188–195	188–195	188–195	185–197
Iodine value (Wiji's method not less than)		170	170	170	170–211
Unsaponifiable matter percent by weight (not more than)		1.5	1.5	1.5	2.0
Acid value not more than	Refined	0.5	0.5	0.5	0.6
	Raw	4.0	4.0	4.0	4.0

- Name and address of the manufacturer
- Name and address of the packer/seller
- Trade name
- Veg/nonveg logo
- Net quantity of the food
- Pictorial representation of the article
- List of ingredients in descending order
- Nutritional information
- Maximum retail price
- Date of packaging
- Lot no., Batch No.
- license no. of manufacturer
- Address of marketing agency (if any)
- Best before use
- Fortification symbol (if any)
- Radiation symbol (if any)
- Genetically modified organism information (if)
- Name and address of the importer (if applicable)
- Any other information required by the regulations

- *Packaging Materials*: The Fair Packaging and Labeling requires that the packaging materials used for linseed and its products meet certain requirements. The purpose of these restrictions is to stop domestic goods from being packaged or labeled deceptively.
- To avoid any legal problems and to give consumers accurate information, producers and packers of linseed and its products must make sure that their labeling and packaging adhere to their country's specific regulation.

8 Specification of Packaging on Linseed (Fig. 1)

- *Linseed meal packed in Multi-walled Kraft paper Bag*: 25 kg Stitched Close with Red Cotton Thread.
- *Labeling Format*: Sticker placed on each individual bag. Details listed: Name of product, Name of Supplier or Customer and Address (if required), NET weight, Pack date, Best By, Line Number, Kosher and Halal logos.
- *Storage and Handling*: Store under cool, dry conditions–ideally around 10 degrees. Do not expose to direct sunlight for extended periods or strong odors. Keep free of pests and insects.
- *Shelf Life 12 months*: When stored in cool, dry conditions away from direct sunlight.

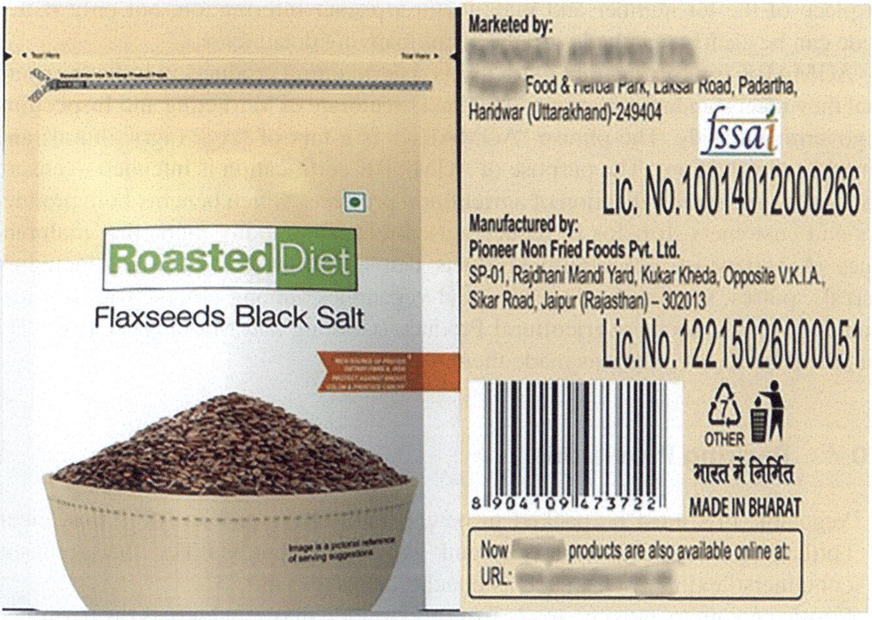

Fig. 1 Designed label for linseed

9 AGMARK Marking Provisions

The Agricultural Marketing Advisor must approve the form in which the grade classification mark is affixed to each container. The following information must be securely and clearly displayed on each container in addition to the grade mark.

- Name of packer
- Place of packing (business address)
- Tank filling No.
- Date of packing in plain letters
- Net weight/volume (wherever applicable)

Note: The date of packing shall be the date when the product is placed in the immediate container.

9.1 Labeling of Non-retail Containers

While most labeling requirements can be met either on the container or in attached paperwork, the product name, lot identification, and manufacturer/packer details must always be marked on the container. A coded identification mark may be used in place of the lot number and manufacturer/packer information, but only if this code can be clearly matched with the accompanying documents.

AGMARK is a certification mark used on agricultural products in India to ensure that they meet standards recognized by the Directorate of Marketing and Inspection, a government body. The phrase "AGMARK" is a mix of "Ag" (agricultural) and "mark" (certification). The purpose of AGMARK certification is intended to ensure the quality and standardization of agricultural products, which benefits both producers and customers. It helps to reduce agricultural commodity marketing malpractices. A variety of agricultural products can be AGMARK certified, including cereals, pulses, vegetable oils, fruits, and vegetables, among others. The certification is governed by the Agricultural Produce (Grading and Marking) Act of 1937 and the rules and regulations made thereunder.

10 Packing Provisions

- Vegetable oils must be packed in new, sound, clean, and rust-free tins, clean bottles, mild steel drums, railway tank wagons, or approved new thermoplastic containers/flexible packs (such as pouches, cans, or jars).
- Plastic containers must be made from food-grade plastic materials, as permitted under the Prevention of Food Adulteration act 1955.
- Vegetable oils shall be packed in the following standard net weights: 100 g, 200 g, 500 g, 1 kg, 5 kg, and thereafter in multiples of 5 kg. Edible vegetable oils may also be packed in volumetric measurements (milliliters/liters), provided the corresponding weight (grams/kilograms) is clearly indicated.
- Contamination-free containers must not include any dangerous or toxic materials that might render the oil unfit for human consumption, either in whole or in part. They must also be devoid of any unpleasant or unattractive odor, fungal contamination, and insect infestation. Packing must be carried out as per the prescribed methods for each type of packaging.
- Although the Food Safety and Standards (Prohibition and Restriction on Sales) Regulations, 2011 require mandatory AGMARK certification for certain items, such as: Blended Edible Vegetable Oil, Fat Spread, in case of Til Oil, Carbia Callosa, Honey dew, Tea, and Ghee FSSAI has prescribed a few conditional restrictions.

11 Common Contaminants, Additives, and Adulterants in Linseed

The usage of numerous food additives added for technological purposes has expanded along with the food processing industry's rapid growth. Because additives prolong the shelf life of the product and preserve its nutritional value, their usage in processed foods has gained validity. Their use reduces the waste of seasonal surpluses, particularly in underdeveloped nations without access to sufficient transportation and modern storage facilities. Additionally, the use of additives can be very advantageous in tropical climates where high temperatures and humidity promote microbial growth and the formation of oxidative rancidity in food. Due to this, there is now widespread concern over food safety as well as unfair commercial practices about quantity, quality, and presentation. But, the deliberate lowering of food quality by the addition or substitution of unreported alternative ingredients, the removal of certain essential ingredients, or both, is known as food adulteration. Usually, this is done to increase the quantity or decrease the price of a certain food product. Customers have been quite concerned about this since it is frequently unwanted from an ethical, legal, religious, or economic perspective (Contamination, 2007). The oils commonly mixed with linseed oil are niger, cotton seed, fish, rosin. and coal oils (Society & Society, 1885).

12 Country-Specific Regulations

Detailed comparison of regulations in key markets (e.g., USA, EU, Canada, Australia).

12.1 Variations in Labeling Requirements Across Different Jurisdictions

According to the WHO Global Strategy on nutrition, physical activity, and health, the food industry should give consumers with clear and consistent food labels and evidence-based health claims to assist them make educated decisions (WHO, 2004). A label performs three functions: providing basic product information, health, safety, and nutrition information, and serving as a marketing tool, marketing and advertising (via label vignettes). India's "Food Safety and Standards Regulations" provide guidelines for food packaging and labeling.

Regulations governing packaging materials vary by area. In Europe, the introduction of Regulation (EC) No. 450/2009 in 2009 boosted market penetration of active and intelligent packaging materials, whereas in the USA, similar materials are included into existing regulations under the Code of Federal Regulation. The European Union encountered issues with diverse legislation, which led to the passage of the Packaging and Packaging Waste Directive in 1994, emphasizing the conflict between environmental protection and economic progress. Rules for food packaging materials are critical in Asia, notably Japan, emphasizing the importance of constantly evaluating and improving rules to handle growing dangers and technology.

12.2 Codex

The Codex Alimentarius, commonly referred to as the "Codex," is a compilation of internationally accepted standards, guidelines, and codes of practice related to food safety and quality. These standards are developed using scientific evaluations conducted by independent expert panels, including: The Joint FAO/WHO Expert Committee on Food Additives (JECFA), The Joint FAO/WHO Meetings on Pesticide Residues (JMPR).

The Codex Alimentarius Commission has set standards for vegetable oils under *CXS 210–1999* Standard. According to the standards for linseed oil, the seeds of many cultivated species of *Linum usitatissimum* that are used to make flaxseed (linseed) oil may be extracted as follows:

(a) Edible vegetable oils are foods that are mainly derived from vegetables and primarily made up of fatty acid glycerides. Other lipids including phosphatides, unsaponifiable components, and free fatty acids that are naturally found in the fat or oil may be present in trace levels in them.
(b) Mechanical processes, such as pressing or expelling, and the use of heat alone are used to create virgin oils without changing the oil's content. They could have been cleaned using basically centrifugation, settling, filtration, and water washing.

12.3 European Union Law

The European Food Safety Authority was established, food safety procedures were established, and basic principles and standards of food law have been set down in Regulation (EC) No 178/2002 of the European Parliament and the Council on January 28, 2002**.** Food law's primary objective is to provide consumers a foundation upon which to make educated food choices and to prohibit any actions that would deceive them.

Directive 2005/29/EC, issued on May 11, 2005, by the European Parliament and Council, addresses exploitative business-to-consumer activities in the internal market. The directive emphasizes various elements related to giving customers information, with the goal of preventing deceptive practices and information exclusions. There should be special regulations pertaining to the dissemination of food information to consumers in addition to the general guidelines against unfair commercial activities.

It is reasonable to maintain the requirement that the statutory nutrition disclosure relates to 100 g or 100 ml quantities in order to make it easier to compare goods in various package sizes. If necessary, it should also permit extra portion-based declarations. Therefore, a nutrition declaration per portion or consumption unit, in addition to the phrase per 100 g or 100 ml, should be permitted in cases when food is prepackaged and specific portions or consumption units are defined. The Commission should also have the authority to establish guidelines for the phrasing of the nutrition declaration per portion or per consumption unit for certain food categories in order to provide equivalent signals about portions or consumption units.

Regulation (EC) No 1924/2006 of the European Parliament and of the Council of December 20, 2006, on nutrition and health claims made on foods, shall govern the voluntary insertion of nutrition or health claims on food labels for the sake of uniformity and coherence of Union legislation.

13 Code of Federal Regulations (21CFR101.9) [Title 21, Volume 2]

13.1 Sec. 101.9 Nutrition Labeling of Oil Including Linseed Oil

- *Fat, total or Total fat:* A statement of the number of grams of total fat in a serving defined as total lipid fatty acids and expressed as triglycerides where fatty acids are aliphatic carboxylic acids consisting of a chain of alkyl groups and characterized by a terminal carboxyl group. Amounts shall be expressed to the nearest 0.5 (1/2) gram increment below 5 grams and the nearest gram increment above 5 grams. If the serving contains less than 0.5 gram, the content shall be expressed as zero.
- *Polyunsaturated fat or Poly-unsaturated (VOLUNTARY)*: A statement of the number of grams of polyunsaturated fat in a serving defined as *cis*, cis-methylene-interrupted polyunsaturated fatty acids may be declared voluntarily, except that when monounsaturated fat is declared, or when a claim about fatty acids or cholesterol is made on the label or in labeling of a food other than one that meets the criteria for a claim for "fat free," label declaration of polyunsaturated fat is required. Polyunsaturated fat content shall be indicated and expressed as grams per serving to the nearest 0.5 (1/2) gram increment below 5 grams and to the nearest gram increment above 5 grams. If the serving contains less than 0.5 gram, the content shall be expressed as zero.
- *Dietary fiber:* A serving's total dietary fiber content is stated in grams, indented, and to the closest gram. However, if a serving has less than 1 gram, no dietary fiber declaration is necessary; instead, the words "Contains less than 1 gramme" or "less than 1 gramme" may be used, and if the serving has less than 0.5 grams, the content may be zero. Nondigestible soluble and insoluble carbohydrates (containing three or more monomeric units) and lignin that are naturally occurring and undamaged in plants are referred to as dietary fiber. The FDA has identified isolated or synthetic nondigestible carbohydrates as having physiological effects that are advantageous to human health.
- *Soluble fiber (VOLUNTARY):* It is voluntary to disclose the amount of soluble dietary fiber in a serving; however label disclosure is mandatory when a claim about soluble fiber is made. Dietary fiber must include soluble fiber.

14 Conclusion

Linseed and its products must be of high-quality and accurately labeled for the benefit of customer safety, legal compliance, and future profitability. Grading based on factors such as moisture content, oil composition, and purity is crucial in ensuring product consistency, while compliance with established quality standards guarantees that linseed and its derivatives, including oil, flour, and supplements, meet industry requirements for safety and performance. Regulatory frameworks established by global organizations like Codex Alimentarius, along with country-specific regulations in markets, such as the USA and the European Union, provide essential guidelines for quality assurance and labeling compliance. Clear and accurate labeling, including nutritional information, allergen statements, and organic certifications, enhances consumer confidence and market transparency. However, challenges such as contamination from pesticides, heavy metals, and microbial agents pose significant risks to product safety, making rigorous monitoring and compliance with regulatory limits necessary. Adhering to standardized quality and labeling regulations allows stakeholders including manufacturers, regulators, and consumers to ensure that linseed products remain safe, reliable, and competitive.

References

Belur, P. D., Iyyasami, R., Sampath, C., & Chandrasekhar, V. (2017). Refining technologies for edible oils. In *Edible oils* (pp. 99–128). CRC Press.

Canadian Grain Commission. (2023). Grain quality and statistics. https://www.grainscanada.gc.ca

Contamination, F. (2007). Code of Federal Regulations (21CFR101.9) [Title 21, Volume 2]. *Food contamination and adulteration*.

Dijkstra, A. J., & Dijkstra, A. J. (2013). Neutralization. In *Edible Oil Processing from a Patent Perspective* (pp. 157–171). Springer.

Dijkstra, A. J., & Segers, J. C. (2007). Production and refining of oils and fats. In *The lipid handbook with CD-ROM* (pp. 157–276). CRC Press.

Farag, M. A., Elimam, D. M., & Afifi, S. M. (2021). Outgoing and potential trends of the omega-3 rich linseed oil quality characteristics and rancidity management: A comprehensive review for maximizing its food and nutraceutical applications. *Trends in Food Science & Technology, 114*, 292–309.

Food and Agriculture Organization of the United Nations (FAO). (2021). https://www.fao.org/publications

Gharby, S. (2022). Refining vegetable oils: Chemical and physical refining. *The Scientific World Journal, 2022*(1), 6627013. https://www.accessdata.fda.gov/scripts/cdrh/cfdocs/cfcfr/CFRSearch.cfm?fr=101.9

Lusas, E. W., Riaz, M. N., Alam, M. S., & Clough, R. (2017). Animal and vegetable fats, oils, and waxes. In J. Kent (Ed.), *Handbook of industrial chemistry and biotechnology* (pp. 823–932). Springer.

Saleem, M. H., Ali, S., Hussain, S., Kamran, M., Chattha, M. S., Ahmad, S., et al. (2020). Flax (Linum usitatissimum L.): A potential candidate for phytoremediation? Biological and economical points of view. *Plants, 9*(4), 496.

Shahidi, S., Mahmoodi, M. S., Komaki, A., & Sadeghian, R. (2022). The comparison of omega-3 and flaxseed oil on serum lipids and lipoproteins in hyperlipidemic male rats. *Heliyon, 8*(6), e09662.

Singh, S. (2021). Developments in the technology of oils and refineries. In *Advances in processing technology* (pp. 189–215). CRC Press.

Society, A. P., & Society, A. P. (1885, October). On the detection of adulterations in oils Author (s): Oscar C. S. Carter Source : In *Proceedings of the American Philosophical Society*, vol. 22, no. 120, Part IV, (pp. 296–299). American Philosophical Society Stable. https://www.jstor.org/stable/982989.22.

United States Department of Agriculture (USDA). (2022). U.S. Department of Agriculture, Agricultural Research Service. https://fdc.nal.usda.gov

World Health Organization (WHO). (2004). https://www.who.int/publications.

Yang, J., Wen, C., Duan, Y., Deng, Q., Peng, D., Zhang, H., & Ma, H. (2021). The composition, extraction, analysis, bioactivities, bioavailability and applications in food system of flaxseed (Linum usitatissimum L.) oil: A review. *Trends in Food Science & Technology, 118*, 252–260.

The manufacturer's authorised representative in the EU is Springer Nature Customer Service Centre GmbH, Europaplatz 3, 69115 Heidelberg, Germany. If you have any concerns regarding our products, please contact ProductSafety@springernature.com

Printed and bound by CPI Group (UK) Ltd, Croydon, CR0 4YY

01/10/2026

02225915-0003